# PRAISE FOR
# *HAITI AFTER THE EARTHQUAKE*

"Paul Farmer, doctor and aid worker, offers an inspiring insider's view of the relief effort." —*Financial Times*

"A day-by-day account of [Farmer's] experience of the disaster, as well as a treatise on why Haiti was particularly vulnerable and how it should be rebuilt. The book's greatest strength lies in its depiction of the post-quake chaos. . . . In the book's more analytical sections the author's diagnosis of the difficulties of reconstruction is sharp."
—*The Economist*

"To his discussion of this receding tragedy, Paul Farmer brings passion, medical expertise, and a long and intimate engagement with Haiti. His account of the year following the earthquake works on three levels: personal, practical, and analytic . . . laden with anecdotes and emotion. . . . Farmer's passionate book . . . [brings] Haiti's appalling tragedy back to the world's attention."
—*Foreign Affairs*

"His honest assessment of what the people trying to help Haiti did well—and where they failed—is important for anyone who cares about the country or international aid in general. . . . Farmer uses the personal triumphs and essays to explain that Haiti's hope for a better future need not be in vain. The international community's failure does not have to continue along the same dead-end path."
—*Miami Herald*

"To humanize what could have been merely an academic study, and as a reminder of why it matters, Farmer and twelve contributors recount their experiences during and immediately after the quake. The recollections of people like Farmer and his colleagues, working around the clock as the bodies piled up, serve as chilling and sad examples of the horrors the world's inequalities can render. . . . Farmer provides an in-depth look at the causes behind Haiti's ills and presents solutions for the country's revival." —*Montreal Gazette*

"A gripping recollection of the quake's ruin, chaos, and despair, and the story of remarkable persistence, hope, and love in the aftermath. Once you've seen Haiti through Paul Farmer's eyes, you'll never see Haitians, or any of the world's poorest people, quite the same way again." —President Bill Clinton

"This is a gripping, profoundly moving book, an urgent dispatch from the front by one of our finest warriors for social justice. With eloquence and wisdom, Paul Farmer shows how we cannot fully comprehend one of the great natural disasters of history without understanding the man-made suffering that Americans and others have inflicted on Haiti. The talented colleagues he enlists here to help tell this story only make it richer and deeper."
—Adam Hochschild

"A valuable book filled with insights. . . . The book is at its best when the emergency and reconstruction efforts are seen through Farmer's filter in his dual roles as a doctor leading an NGO and as U.N. deputy envoy for Haiti." —*Philadelphia Inquirer*

"*Haiti After the Earthquake* is a captivating book about not just what has happened in Haiti in the past eighteen months but why recovery has been so difficult, and how the next unnatural disaster can be prevented. It is a story of the extraordinary strength and courage of the Haitian people, and of their great need now and in the years to come. . . . Paul Farmer has written an empathetic, critical, and informative analysis of the modern aid structure, Haiti, and how the

two must be reconciled if the Western Hemisphere's poorest nation can ever hope to stand on its own."
—*Washington Independent Review of Books*

"While Farmer's book contains valuable insights into how to improve humanitarian aid both in Haiti and in general, it is most powerful when he presents stories of individual projects in Haiti, or patients he encountered after the quake." —*Daily Beast*

"Through the sharing of his experiences and the essays of fellow relief workers and survivors, the book serves as both a first draft of history and a call to action for rebuilding a country devastated by natural and unnatural disasters. . . . Farmer deftly tells the story of his multiple roles—doctor, administrator, and diplomat. . . . His writing remains accessible, revealing hope amid criticism, and providing touches of humor in a unique personal narrative. . . . Readers will empathize with his anger over Haiti's suffering as well as appreciate his insistence that the disaster should open the way for serious development and rebuilding in a country long ignored."
—*Madison Capital Times*

"Farmer demonstrates his deep love for Haiti while at the same time pushing for the drastic foreign and domestic reforms needed to rebuild this troubled nation. Highly recommended for anyone interested in learning more about the history of, and recovery efforts in, Haiti." —*Library Journal*, starred review

"A searing firsthand account of the earthquake and its aftermath. . . . An eye-opener of a report and a wake-up call that change is needed."
—*Kirkus Reviews*

"Paul Farmer has written an essential book for understanding the country that was shattered by the earthquake of January 12, 2010. . . . The uniqueness of Farmer's written contribution to this new stage of Haiti's history is the piercing historic and social/political dimensions he offers to the reader. He brings to its pages a deep examination of

Haiti's vulnerability to the devastating blow it suffered and the sharp shift in policies and practices now required if the country is to move forward. In so doing, he offers insights into why, eighteen months later, the relief and reconstruction effort is bogged down."
—*Globe & Mail*

"Farmer, currently UN deputy special envoy for Haiti, offers candid insider analysis of what is truly required for a healthier, just, and sustainable Haitian future. Farmer's clarion and moving chronicle is followed by powerful essays by other doctors, community organizer Didi Bertrand Farmer, author Edwidge Danticat, and radio journalist and UN advisor Michele Montas-Dominique, who writes, 'Through coups d'état, hurricanes, and earthquakes, we have been rebuilding Haiti, seemingly from scratch, for two hundred years.'" —*Booklist*

"*Haiti After the Earthquake* is a beautiful, harrowing illumination of the greatest natural disaster of our times, and the complex history—and structural violence—at the root of Haiti's tragedy. The narrative is both personal and national, giving voice to a collective experience of grief and profound loss. Paul Farmer's fine scholarship, natural leadership, and deep love for the country and people of Haiti shape each page of this remarkable text, a gift to all of us who are privileged to work there." —Ophelia Dahl

"This important new book connects us all to the tragedy in Haiti, to what came before, and to what must follow if we are to fulfill the promise of recovery and reconstruction. Paul Farmer and the other contributors together lead us through the events of January 12, 2010, and their aftermath—teaching us, in the process, about the natural and unnatural disasters that have befallen a people and a nation."
—Michaëlle Jean, former governor general of Canada

# Haiti

## after the earthquake

# *Haiti*

## *after the earthquake*

═══════

# PAUL FARMER

*Edited by Abbey Gardner and Cassia Van Der Hoof Holstein*

WITH

*Joia S. Mukherjee • Edwidge Danticat*

*Michèle Montas-Dominique • Nancy Dorsinville*

*Didi Bertrand Farmer • Louise Ivers • Evan Lyon*

*Dubique Kobel • Naomi Rosenberg • Timothy T. Schwartz*

*Jennie Weiss Block • Jéhane Sedky*

PublicAffairs

*New York*

"The Dead," from *Questions About Angels*, by Billy Collins, ©1991. Reprinted by permission of the University of Pittsburgh Press.

Hardcover first published in 2011 in the United States by PublicAffairs™, a Member of the Perseus Books Group
Paperback first published in 2012 in the United States by PublicAffairs

PublicAffairs books are available at special discounts for bulk purchases in the U.S. by corporations, institutions, and other organizations. For more information, please contact the Special Markets Department at the Perseus Books Group, 2300 Chestnut Street, Suite 200, Philadelphia, PA 19103, call (800) 810-4145, ext. 5000, or e-mail special.markets@perseusbooks.com.

Editorial production by *Marra*thon Production Services. www.marrathon.net
BOOK DESIGN BY JANE RAESE
Text set in Apollo

The Library of Congress has cataloged the hardcover edition as follows:
Farmer, Paul, 1959–
    Haiti after the earthquake / Paul Farmer ; with Joia S. Mukherjee . . . [et al.].—1st ed.
    p. ; cm.
    Includes bibliographical references and index.
    ISBN 978-1-58648-973-1 (hardback)—ISBN 978-1-58648-974-8 (electronic)
    1. Emergency medical services—Haiti. 2. Earthquakes—Haiti. I. Mukherjee, Joia.
    II. Title. [DNLM: 1. Earthquakes—Haiti—Autobiography. 2. Relief Work—Haiti—Autobiography. 3. Public Health Practice—Haiti—Autobiography.
    4. Socioeconomic Factors—Haiti—Autobiography. WA 295]

RA645.7.H2F37 2011
363.34'95097294—dc23
                                                                    2011014000
ISBN 978-1-61039-098-9 (paperback)
ISBN 978-1-61039-207-5 (paperback e-book)

10  9  8  7  6  5  4  3  2

*To Al and Diane Kaneb,*
*and all those who stand with the Haitian people*

*Then Jesus cried out again in a loud voice and breathed his last.*
*At that moment, the curtain of the temple was torn in two,*
*from top to bottom. The earth quaked, and the rocks were split.*
*The centurions and those with him who were keeping watch of Jesus,*
*saw the earthquake and what took place and they were terrified ...*

—Matthew 27:50–52, 54, Palm Sunday Liturgy


*The dead are always looking down on us, they say.*
*While we are putting on our shoes or making a sandwich,*
*they are looking down through the glass bottom boats of heaven*
*as they row themselves slowly through eternity.*

*They watch the tops of our heads moving below on earth,*
*and when we lie down in a field or on a couch,*
*drugged perhaps by the hum of a long afternoon,*
*they think we are looking back at them,*
*which makes them lift their oars and fall silent and wait,*
*like parents, for us to close our eyes.*

—The Dead, Billy Collins

# CONTENTS

# NÈG MAWON

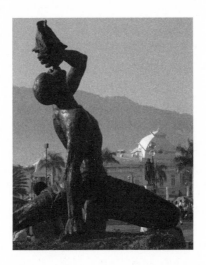

*H*aiti *was founded* by a righteous revolution in 1804 and became the first black republic. It was the first country to
break the chains of slavery, the first to force Emperor
Napoleon to retreat, and the only to aid Simón Bolívar in his struggle
to liberate the indigenous people and slaves of Latin America from
their colonial oppressors. Tragically, this history of liberty and self-
determination has drawn two centuries of political and economic ire
from powerful countries resulting in policies which have served to
impoverish the people of Haiti.

Feared by Thomas Jefferson for their successful uprising; extorted
by France in 1825 for 150 million francs to compensate the loss of the

Empire's "property"—both slaves and land—(a debt the Haitian people completed paying, with interest, more than a century later); occupied by the U.S. military between 1915 and 1934 to stifle European influence in the Western Hemisphere; and disrespected in their quest for democracy by an unrelenting series of dictators and coup d'états backed by Western countries: the free people of Haiti have been continually re-shackled politically and economically.

In the wake of the January 12, 2010, earthquake, Haiti's history of unrelenting struggle for justice is its greatest resource. This history, as Haitians remind us, is what makes Haiti mighty: mighty without material wealth, without natural resources, without arable land, without arms.

Amidst the rubble of the houses, buildings, and schools, and in front of the once grand National Palace, stands Nèg Mawon—the symbol of Haiti. Nèg Mawon at once embodies the marooned man, the runaway slave, and the free man. He symbolizes the complex history of the Haitian people: stolen from Africa, marooned on an island and liberated through a brave and radical revolution. Shackles broken, machete in hand, the free man does not hide; rather he blows a conch to gather others to fight for the freedom and dignity of all people. For the self-evident truth—that all men are created equal. Nèg Mawon is the indefatigable spirit of Haiti's people, a people profoundly and proudly woven to their history.

When I arrived in Haiti on Thursday, January 14, 2010, I asked my friend who was driving, "Koté Nèg Mawon"—where is the free man? "Li la" he said—he is here. And as we rounded the corner behind the Champs de Mar, the plaza in front of the devastated palace where thousands had already made their homes—and remain today—there, rising from the dust of the still trembling earth, stood the statue of Nèg Mawon. I was drawn by the image out of the car and as I stood, weeping, an old woman put her arm around me; she too was crying. I said, "Nèg Mawon toujou kanpé!!"—the free man is still standing!! And she replied, powerfully, "Cheri, Nèg Mawon p'ap *jamn* krazé"— my dear, the free man will *never* be broken. It is with this surety that we must stand with Haiti, a country whose spirit and people will never be broken, and work in solidarity toward the future the Haitian people deserve.
                                                              —*Joia S. Mukherjee*

# Haiti

*after the earthquake*

# WRITING ABOUT
# SUFFERING

*S*ome years ago, after two decades of witnessing and writing
about epidemic disease and violence of all types, I set out to
write a book based on some lectures about violence and
medicine that I'd given at the University of Rochester. The title of
the book was going to be *Swords of Sorrow*, from a Gospel line (Luke
2:35): Mary learns that her soul will be pierced by a "sword of sorrow" because she is willing to be a vessel of grace. I liked the alliter-
ation. But I never finished that book. What was the point, I worried,
of writing another book about the suffering caused by war and
genocide and other misfortunes natural and unnatural?

I thought again about that truncated project shortly after an earthquake struck Haiti's capital city on January 12, 2010. Preliminary estimates of the dead ran to six figures. The immediacy of rescue and
relief soon gave way to a series of questions about the dimensions of
what had happened, about why Haiti had been particularly vulnerable to such a disaster, and about how to respond to the unfolding
"humanitarian crisis" (to use the jargon of the day). Suffering is
never just pure suffering; it occurs in a particular place and time. My
book would have examined histories of suffering in Haiti,
Guatemala, and Rwanda—Haiti being the place that has taught me
the most.

Knowledge of Haiti might not help a trauma surgeon attend to
broken bodies pulled from the rubble. But deep familiarity with the
place helped frame answers to some of the questions posed above

and also helped guide actions in the aftermath of the quake and during the reconstruction that would follow. The relevant knowledge needed to be historically deep (because the damage caused by the quake and the responses to it were rooted in Haitian history) and geographically broad (because Haiti had for centuries been caught up in a transnational economic and political web, a condition very much on display before and after the quake). This may sound academic. I didn't want to write a dispassionate study of the Haitian earthquake. Instead, I wanted to offer an account of a difficult time; to bear witness.

Bearing witness surely has a certain value, especially if it is linked to goodwill efforts to prevent unnecessary suffering caused by war or disease or insufficient preparation for natural disasters. Documentation by eyewitnesses can serve to inform people who are not on the scene but are in a position to help or hinder subsequent interventions. But was it appropriate for a physician, an American at that, to speak for the victims? Many in academia would argue vehemently that only the victims could speak for themselves, and that anyone who presumed to speak on their behalf would rob them of their agency. However, this is not always true: as far as the earthquake goes, the chief victims' voices were stilled forever. Seeking to "echo and amplify" (to paraphrase Haiti's former President Jean-Bertrand Aristide) the voices of those we encountered as well as those silenced was and remains our principal interest in writing about violence of all sorts.

I use *we* and *our* here because, a few months after the quake, a small group of friends and coworkers decided to put together an account of that terrible time. We've done our best to offer an honest rendering, even though no one had stopped to take notes amidst the maelstrom. It is also our desire to broadcast the voices of those most affected.

This book faces the same problems I encountered in writing *Swords of Sorrow*. In addition to clichéd (and overly academic) concerns about voice and representation, serious challenges are involved in seeking to write and complete a book in a few months. These challenges are heightened by publishing such a book in English because the primary victims of the quake do not speak English (or speak it less well than they do other languages).

We've tried to address these challenges in the structure of this book, which includes my own account along with a series of brief essays, photographs, and one drawing by friends, family, and coworkers. I describe the aftermath of the earthquake as experienced by a physician working alongside colleagues in Port-au-Prince and central Haiti both immediately after the quake and in subsequent months. I double back to revisit my personal history in Haiti, and that of Partners In Health and its Haitian sister organization, Zanmi Lasante, over the past twenty-five years.

This quarter-century has been, for us, one of satisfying growth in spite of disappointments and the dashing of many of the hopes awakened by the fall of the Duvalier dictatorship in 1986. If this book has a central metaphor, it's one taken from clinical medicine: the earthquake can be understood as an "acute-on-chronic" event. It was devastating because a history of adverse social conditions and extreme ecological fragility primed Port-au-Prince for massive loss of life and destruction when the ground began shaking on January 12. For this reason, the account is not linear but rather follows clinical logic: it explores the acute-on-chronic disaster that occurred on January 12 and its origins in Haiti's troubled history.

A sound account of the quake must go deep into Haiti's history to illuminate what caused the chronic disabilities, engendered over five centuries by transnational social and economic forces with deep roots in the colonial enterprise. Haiti was born of resistance to this enterprise, and therein lies both the strength and disability of the new polity—the reactive and reticulated pattern of growth registered in the nineteenth century and in the past one, when Haiti became anchored more formally in the "American hemisphere" through a nineteen-year military occupation by its oldest neighbor. When the U.S. Marines withdrew in 1934, they left a superficial calm and a social class that relied heavily on the army as the arbiter of political transitions.

Historians often claim that their discipline reveals the significance of current social processes, and they are right: the decades preceding the quake set the stage not only for what occurred during the acute event but also for the challenge of reconstruction. Following a brief review of Haitian history—which is, necessarily, a review of the history of the New World—we return to the challenge of reconstruction after the temblor of 2010. In the years before it, we saw that Haiti had become a veritable "Republic of NGOs," home to a proliferation of goodwill that did little or nothing to strengthen the public sector. Thus did clinics sprout up without much aid to the health system; thus did schools arise by the hundreds even as the Ministry of Education faltered; thus did water projects appear even as water security (like food security) was enfeebled.

This was the situation pre-quake, as described in this book. Efforts to rebuild after the quake needed to draw on the sudden attention of the world and the generous promises and pledges to craft a new way of doing business that did not further weaken the Haitian government. It's hard to imagine public health without a public sector, and the same could be said for public education and public works. And so this book recounts efforts to stand up a "recovery commission" to address the dysfunctional system of humanitarian aid that, good intentions aside, has become another obstacle to Haiti's recovery and sovereignty.

It's the argument of this book that rebuilding capacity—public or private—in Haiti requires sound analysis of what, exactly, has gone so wrong in the previous four decades. To accomplish this—what doctors call diagnosis and prescription—we've had to abandon anxieties about representation and about intruding in the text both as narrators and as characters. Every account is personal. Most of those who contributed to the relief efforts described here are not included (though we've tried to thank some of them in the acknowledgments). We've also sought to focus on the shortcomings of the quake response, rather than the victories.

In academic circles, few rewards are given for this sort of candor, or for failing to include all the key actors on the scene. But knowing that a quarter of a million voices were silenced on a single night and that more recent problems (such as cholera) are part of the same tragedy encourages us to offer these personal and place-specific narratives.

Whether these narratives are termed "history's first draft" or simple first-person accounts, they constitute our collective effort to recount and account: to recount what happened before it slips from our memories and to account for what placed Haiti, a country we all love, at such extreme risk well before January 12, 2010.

This book, with all its limitations, is offered as a humble tribute to those who perished that day, to those who live on with their injuries, visible and invisible, and to those who continue to stand with the Haitian people. Among them are the tens of thousands who responded to the suffering caused or worsened by the earthquake, including those who supported, quietly and from afar, the imperfect efforts described in these pages.

# 1.

## THE CATASTROPHE

*O*n January *13*, the day after an earthquake struck Haiti's capital, I finally got through to Dr. Alix Lassègue, the medical director of Port-au-Prince's largest hospital and a longtime friend. The hospital's real name is l'Hôpital de l'Université d'Etat d'Haïti, but most people call it the General Hospital. I began trying to reach Lassègue a couple of hours after the quake. His cell phone number, like all the other numbers I tried, led to a recorded message or an ominous buzz. From what we knew at the time, the hospital was smack in the middle of the quake zone. The facility sat among a dozen government buildings, including the medical and nursing schools, and we could see from live reports that most of those buildings had collapsed—during business and school hours. It was clear that our work as health providers in Haiti would be changed forever.

So now what? It was hard to know how to prioritize anxieties, and as a doctor, I thought immediately of the General Hospital. It wasn't hard to imagine the enormity of need in this struggling public facility which had, in the best of times, too many patients, too few staff, and far too few resources. After dozens of tries, it was almost a shock when I connected to Lassègue on a colleague's cell phone.

"What do you most need?" I asked.

Lassègue would hear this question again and again over the next weeks and months, usually with scant practical outcome, but this

6

was early in the game—less than twenty-four hours after the quake. Of course he needed just about everything, including electricity, supplies, salaries, and medications; the hospital had been scrambling for all these even before the quake. He gave me a long and fairly specific list. He needed materials and labor to repair the damaged parts of the hospital, and engineers able to assess the structural integrity of the buildings still standing. He needed help trying to save the lives of those still trapped under collapsed buildings abutting the hospital grounds, including not only the nursing school next door—"a total loss, I fear, and all in it"—and nearby federal buildings, but also houses, businesses, and schools. "It's much worse than we thought," Lassègue said. "Just managing proper disposal of the bodies is overwhelming us." He needed help moving casualties out of the courtyards and into the morgue but couldn't do that because the power was down. ("Why move bodies into the morgue," he asked, "without means of preserving them?") I didn't say much during the call because I'd never contemplated such problems.

Lassègue kept talking. "What I need most," he concluded, "are surgical teams—surgeons and anesthesiologists and nurses and post-op care and medications. And generators." It was a relief to hear these specific requests, because they were needs we could address. I promised to get the word out and to join him as soon as I could, but our connection was lost and I'm not sure he heard the last bit.

I'd been to the General Hospital many times over the previous twenty-five years, usually with a heavy heart. When we at Zanmi Lasante sent our patients to Port-au-Prince, it was never good. They needed something we couldn't provide in central Haiti—usually a diagnostic test or procedure. Often, these patients had already been to the General Hospital or to some other facility in the city. They were almost always people who needed medical care but had been effectively shut out from receiving it because they were poor and couldn't pay the fees most clinics and hospitals demanded for consultations, lab tests, and medications. "Free care" was never free because even the most basic services had hidden costs. The General Hospital was surrounded by scores of small for-profit private pharmacies and labs that counted on referrals and income for the sale of everything from surgical gloves, sold by the pair, to the most basic medicines and lab tests.

The dire need of Haiti's destitute sick for even basic medical services was the reason we'd founded Partners In Health and Zanmi Lasante a quarter century ago. These organizations had grown significantly in the decade before the quake: our Haitian colleagues—numbering in the thousands—ran a dozen public hospitals stretching from the Dominican border to the coast at Saint-Marc. For many poor Haitians, these hospitals had become a last line of defense, and we tried never to refer patients to other facilities unless absolutely necessary. When we had no choice but to refer them, we would try to send patients along with any medicines or supplies they might need—from antibiotics to intravenous solutions to gloves for their examining physicians—as well as some cash. We also sent a doctor or nurse to accompany them, because in our experience, too many patients sent elsewhere were simply, in medical jargon, "lost to follow-up." In the United States, the expression "lost to follow-up" means that a patient in question cannot be reached for the continuation of care. But in the case of Haitian public hospitals, without reliable partners to help with resources ranging from staff to medication to electricity, patients were sometimes lost to follow-up within the facilities themselves. In years past, I'd visited patients in the General Hospital who'd been occupying a bed for days and hadn't yet seen a qualified physician. I'd also seen patients who'd gone without a proper meal in days. (Their families were expected to bring food.)

I do not mean to disparage the General Hospital. As the years went by, we had more and more sympathy for the country's largest public hospital and for those running it. For the most part, these Haitian health professionals were doing their best but could not function without proper salaries and without the tools of our trade. Some senior doctors there were as talented as any I'd met in hospitals at Harvard and other parts of the world. And many had showed up within hours of the quake. Indeed, one of the constants in the days after the earthquake was the presence of Dr. Lassègue and the chief of nursing, Marlaine Thompson.

But the entire Haitian health system was underfunded, and its flagship hospital was in sorry shape. The shortcomings of the hospital could be readily traced to a lack of funding and the imposition of a fee-for-service model in a country where the majority of people, and certainly those most at risk for illness and injury, didn't have money.[1] Although a key function of a university hospital is to train health care professionals, the lack of resources to run the hospital or pay workers made it a difficult training environment. Before the quake, the General Hospital was rocked by strikes and work stoppages; key supplies were often out of stock. Some friends of the hospital had taken small steps to help colleagues there provide better services, including supplying meals to inpatients—especially to those admitted with some complication of malnutrition.

The shortage of trained clinicians able to provide care to the poorest patients remained an enormous problem; doctors and nurses left for other countries or were siphoned off to better-equipped and better-paying nongovernmental organizations and private hospitals. Given the weakness of the public-sector hospitals, and the faltering "flagship" public hospital, many of our supporters wondered why we sought to direct attention there in the hours after the quake. Why not aid the private (and NGO) hospitals instead? Most of those NGOs and hospitals were not mandated to provide care for all comers. Even if they'd been established to help the poor, they had no binding obligation—legal or otherwise—to open their doors to every patient needing medical attention. As mediocre as it was, the General Hospital remained Haiti's provider of last resort. And it was smack in the middle of the quake zone. We knew from the beginning, from the hours after the quake, that the hospital would soon be overrun. That's why we promised to help.

Within a day of making that promise, I hitched a ride, with surgeons and other doctors, on one of the first private planes bound for Haiti. Although my recent trips to the country had been as a UN Deputy Special Envoy, a volunteer post under Bill Clinton, I made it clear that I was making this trip as a private citizen and as a doctor. Traveling there "under the radar" on behalf of the United Nations had been difficult in previous months. But January 12 changed that.

The UN headquarters had collapsed in the quake, and most of its leadership was unaccounted for. No one in that beleaguered institution was likely to object to violations of protocol.

I was soon reunited with many of my colleagues from Zanmi Lasante and Partners In Health, most of them doctors working in Haiti: Louise Ivers, an infectious disease specialist who weathered the quake as the only physician in sight in the midst of dreadful losses and injuries in a hard-hit part of town; Joia Mukherjee, the medical director of Partners In Health; and David Walton, an internist and former student who'd worked in Haiti for a decade or more. Claire Pierre, an internist who'd grown up in Haiti and then trained in the United States, flew in with me and rarely left my side in the first days. All were volunteers from Harvard.

I haven't yet mentioned by name many of my Haitian coworkers. Most of them were fully engaged, a few at the General Hospital but most in the hospitals and clinics that we'd built up over the preceding years. These facilities were situated north and west of the epicenter, and from day one, my colleagues were preparing for waves of injured survivors fleeing the quake zone. By day three, the first wave had already crashed upon them.

There was so much to be done. But by day three, when we finally reached Port-au-Prince, we'd already missed two days to help save lives. Now we were surrounded by thousands of survivors—but many wouldn't be with us long without the right care. The only gratifying moments in those first few days came from two sources: pulling people alive from under the rubble (there were far too few of these "saves") and making sure that the injured received proper medical care (this occurred much more often).

As doctors and nurses, we were grateful to offer services to the injured, perhaps in part because the extent of the destruction made other needed activities, such as clearing debris or housing the homeless, seem overwhelming. Surely those tasks might be postponed for a few days at least, while we attended to the injured and tried to save lives? But from the beginning, we knew there were no simple answers. We could tend to the injured, but what about the homeless? We could treat the sick, but what about burying the dead? We could insert intravenous lines, but what about slaking, with clean water, the thirst of millions?

In those first few days after the quake, it seemed almost sacrilege to think about anything other than succor; the hard and inevitable work of reconstruction was difficult to even contemplate. And so we focused on alleviating the suffering right in front of us.

But for those not new to Haiti, the big picture of rebuilding was always in the back of our minds, even as we tended to the injured and the dying. This had been our modus operandi at Partners In Health and Zanmi Lasante for decades: to struggle to serve those right in front of us even as we struggled to think about the big picture. We sought to provide modern medical care and social services—schooling, housing, food and water, security, jobs—to neglected rural areas. But the temblor had struck the heart of the city. Although we wanted to help, where in the city should we go? Spontaneous settlements were springing up in every open space, and the sick and wounded were everywhere. We had little time to think.

Dr. Claire Pierre and I, and soon other reinforcements, were left to keep a promise: one place where help was clearly needed was Haiti's largest hospital. We weren't the only ones to reach this same conclusion. Already cluttered on day three with the injured and dying, the General Hospital was a scene of enormous confusion. Relief workers arrived by the dozens and casualties by the hundreds. With no electricity in the morgue or anywhere else, the entire place smelled like a charnel house.

There was never enough time, in those first days, to take stock, but we soon knew that both relief and recovery would be hampered by losses in the medical community. As Dr. Lassègue had said, the nursing school had collapsed during class, killing students and faculty alike. The Ministry of Health had been destroyed, too. Many clinics and hospitals in the city were down. The state medical school and hospital, the country's chief teaching facility, were badly damaged. Even for seasoned physicians, the quake zone was a horrifying scene. But more and more volunteers were streaming in to help.

Three days after the quake, the General Hospital campus was un-recognizable: the central courtyard, like the other open spaces in the city, was covered (or being covered) with tents and makeshift lean-tos fashioned from sheets and pieces of plastic, under which lay the injured and (if they were lucky) surviving family members and friends. Also there, although I was too dazed to see them, were al-most fifty children with disabilities: the hospital's unaccompanied minors, most of them orphaned in every sense of the word. We'd been trying to relocate them to a safe haven outside the city for weeks, but the quake found them still in the General Hospital. (I re-membered these children only many hours later, at three or four in the morning, and could only hope that someone else on our team had a plan to get them all to safe haven.)

We soon learned that simply keeping track of patients within a single hospital was a full-time job. Although the courtyards were packed, most of the wards were half-full: patients and staff were afraid to go into even ostensibly undamaged buildings. They had their reasons. For days, aftershocks had rolled through the city.[2] Ru-mors of approaching aftershocks emptied several of the wards as ter-rified and sick patients ripped IVs out of their arms in a rush for open space. The anxiety hung over the hospital, like the smell, and made delivery of medical care even more difficult.

This infectious anxiety endured for weeks, as did the aftershocks. To offer an example: late one evening, about a week after the quake, I spent the better part of an hour trying to convince a gasping, skele-tal young woman, her lungs half-consumed by tuberculosis, not to join the exodus that had emptied the wards after yet another after-shock. We were both inside when the shaking began, and I remem-ber putting a hand out to steady her oxygen tank, which weighed almost as much as she did. Never had I imagined such a scene: grasp-ing the top of a heavy tank inside a trembling building and trying to comfort a patient, while wondering whether the whole place was about to come down.

The patient's name was Natasha, and she was alone except for a young man sitting on the bed next to her. I assumed he was a family member, or perhaps a nurse's aide. It turned out that he was a Good

Samaritan who'd never met Natasha before. He had just traveled from a town south of Port-au-Prince with his own sister, badly injured when the quake destroyed their modest house. His sister had died a few hours before, he said, and he'd not yet decided where to go. So he lay down, alone in a fog of grief, in an empty hospital bed. And then the ground started to shake again. He leapt up to join the general exodus, but saw Natasha straining against her lifesaving contraptions, including the oxygen tank. He stayed in the building and did his best to calm her. Blood was seeping from around the IV catheter in her arm; panicked, she was also tugging against the tube that piped oxygen into her nose. Claire Pierre and I arrived just then and begged him to stay with her until we could find a staff member to assume these duties. They were both there the next day, still unassisted, but by then he was sitting next to her, reading from a well-thumbed Bible. He had also gone out into the fractured streets and found her something to eat.

———

Staff shortages at the General Hospital and elsewhere in the quake zone led some to assume that Haitian doctors and nurses had fled after the quake, unwilling to help. Our experiences suggested a different conclusion. Despite nursing their own wounds and losses, many Haitian health professionals were, in fact, back on the job within days or even hours. One assessment by an emergency medical aid group suggested that 95 percent of public-sector health workers had returned within one week of the quake.[3] What was missing, in addition to the hospitals and clinics in which they worked, was decent pay. How could they take care of their families, or purchase and maintain the equipment they needed to do their jobs?

The consequences of a longstanding lack of investment in medical infrastructure and training were obvious: manifest, for example, in quarrels about who would take care of the sick and wounded at night. Many relief workers blamed security protocols: they couldn't stay at the General Hospital at night without proper security, they said. But the hospital had never had funds for security. Most Haitian employees were not as concerned about security as they were about salaries. We all gave thanks for the Good Samaritans who struggled to save lives after the quake, even as we struggled with chronic problems such as low public-sector wages and lack of supplies.

Giving thanks for Good Samaritans was one thing; coordinating them, quite another. On day four after the quake, it was clear that the wounded city was mobbed with rescue and relief workers. More medical care was available in urban Haiti than ever before. The coalition brought together by the disruptive force of January 12 included a veritable horde of highly trained health professionals, most from North America (including hundreds of Haitian-Americans) and Europe but also many from Cuba and across Latin America and from countries as far away as Israel, Japan, and China; Haitian health providers who had never or rarely left Haiti, most of them touched directly by the quake and already teetering between gratitude for and resentment of better trained and better equipped teams who, while volunteering in Haiti, had paying jobs at home; the recently injured, some minority of them long spared the risks of premature disease and death endured by Haitians living in poverty; the UN survivors (the peacekeepers in their barracks were largely spared the fate of the civilians in the UN headquarters, which had collapsed in the quake); and of course the people and patients we knew best, the rural and urban poor. There were also sudden appearances by celebrities, including some, like Sean Penn, who came with cash and supplies and settled in to stay. Never in my wildest dreams could I have imagined being smack in the middle of such a life-and-death mix, much less in a post expected to bridge such disparate worlds. (Isn't that what envoys do?)

But such was our role and so were our tasks. As Dr. Lassègue predicted, one of the biggest problems was where to send patients in need of advanced surgical care. Some could be sent to the Partners In Health–affiliated hospitals in central Haiti, although our surgical capacity was limited; some could go to the new MASH units[4] in the city, such as those erected near the airport by the University of Miami and the Israeli Defense Forces, although nursing and follow-up care there was limited. But for many, we didn't yet have a plan. Even though thousands of relief workers were on hand, we were all waiting anxiously for the arrival of reinforcements.

What passed for Haiti's most important teaching hospital was still, despite the destroyed buildings around it, receiving more and more of the injured: people from south of the city and those lucky few rescued after days under rubble. We knew some reinforcements would soon be steaming into harbor in the form of a giant floating hospital. A week and a day after the quake, the USNS *Comfort* arrived, an oil tanker refitted with one thousand beds (including almost a hundred intensive care beds), twelve operating rooms, a large and well-trained staff assisted by scores of volunteers, and diagnostic equipment (including CAT scanners).[5] Even before the *Comfort* was stationed in the Bay of Port-au-Prince, helicopters wheeled overhead, some of them starting to ferry patients from on-land hospitals and other staging areas to the ship.

The *Comfort* towered over an armada of craft from a dozen or so countries in the harbor, including the USS *Carl Vinson*. It wasn't the English Channel before Normandy, but Haitian waters hadn't seen such traffic since Napoleon's failed attempt to retake Haiti in 1803.

Using the *Comfort* effectively, however, posed problems. The difficulties of coordination were clear enough within the General Hospital; now its leaders also had to manage the surfeit of goodwill offshore. Everyone wanted to help, but no one knew exactly what to do. Each of the many tents erected by NGOs in the hospital courtyards became its own semi-autonomous world.

In one tent, two dozen cots were packed into a space the size of a suburban kitchen. The patients on these beds were mostly quiet, with x-ray printouts clipped to the end of their beds; a few were groaning in pain and, post-op, needed nothing more than pain meds, which were in short supply. Most still wore clothes they'd been wearing when the quake hit, though pieces had been sheared away to expose their injuries: a broken leg here, a crushed arm there. Many had multiple fractures, and some had already undergone amputations. Family members often hung close to patients, doubling the number inside the small tent.

A group of nurses from Boston, sweating in the close heat, managed to keep things together—even though they didn't speak a word of Creole. These nurses were among the unsung heroes of the first weeks after the quake. Occasionally a surgeon—in this tent almost always an American—would come to check on a patient with whom he or she could not converse but whose life could be, and often was, saved by surgery. A few Haitian nurses' aides were working in the tent, but they spoke no more English than the patients did. We were lucky enough to have a few young but experienced Harvard doctors—one, in addition to Claire Pierre, was an American internist, Evan Lyon— who spoke fluent Creole and performed superhuman feats of translating inside and outside the tents, while also providing medical care.

I watched my former trainees (and there were many others, Haitian and American) with pride and gratitude. Claire could not be dissuaded from working twenty hours a day, taking no time to mourn the loss of many lifelong friends or the fact that her mother's home had been flattened, taking with it nearly every memento of her childhood. Evan stuck close to Lassègue, trying to help manage the influx of volunteers, some of them prickly, while nursing his own grief. (After a dozen years with Partners In Health, he'd lost friends, too.)

Claire and Evan were soon joined by a handful of medical residents from Boston, one of them Haitian-American and all of them willing to work on the logistics of connecting the disparate worlds of the patients, Haitian providers (from homeless, hungry medical students to returning nurses), volunteers, and even the military. The U.S. Air Force 1st Special Operations Wing took over coordination of the airport within days of the quake; working with them afforded the only means by which we could airlift patients to the ship or other remote sites.[6]

It was, for all of us, an entirely unprecedented circumstance. We were never sure what to do and were left with doubts about "disaster-relief expertise," even when those we encountered proclaimed surety. We wanted to be rescued by expertise, but we never were—this was the long, hard lesson of the quake.

To give readers a sense of what it was like in those first few days after the quake, at least for some of the doctors and nurses and patients, let me describe the events of a single afternoon and evening at the General Hospital. At least I believe it was a single night, a very long one, although none of us were taking notes. My guess is that it was day eight after the quake, because the *Comfort* was steaming into port and tents dotted the hospital grounds. These tents—a Red Cross tent, a Dartmouth tent, a Médecins Sans Frontières tent, and on and on—were at times like fractious federations. (There were even Scientologists in bright yellow t-shirts, though I didn't know how to explain to my Haitian colleagues what they were doing because I hadn't a clue what it was.)

In one tent, I spied a Haitian doctor standing anxiously over a thirty-four-year-old man who thought he'd escaped serious injury when his parents' house collapsed around him but now presented in respiratory distress. He looked whole but was gasping for breath. I was surprised when he addressed me by name and in English: "Dr. Paul, I know you from Cange. Help me, please. I can't breathe!"[7] This was the first and only time a patient there addressed me in English, and I immediately recognized him as the son of an acquaintance from Port-au-Prince. I had stayed many times with my closest Haitian friends, Father Fritz and Yolande "Mamito" Lafontant, in a house across the street from the one the patient's father was building in a neighborhood called Christ-Roi. (Mamito and Father Fritz had taken me in as a volunteer in 1983 and would later help found Zanmi Lasante and Partners In Health.) Much of the area, including the young man's large stone-and-cement house, had been leveled by the quake, while the Lafontants's house, though damaged, was still standing.

"How are you? What happened?" (I responded in Creole, not wishing to burden the man with a language that his wife, standing by his side, did not understand and which he spoke imperfectly even when not short of breath.)

His story came tumbling out in shreds: part of a wall had fallen on his legs; it took him an hour to free himself, but he was soon up and helping others in the neighborhood. "I felt okay," he said, "but my right leg hurt." He touched his right thigh. "It was only three days later that I suddenly couldn't breathe." The gasping itself was unnerving; his oxygen-saturation level suggested he should not be able to speak at all. I asked one of the Boston nurses, from Children's Hospital, to give him morphine, which pretty reliably eases such respiratory distress. What we really needed was to get him transferred to the *Comfort* and hooked up to mechanical ventilation—a "breathing machine," a procedure that would have been step one in a properly equipped hospital—while we tried to figure out what was wrong with him. But it was almost dark when he arrived, and the choppers needed to get him there were grounded for the night.

A physical exam revealed a high fever and minor abrasions on his legs. (Even these can be portals of entry for infection.) He'd been treated with antibiotics in another facility—the General Hospital was the third one in which he'd sought care—but an x-ray suggested severe pneumonia. We gave him a broad-spectrum antibiotic, and tried to treat him for blood clots that might have traveled from the large veins in his legs to his lungs. But we didn't have the right formulation of blood thinner on hand.

In minutes, the morphine kicked in and he was feeling well enough to ask, in one of his first complete sentences, for something to eat. His oxygen-saturation reading had improved some, but we still wanted him out of the tent and onto the *Comfort* as soon as possible. Although the morphine was responsible for his improvement, it wouldn't last long, nor would it treat his problems at their root. Fearing he wouldn't survive the night without mechanical ventilation, Evan and others tried to line him up for transfer.

We had many other patients to see that night. A slight elderly woman at the other end of the tent was wracked by the spasms of tetanus—the first of many cases we would see that week and the next. White-haired and weighing about ninety pounds, she had tears rolling down her cheeks. Every few minutes she would go rigid with potentially bone-breaking and suffocating spasms. The slightest stimulus triggered them; she needed to be in a dark, quiet room. But that would move her far away from medical care because, with frequent aftershocks shaking the foundations of the hospital, no one wanted to work inside.

At one point, I ducked outside for a breath of fresh air, and saw a young woman, perhaps twenty-five, lying on a stretcher outside, all alone in the pitch dark. Had she died? No, she was breathing and warm to the touch. I said hello and asked how she was feeling; she raised her hand and said, simply, "I think my legs are broken." I looked at an x-ray that had been tucked under her feet: both of her femurs were fractured high up, near the pelvis. I asked if she'd received anything for her pain; she had not. She had no family present—that was clear. She feared that her parents and infant daughter had perished. "The roof fell on us," she said and began to weep quietly. The best feeling I had during that wretched evening was bringing her pain medications, which soon led to what might have been her first sleep in days.[8] Her orthopedic injuries could be repaired, but as far as the emotional ones, who knew?

On one of those first days, Ophelia Dahl, the director of Partners In Health, had come down in a plane full of supplies and surgeons. She had also been working in Haiti since 1983, and it had changed her life as it changed mine. She was at the General Hospital that night, if memory serves. "Why aren't there more pain meds?" was one of her first questions. She was headed up to central Haiti to check on our teams there but was spending the night in the city. Ophelia and I were surveying the spectacle in the hospital—the misery and the pain, but also the mercy and compassion—and thinking the same thing: why Haiti?[9]

As would be the case on many evenings, we had no shortage of work and no reason to leave, except if we didn't we would be exhausted and useless the next day. I tried to corral my coworkers into rest. It was almost midnight, and we'd made some progress: we'd secured for the young man in respiratory distress the promise of a transfer to the *Comfort* by helicopter at daybreak; the old woman with tetanus had received antibiotics and heavy doses of diazepam (she would make it, I thought, if she didn't require mechanical ventilation); a number of patients with major trauma were now, like the young woman alone in the dark, resting thanks to pain meds.

As we prepared to leave, I heard an argument breaking out in English. A couple of Haitian-American doctors were yelling at some incredulous American surgeons. They were clashing over control of the operating rooms, which had never attracted much interest during all the years that poor Haitians in need of surgical interventions died unattended, even in this hospital of last resort.[10] One of the surgeons seemed to want me to referee the argument, but although there was much to say, it seemed the very worst place and time to say it. No one had energy to mediate disputes. So I hid in Claire's mother's car, waiting for Ophelia, Evan, and the others, until we finally left the hospital for houses further up the hill, away from the worst damage. We were spent. As our car climbed through a wrecked and darkened neighborhood, a dog darted in front of us and we heard a thud. No one said a word.

Most of my colleagues were staying with Claire's extended family. (Her godmother had taken in scores of volunteers and newly homeless family members, including Claire's mother.) But I headed back to the wooden (and thus safer) house of close friends in Pétionville, arriving shortly after midnight. They lived far above the heat and odor of the vast, blacked-out city below. My host Maryse had even put flowers in my room, as she always did. There was a bottle of water by my bed and, aside from the white noise of a whirring fan, blessed silence.

But I couldn't sleep. In the dim reaches of misery, insomnia is a constant companion, especially when twenty-first-century people die of nineteenth-century afflictions—minor injuries and simple fractures as well as pneumonia, tuberculosis, and other infections, such as tetanus, preventable with a vaccine available for pennies. I was pursued by the sights and smells and sounds of the day: the unrelieved pain; patients and doctors sprinting outside during an aftershock; the young man in respiratory distress (Had we given him everything that might tide him over until he reached the ship? If only we had more blood thinners and the right lab equipment!); the arguments and competition between different dispensers of "disaster relief" over the privilege of looking after people who had long been neglected; the grief of my former students (among the most competent of the lot, but they too were spent); the solidity of the hospital's Haitian leadership; the unrelieved pain (Why didn't we have, at the very least, more analgesia for those with awful trauma?); and pervading all, the charnel-house odor from the morgue and under the rubble. I tried especially to forget the morgue. But counting sheep kept turning into the grim process of counting the dead. I even thought of the hapless dog. The image of the man who couldn't breathe was still with me as dawn approached. (Had he survived the night? Surely the floating hospital could save him?)

Hanging on to this hope, I fell into a deep sleep. But after just an hour or so, I was shaken alert by a large aftershock. The wood of the house strained and creaked; the paintings in the room tilted; the water bottle at my bedside started to tremble. My host yelled for us to "get out of the house right now!" The sun was coming up, and I watched impassively as the water bottle fell to the floor. I heard those in the house scrambling to get out, and saw, in my mind's eye, the crushed limbs of people trapped in countless other houses during the quake. I knew I should move and thought of my children, who had spent the recent holidays in Haiti but, by the grace of God, had been spared the fate of so many a few days after they left. It would have been prudent to bolt down the stairs and into the street.

But I didn't move a leaden muscle and did not wake again until the sun was high in the sky.

# 2.

=

# PRAXIS AND POLICY
## *The Years before the Quake*

*A*lthough *many of those* who came to Haiti right after the quake claimed to have expertise in disaster relief, there was ample reason for skepticism. From the beginning, we struggled to help the injured and otherwise afflicted, but it wasn't always clear what needed to be done. We continued in this emergency mode for days, furnishing direct care to the injured and displaced, while trying to make (or help others make) decisions about the coordination and delivery of services. This tension was everywhere: on the one hand, a particular injured or sick person, but on the other, decisions about shelter or clinical services for hundreds of thousands of displaced people. Most of the policy decisions were, of course, not being made by physicians. But never before had my medical colleagues been pushed to think harder about challenges so far removed from clinical care.

In many ways, however, this tension—between serving those right in front of you and seeking to reduce the longer-term risk of others ending up in front of you—has been the chief tension of my work for years. This tension has animated the work of my students, trainees, and coworkers, too, because poverty and inequality are the drivers of most of the diseases and misfortunes we see. Even an

earthquake is not only a "natural" disaster, just as the destructive-
ness of Hurricane Katrina and the storms that struck Haiti in 2004
and 2008 were influenced by many factors besides weather. These
events reveal the social roots of disaster.[1] It's an undisputed fact that,
even before the quake, Haiti, Latin America's first independent nation, was plagued by political, economic, and ecological fragilities.
Part of this book's project is to examine how Haiti and its institutions
became so weak: to lay out the history of the chronic ailment. The
other main topic of this book—beyond an account of the quake—is
this tension between praxis and policy: the struggle between direct
service, which is what doctors are supposed to provide, and policy,
which is what politicians and legislators are supposed to formulate
with, in theory, the guidance of the citizenry they represent.

For years, I'd sought to face this challenge through direct service
to the poor—especially those affected by infectious diseases—and,
as a professor at Harvard Medical School, by writing and teaching
about the large-scale forces that shape vulnerability to suffering
and premature death. This dual mandate is, as I've said, a fact of life
for my students, trainees, and for all my colleagues at Partners In
Health. We work in a dozen nations—including the United
States—where the poor suffer disproportionately. During my first
decade in Haiti, I mostly left policy alone, except to critique it. In
books and articles, my colleagues and I sought to bridge the gap between service and policy or at least to help inform policy discussions. But writing for an academic audience is not the same as
sitting through policy meetings and diplomatic conferences. Academic physicians, including those in the field now called social
medicine, would be hard-pressed to show concrete ways in which
research and writing shape health policy or lead to improved implementation of services.

Health care does not exist in a separate universe from politics. Fiscal policy, infrastructure, wages, taxation—all affect the practice of
medicine, and we learned, over the years, that seeking to improve
health policy was one of the best ways to defend the modest gains
we'd achieved for our patients. This effort to link praxis and policy

started at the local level. For example, our work with Haiti's national tuberculosis and AIDS programs in the late eighties began in a handful of towns and districts. A few years later, thanks in large part to Dr. Jim Kim, another founder of Partners In Health and then also a Harvard faculty member, and to Dr. Jaime Bayona, a Peruvian colleague, we became more engaged in international health policy debates about tuberculosis, including the more difficult-to-treat forms of drug-resistant tuberculosis. "Difficult-to-treat" did not mean "untreatable," we argued, again and again, in meetings and in obscure medical journals.[2] Unlike many in the international agencies we sought to persuade, we had direct clinical experience treating patients with drug-resistant tuberculosis, and we could claim some degree of authority thanks to high cure rates in Haiti and Peru.

These debates led us to Russia, which was facing epidemics of drug-resistant tuberculosis, as the United States had faced a few years prior. In Russia and elsewhere in the former Soviet Union, these epidemics were large and were proving especially deadly inside prisons.[3] The financier-philanthropist George Soros had donated more than twelve million dollars to provide tuberculosis care in Russian prisons. He'd asked our team to help because conventional treatment approaches were failing to cure patients with drug-resistant strains. But the program as conceived still did not have enough financing for second-line medications (needed to treat drug-resistant tuberculosis) or enhanced lab capacity, which would permit clinicians to discern which patients needed such drugs. When we asked Soros for more money, instead of saying yes, as we expected, he said no. It would be a mistake, he explained, to let governments off the hook.

It was this work (and Soros himself) that led me in the 1990s to visit the White House, where Hillary Clinton became a patron of our efforts to raise the standard of tuberculosis care in Russian prisons and elsewhere. (TB was not a regional epidemic, but a global threat.) She soon also became a friend and mentor. Over the next decade I saw firsthand how high-level policy interventions could open up new—and sometimes vast—possibilities for improved delivery of services to the poor and marginalized. In one prison in western

Siberia, we worked with the Russian Ministry of Justice, to bring case-fatality rates from 26 percent (more than a quarter of those on treatment died) to close to zero within two years.[4] The drugs were expensive, but they worked, and better planning and pooled procurement would drive costs down further. In its first year of operation, the Gates Foundation supported an ambitious program to scale up these complex interventions in Peru while also augmenting efforts in Russia.

The tuberculosis pandemic was one complex health problem among many, and neither Russia's prisons nor Lima's slums were the world's poorest settings. Other epidemics were spreading in Africa, even as science gave us new tools to fight them. By the close of the millennium, it was obvious that we needed a radically different approach to the health problems of the poor. Existing models were premised on the idea that public health and medicine should be cheap. But these anemic approaches wouldn't do much to lessen the burden of disease on the poor. Those on the front lines encountered millions with AIDS and tuberculosis and malaria, and also every imaginable cancer and noncommunicable disease. Because these patients were poor before they became sick, we needed something other than fee-for-service models. We also needed heavy investments in infrastructure, training, and direct services, especially for the bottom billion—the poorest and most marginalized. Implementation was the biggest challenge—and figuring out how to finance it.

AIDS was not only the leading cause of adult death in many of the places we worked; by the year 2000, it surpassed tuberculosis as the world's leading infectious killer. As we showed in central Haiti, effective diagnostics and therapeutics for AIDS could be delivered to even the most destitute sick with the help of community health workers.[5] But few seemed interested in funding AIDS care in poor countries. Policy debates pitted prevention against care—as if these were competing priorities rather than complementary ones—and many thought doing both would be too expensive. Partners In Health had been able to finance AIDS treatment in central Haiti because of the generosity of people such as Tom White, a Boston contractor who had given us millions of dollars over the years. But dependence on angel investors wasn't going to save millions of lives in Africa, much less integrate prevention and care and strengthen weak health systems. "You need billions, not millions, of dollars," Jeff Sachs, a development economist and colleague at Harvard, observed.[6]

In December 2000, Sachs and his wife, Sonia, a pediatrician, came to central Haiti to meet some of our AIDS patients, most of whom were flourishing with the help of antiretroviral drugs—the very drugs that many health policy experts argued were too difficult to administer in such poverty-stricken settings. On the spot, Sachs promised to work with the United Nations and several governments to create new funding mechanisms to respond to AIDS, tuberculosis, and malaria, three diseases that by 2001 were claiming six million lives a year. He kept his promise. I was lucky enough to travel to New York with the Haitian delegation, led by another health advocate, First Lady Mildred Aristide, to the first UN general assembly on AIDS. We collectively pushed for new resources to respond to what was then a fairly new and now global threat. A group of Harvard faculty also published a consensus statement arguing that AIDS care and prevention needed to be integrated in the settings hardest hit by the disease.[7]

A year later, with the help of Sachs and many others, including heroic AIDS activists, the Global Fund to Fight AIDS, Tuberculosis, and Malaria was born. One of the Global Fund's first major grants went towards AIDS programs in Haiti. That same year, a group of physicians lobbied the new U.S. administration to pursue the same agenda, and before long, George W. Bush launched the U.S. President's Emergency Plan for AIDS Relief. Together, these two programs brought billions of dollars to bear on the neglected diseases of the poor, and saved—no exaggeration—millions of lives. We believed that these disease-specific programs could, if designed properly, be used to strengthen health systems generally, as they had done in central Haiti.[8] Jim Kim left Harvard for the World Health Organization to pursue this vision—bringing better medical services to the world's bottom billion—on the level of global policy. (Jim later became president of Dartmouth College and was responsible for Dartmouth's significant presence in Haiti in the first weeks after the quake.)

It was during these years, when I was shuttling between Haiti and Harvard, that President Clinton launched the Clinton Health Access Initiative (CHAI) and became another mentor and colleague. At an AIDS meeting in Barcelona in the summer of 2002, he made plans to come to Haiti and encouraged us to work in Rwanda. "You watch," he predicted then, "Rwanda will become a model of smart development." Shortly thereafter, Ira Magaziner, the other driving force behind CHAI, also visited AIDS patients—many of whom had to all intents and purposes risen from the dead after receiving the right treatment—and facilities in central Haiti.

By 2003, when President Clinton arrived to announce his foundation's intention to help out in Haiti, we were ready to extend our work throughout the center of the country. Indeed, we'd already started and had a crackerjack Haitian team led by Fernet Léandre, Maxi Raymonwille, Loune Viaud, and many others. It was about that time that Louise Ivers, David Walton, Evan Lyon, and Joia Mukherjee, introduced earlier, joined the Haiti team to scale up our efforts within the public sector health system. With support from the Global Fund, we designed our effort to help not only AIDS patients but all patients, and to focus on prevention at the same time. The idea was to work in public facilities (such as the General Hospital, which is where Clinton made his announcement), rather than competing with or supplanting them. The Haitian government was squarely behind the plan. I was as enthusiastic as I'd ever been about linking direct service to training (at Harvard and in Haiti) and research that might inform health policy.

We'd also launched, with Cuban colleagues and the Aristide Foundation, a new medical school that would focus on improving the health of the Haitian poor, especially in rural areas.[9] (The great majority of Haiti's health professionals worked in Port-au-Prince.) We were set for a good decade, I thought, and so did our students and trainees at Brigham and Women's Hospital (the Harvard hospital where I trained and where we'd launched training programs for young doctors committed to global health).

But then came the February 2004 coup in Haiti, which further weakened the public health infrastructure.[10] Haiti's president and his wife, our staunchest advocates in the fight against AIDS, were spirited away to the Central African Republic in a way that resembled nothing so much as the "extraordinary renditions" of suspected terrorists described in the popular press. Haiti's elected government was replaced by a group of unelected officials (unelected by Haitians, in any case), and the Prime Minister, Yvon Neptune, was tossed in jail without charges. It was a dispiriting time, in large part because of the lies and distortions that figured prominently in many official policies, including some of my own country.

Although the Global Fund efforts went forward, the Clinton Foundation declined to work in Haiti under the régime installed after the coup (an honorable gesture, which made absolutely no impression on the de factos, as they were called). Instead, the Clinton Foundation urged Partners In Health to launch a major rural health initiative in Rwanda with the national government's health authorities. I'd visited Rwanda before and admired its governance, born of horrible circumstances and still subject, at the time, to legitimate critique and negative propaganda (some of which came from France, some from surviving architects of the 1994 genocide, but also some from more credible voices in human rights circles). In the fall of 2004, we made a long-term commitment to begin a comprehensive rural health initiative in Rwanda.

From 2005 on, we continued to expand our work in the public hospitals across central Haiti, while some of us, including leadership from our Haiti team and Harvard Brigham colleagues, began setting up shop in southeastern Rwanda. We were first dispatched to a long-abandoned hospital in an area of former national parklands where as many as 60 percent of the population had been displaced, at one point or another.

It was satisfying work. By the summer of 2008, it was easy to see the power of good public health governance when linked to funding and to decent implementation capacity. Working with the Rwandan Ministry of Health (which had also received support from the Global Fund) and the Clinton Foundation, Partners In Health recruited and trained two thousand health workers, rehabbed a dozen clinics, rebuilt two hospitals, and broke ground on a third. (We'd been sent to three of the four districts in Rwanda that lacked any working district hospital; the country has thirty districts.) If the work remained on track, we would soon be serving as large a population in Rwanda as we served in Haiti, where the effort had taken two decades.

But Haiti exerted a hold over us all, and we felt it more sharply in times of trouble. The country had known plenty of troubles, even compared to Rwanda, and the situation was about to get worse. During these years, I flew between Haiti, Harvard, and Rwanda, and my family moved to Rwanda's famously spotless capital city of Kigali in 2006. Kigali was in many ways the mirror opposite of Port-au-Prince. Although Haiti's capital in 2007 was no longer being termed "the kidnapping capital of the world," as it had the year before, progress there was slow.[11] Haiti was disheveled and disorderly and unsafe. The de facto government had been replaced by one led by René Préval, Aristide's former prime minister, but his government was unable to find firm footing. In April 2008, a worldwide spike in food prices (which had almost nothing to do with Haitian policies and more to do with biofuels and U.S. and European agricultural subsidies), commodity speculation, and lopsided trade policies, led to riots throughout Haiti; attacks on UN peacekeepers stationed there resulted in several deaths, most of them Haitian. Yet another government collapsed, and for months the country had no prime minister because the Haitian parliament refused to ratify the proposed successor, Michèle Pierre-Louis, an economist who had worked on education initiatives and headed up George Soros's foundation in Haiti.

The riots and political impasse had shaken the eight-thousand-strong UN establishment in Haiti. Leadership in the local UN offices and in New York pushed for a shift of focus, from peacekeeping and policing to what some called "human security"—decent jobs, food security, education, access to clean water, and medical care. From Rwanda, where we'd experienced the effect of that country's commitment to development and human security, we cheered this shift.

Late August of 2008 found many of us in Rwanda, when, during a visit from President Clinton for the groundbreaking of a new hospital, we got more bad news from Haiti. Another hurricane (on the heels of two before it) had struck northwest Haiti and Cuba with great loss of life in Haiti (but almost none in Cuba, which had evacuated more than a million citizens from harm's way).[12] Haiti's third largest city, Gonaïves, was under several feet of water. I headed back there and, on September 6, hours after returning from the drowned city, drafted a letter to our supporters. I'll quote it at length because the sentiment that "Partners In Health is not a relief organization, but we'll do whatever we can to help" would prove relevant again only fifteen months later. So too would our understanding of the sharp limitations on Haitian officials who lacked the resources to respond to such circumstances. Here is the letter as it was posted:

> I am writing from Mirebalais, the place where our organization was born, having just returned from Gonaïves—perhaps the city hit hardest by Hurricane Hanna, which, hard on the heels of Fay and Gustav, drenched the deforested mountains of Haiti and led to massive flooding and mudslides in northern and central Haiti. A friend of mine said this morning: "I am 61 years old, born and raised in Hinche. I have never seen it under water." Gonaïves, with 300,000 souls, is in far worse shape, as you'll see from the other pictures I append. The floodwaters in Hinche are dropping, but as of 5 P.M. last night, when we left Gonaïves, the city was still under water. And hurricanes Ike and Josephine are heading this way as I write.
>
> Everyone copied on this note has already heard, most probably directly from PIH, about these storms and their impact on Haiti. I apologize for writing again and for asking my own colleagues and friends to consider sending more resources—we need food, water, clothes, and, especially, cash (which can be converted into all of the above)—so that Zanmi Lasante, and thus all of us, can do our part to save lives and preserve human dignity.
>
> The need is of course enormous. After twenty-five years spent working in Haiti and having grown up in Florida, I can honestly say that I have never seen anything as painful as what I just witnessed in Gonaïves—except in that very same city, four years ago. Again, you know that 2004 was an especially brutal year, and those who work with Partners In Health know why: the coup in Haiti and what would

become Hurricane Jeanne. Everyone knows that Katrina killed 1,500 in New Orleans and on the Gulf Coast, but very few outside of our circles know that what was then Tropical Storm Jeanne, which did not even make landfall in Haiti, killed an estimated 2,000 in Gonaïves alone. . . .

We're faced with another round of death and obliteration. Haiti's naked mountains promise many more unnatural disasters. We know that a massive reforestation program and public works to keep cities safer are what's needed in the medium and long term. But there's a lot we can do in the short term to help out with disaster relief.

None of us regard Partners In Health as a disaster-relief organization. Together, we've built Partners In Health—meaning the network of locally directed organizations working in ten countries—to serve a different cause. We wanted to attack poverty and inequality and bring the fruits of modernity—health care, education, et cetera—to people marginalized by adverse social forces. It seemed likely, as reports came in this week, that many other institutions and organizations would be far better able to respond to the aftereffects of storms and floods. I'd been told, as the American Airlines flight passed over flooded Gonaïves, that the city was cut off from outside help, but even as I heard this, I knew that our own colleagues were there, volunteering what meager resources we had on hand, and a few hours later I was there, too. I was hoping that we'd find that the city was receiving the expert attention of organizations trained to do disaster relief. So imagine my surprise, yesterday, when I discovered that very little in the way of help had reached Gonaïves or the other flooded towns along the coast.

Although it's not true that Gonaïves cannot be reached by vehicle, it is true that the city center is still under water, and that the road into the city is well and truly flooded. Between Pont Sondé—the only way to the coast (since the major bridge between Port-au-Prince and Gonaïves is out, as is that to the north)—and the flooded city, we saw not a single first-aid station or proper temporary shelter. We saw, rather, people stranded on the tops of their houses or wading through waist-deep water; we saw thousands in an on-foot exodus south towards Saint-Marc.

We saw a couple of UN tanks rolling through the muddy water over these streets, some Cuban doctors, and two Red Cross vehicles (one of them stuck in mud at least 10 miles from the city), and heard and saw helicopters overhead. But for the most part the streets were full of debris, upside-down vehicles, and dazed residents looking to get out before the next rains. Our friend Deo from Burundi was there and said it reminded him of nothing so much as what he'd seen there, and in Rwanda, at the time of the genocide in 1994—long lines of people carrying little more than their children, goats, and balancing sodden bags and suitcases on their heads.

A speedy, determined relief effort could save the lives of tens of thousands of Haitians in Gonaïves and all along the flooded coast. The people of that city and others have been stranded without food or water or shelter for three days and it's simply not true that they cannot be reached. When I called to say as much to friends working with the U.S. government and with disaster-relief organizations based in Port-au-Prince, it became clear that, as of yesterday, there's not a lot of accurate information leaving Gonaïves, although estimates of hundreds of deaths are not hyperbolic. We had no cell phone coverage there and had to wait until last night to call people in Port-au-Prince. One sympathetic American friend, following up on our distress calls about the lack of relief, told me this morning the retort she'd heard from an expert employed by a UN-affiliated health organization: "Three days without water is nothing. People in southern Haiti affected by Gustav went ten days without water."

No human can go ten days without water. Food, perhaps. But not water. So we can expect that the people you see in these photographs, which I took by borrowing the digital camera of a Zanmi Lasante employee from Gonaïves (whose family, like all those you see, lost everything), are at great risk of falling ill with water-borne illnesses. There is also a lot of dead livestock floating down the streets of the city. The stench is overwhelming.

We are familiar with a lot of the Haitian officials charged with responding to this tragedy, which is, agreed, widespread. They showed up in Gonaïves: the district health commissioner, who is from the city and felt lucky to have avoided drowning; the coordinator of the government's disaster response; nurses and doctors we've known over the years. They are doing the best they can with scant supplies. They are tired, thirsty themselves, hoarse-throated. Even Haiti's newly appointed Prime Minister, on her first day on the job, showed up this morning in Mirebalais, keeping a promise she made many months ago, long before she was directly involved in politics. She now has to install a new government, perhaps this afternoon, and respond to multiple disasters at once. These people, who are trying to help their fellow Haitians, deserve our help.[13]

I wrote this letter a few hours before Ike, the fourth storm, hit Haiti. Pierre-Louis' first official visit was to the shabby Mirebalais hospital, which sat in a place everyone called *lòt bò latem*—"on the other side of the river." The bridge connecting the town center to the hospital was also the span that connected central Haiti to the coast. A modest bit of infrastructure, the bridge was nonetheless a key artery. (Although there's no reason that the new prime minister would pause to make such an observation any more than might any of those accustomed to crossing it.) But that night, as Hurricane Ike drenched central Haiti's deforested mountains, a flash flood hit a UN base (home to a battalion of Nepalese peacekeepers) and swept scores of empty cargo containers into the river. The containers—with "UN" marked in huge black letters—struck the Mirebalais bridge with enough force to bring it down, and the Central Plateau was cut off from the coast for months. The only way to reach the hospital was in dugout canoes.

This letter became Partners In Health's first online appeal. (The generous response to this letter would later be dwarfed by the heartening response to our appeals after the earthquake.) After returning to Harvard, I forwarded the Gonaïves letter to a number of current and former U.S. government officials. We heard back from several of them, including President Clinton, who called within hours of receiving the appeal. He underlined the need to link palliation of suffering—disaster relief—with strategy and longer-term investments to grow Haiti's economy. To paraphrase his comments: "What can I do to help? We have to provide relief, but we need to focus on the big picture: Haitians need more and better jobs, and perhaps some of them could be in reforestation and public works, like during the American Depression." Clinton called as I was about to begin a lecture at Harvard Medical School, and I thought, once again, about how disparate were the worlds we spanned: Haiti and Harvard, New York and rural Rwanda.

Clinton had been in northern Rwanda for a hospital's ground-breaking. But while there (with his daughter Chelsea), it seemed he spent more time talking about Haiti than he did about our medical work in Africa. (By then, we were working together not only in Rwanda but also in Malawi and Lesotho.) After the hurricanes, we made plans to meet in Haiti and to travel to Gonaïves together within the next month or two.

With food riots, storms, the collapse of a shoddily built school full of kids,[14] and an entire city and some of Haiti's most fertile regions under water (which led, in part, to widespread hunger across the country), 2008 seemed apocalyptic. Few imagined that something much worse was in store.

---

I was still trying to think and write and teach about health and development. Any doctor practicing in Haiti knew very well that the country's refractory poverty, worsened each year by political instability, unfair trade policies, and environmental disasters, rendered our patients sick. In other words, large-scale forces beyond the traditional scope of clinical medicine were the chief drivers of illness and misfortune among the poor. The story was similar everywhere we worked, from Russia to Rwanda: our patients needed jobs. Most would have been happy with almost any kind of steady employment. The jobs we'd created over the years were mainly for community health workers. They had long been paid too little in part because of the social fiction, encouraged by influential economists and policy mandarins, that such workers should be unpaid "community health volunteers." Development experts (themselves compensated) claimed it was not "sustainable" or cost-effective to pay community health workers.

For years, we'd encouraged medical students to listen to their patients. The more I listened to patients, the more I revised my views on the matter of jobs. In a book written almost two decades previously, I railed against the offshore assembly industry in Haiti, which, it had seemed then, did little more than exploit grotesque differentials in labor costs.[15] In 1971, Eduardo Galeano noted "the wages Haiti requires by law belong in the department of science fiction," and nothing that had happened there since changed my mind about the imperative of decent pay and better conditions for workers.[16] But scores of Haitians were fleeing the depleted countryside, where we worked, for the Dominican Republic or the often-illusory promise of factory jobs in Port-au-Prince. Again, these forces, many of which originated far from Haitian soil, were beyond the control of those buffeted by them. President Clinton himself had publicly apologized for pushing legislation that undermined Haitian rice production: U.S. agricultural subsidies meant that Haitian farmers could not compete with U.S. agribusiness.[17] Haiti, once the world's leading exporter of sugar, was also now a net importer of subsidized sugar from the United States and elsewhere.

Haitian agriculture continued to be hammered by the forces of nature, by the punishingly unfair political economy (to use an old-school term), and by the simple fact that few young Haitians wanted to work in a sector that offered diminishing returns. Those who did want to farm had no access to credit, good seeds, fertilizer, or the tools of their trade. Addressing these problems required massive pro-poor investments in agriculture, which would do more to alleviate Haitian poverty than fifty thousand new assembly jobs. But did development need to be a competition for scarce resources when all other parts of the Haitian economy needed investments, too?

Deforestation was a case in point. Halting or reversing the steady disappearance of Haiti's forests would reduce the risk of floods and avalanches and erosion but would require multiple interventions at once. Everyone knew, for example, that Haiti needed a new energy source, at least for cooking, that left the few remaining trees standing. Rural people felled trees to make charcoal, which they used for their own daily needs and sold as a cash crop. Alternative cooking energies wouldn't solve the problem unless they truly became available to all and unless simultaneous investments were made in agriculture, food-processing plants, and fair trade.

Just after the fourth storm struck, I wrote in the *Nation* that progressives needed to spend more time thinking about how to expand the Haitian economy by improving conditions for smallholder farmers while creating new job opportunities in manufacturing and public works (and, of course, in health care and education). Allow me to cite the *Nation* essay at length as it shows why doctors who listen to their patients can find themselves far afield from clinical medicine, and why it's important to understand Haiti's history in seeking to make (to use medical jargon) a diagnosis and treatment plan. Because Haiti's new prime minister took office on the day of the fourth storm, I started by referring to the challenges before her. These were rooted in Haiti's history:

> Pierre-Louis, an economist new to politics, knows that these disasters are not purely "natural." She also knows that the rural poor cut down trees to make charcoal because they have no choice. Only alternative fuels and reforestation, linked with other public works, and thus jobs, can reverse Haiti's deforestation. Jobs outside the agricultural sector are urgently needed if reforestation is to happen. This should make progressives slow to disparage new jobs in the tourist and apparel industries, dealt severe blows by the political unrest of the recent past.
>
> That Haiti is a veritable graveyard of development projects has less to do with Haitian culture and more to do with the nation's place in the world. The history that turned the world's wealthiest slave colony into the hemisphere's poorest country has been tough, in part because of a lack of respect for democracy both among Haiti's small élite and in successive French and U.S. governments. During the first half of the nineteenth century, the United States simply refused to acknowledge Haiti's existence. In the latter half, gunboats pre-empted diplomacy. And in 1915 U.S. Marines began a twenty-year military occupation and formed the modern Haitian army (whose only target has been the Haitian people). After the fall of Duvalier in 1986, Wash-

ington continued to support unelected, mainly military, governments. Indeed, it was not until after 1990, when Haiti had its first democratic elections, that assistance to the government was cut back and finally cut off. The decay of the public sector—through aid cutoffs and neoliberal policies—is one of the chief reasons Haiti, unlike neighboring Cuba, is unable to respond to hurricanes with effective relief.

Haiti needs and deserves a modern Marshall Plan that rebuilds public institutions and creates jobs outside of the worn-down agricultural sector. Without one, it will have a hard time surviving the hurricane season. And next year will be worse.[18]

It was an easy prophesy: next year would be much worse. Through Zanmi Lasante, Partners In Health had created thousands of jobs in health care and education, and quite a few in construction, but we worried that they were not generative enough. What would a Marshall Plan for Haiti look like? Again, the agricultural sector needed massive investments to make farming more remunerative. Reforestation efforts also needed to be linked to real incentives for Haiti's smallholders. But what else deserved more support? Something in light industry, outside the perilously crowded and fragile capital city? What about fish farming? Support of women entrepreneurs? We turned to a small group of Partners In Health supporters with business experience and challenged them to launch a project called "1,000 Jobs for Haiti." With their help, we created many pro-poor jobs in central Haiti.

But Haiti needed millions, not thousands, of decent jobs, and this meant intervening at a policy level. When Hillary Clinton accepted the job of Secretary of State, in January 2009, I was faced with an entirely new dilemma: should I join the government and work with her full-time on development issues? Red flags came up as I contemplated the role. Some of the people I conferred with raised doubts about my working full-time on policy. Others suggested that my work for Partners In Health, for which I'd always been a volunteer, might be seen as a conflict of interest rather than relevant experience. Even more troubling was another open question: Would I have to give up clinical medicine and teaching? I would surely have to give up a certain freedom of expression in a highly partisan environment that was unpleasant for the conflict-averse. I couldn't imagine a life without clinical work, teaching, and writing whatever I felt was right; nor could I imagine a life without volunteer work for the destitute sick. Harvard Medical School had given me that freedom, and for perhaps the first time in my life I understood what a gift it was to be in academic medicine.

It was at this time, as I struggled with a decision that had been made public against my will,[19] that President Clinton accepted the honorary post of UN Special Envoy for Haiti. He knew how anxious I was about failing to be the sort of effective bureaucrat that our government and the development enterprise deserved. He asked me to be his deputy at the United Nations, which had a huge, largely military, presence in Haiti. I would share the rank of UN undersecretary-general; each of us would be paid a dollar a year. This meant I would not have to give up my teaching and clinical work but might still have a voice in policy discussions about Haiti. I sought the approval of the dean of Harvard Medical School, who offered it without reservation. "You are linking research and training to service, and you involve your students and trainees," he told me in August 2009. "That's what global health needs to be about." My chief at Brigham and Women's Hospital was supportive for the same reasons.

Jeff Sachs helped me try to recruit Garry Conille, a Haitian physician schooled in the ways of the UN, to head the team. But Conille was otherwise occupied, the UN told us. I insisted on bringing Haitians onto the team—none had been proposed—and colleagues at Partners In Health and the Clinton Foundation, led by Laura Graham, Clinton's current Chief of Staff. Graham was a force of nature: she invested uncountable hours in every issue she worked on. The bureaucratic challenges in this arena were significant, but a young Egyptian journalist, Jéhane Sedky, who had worked with Clinton in his previous role as Special Envoy after the 2004 tsunami, knew the ropes; she helped Jennie Block, a theologian and friend, and me pull together a team to help Clinton stand with Haiti. Our focus would be to "build back better" from the 2008 storms by pushing for long-term investments in sustainable development. We also sought to address sharp deficits in public health and public education. Foreign assistance needed to be built back better, too, and our little team shared another aspiration: to move the focus from military assistance to development assistance, from security to human security, towards freedom from want.

Three weeks later, I made my first trip to Haiti as a diplomat. Such travel was an experience familiar to President Clinton, but was, after hundreds of trips to Haiti, new to me. I moved about in an armored car and in a motorcade; I had a bodyguard (a Haitian-American policeman from Atlanta, who politely termed himself "a personal protection agent"). Clinton counseled me to focus on two broad agendas: the medical and public health issues I knew best but also the economic issues that influenced who got sick and who did not. I later learned that my trip had merited press coverage in the Miami *Herald:*

> A prominent Harvard doctor and Haiti advocate completed his first visit to the Caribbean nation Tuesday in his new capacity as the United Nations' deputy Special Envoy.
>
> Paul Farmer made the five-day visit as part of a follow-up trip that UN Special Envoy Bill Clinton made last month to Haiti, which suffered extensively last year because of back-to-back storms, food riots and a nearly five-month political crisis. The trip's goal: gauge how best to support the Haitian government in its national recovery plan.
>
> During his visit, Farmer met with Haitian President René Préval and Prime Minister Michèle Pierre-Louis and other government officials, as well as with business leaders and representatives from the UN and nongovernmental organizations. Farmer also visited the Central Plateau region and Cap Haïtien, Haiti's second largest city, where he met with local leaders and tourism officials.[20]

This all sounded good, and I believed in the mission. Haiti had a terrible reputation internationally for dozens of reasons, most of them wrong. But it wasn't possible to claim that anti-Haitian propaganda was based purely on fantasy. After the public meetings mentioned in the press, I dragged the UN security team to visit the widow of a friend and colleague. Our lead surgeon, Dr. Josué

Augustin, had been murdered in Hinche on August 31. (Although I struggled to believe it was murder, and not an accident, what meager forensic evidence we had was clear enough.) It was impossible to begin a cheerleading campaign for Haiti as a safe place to invest when a protégé had been killed that same week. I wrote a eulogy for Josué:

> All of us are still reeling from the loss of Josué Augustin, whom we have known as student, intern, resident, colleague, and friend. Above all, we knew him as Dr. Josué, a level-headed and thoughtful surgeon and the driving force behind our collective efforts to make sure that surgery did not remain the "neglected stepchild" of our work in Haiti. Josué combined a rigorous pragmatism with a broad vision of what could be done to improve complex medical services, and surgery especially, in settings in which such endeavors are too often dismissed as impractical, not cost-effective, or even (absurdly enough) unnecessary. What this meant in terms of everyday practice was that he was there to round on patients, to scrub in, to organize a team of people (many of them from rural Haiti, others from far away) to provide care to those who would otherwise not have it. What this meant in terms of his own agenda was that he was always willing to engage people from all over the world (and especially from the United States and Cuba) who believed in his mission. It meant he was willing to go to where the pathology was, whether that meant Cange, Boucan Carré, Saint-Marc, Belladères, Petite Rivière de l'Artibonite, Lascahobas, or Hinche, where he was taken from us, and from his family and patients, just last week. What this means for us, beyond our grief, is that we must fight hard to make sure that Josué's vision of equitable surgical services for the poor is one that remains front and center, not just in Haiti but in those other regions, regions full of people in need, too readily written off as unsuitable for surgery. We honor Josué by making sure that such an important mission outlives him or any other one person.

Although uncomfortable with the heavy protocol, which was often completely over the top, I settled into a good working relationship with the UN Haiti team. This group of eight or so people led a staff of several thousand, most of them military peacekeepers. My chief interlocutor was the Secretary-General's special representative, an old-school diplomat named Hédi Annabi. We got along well despite different views on Haitian politics. A native of Tunisia, Mr. Annabi had been working in tough settings for decades. He was courtly and reserved, spoke several languages fluently (Creole not among them, as he once pointed out sharply when I began speaking to President Préval in the Haitian language), and followed protocol to the letter. When he invited me to address him by his first name, I did, but felt impertinent.

Annabi's second-in-command was a tall man named Luis da Costa, who was to my thinking very Brazilian: warm and witty and unreserved. By nature a peacemaker, he sought to patch over debates and discord, the coin of the realm everywhere the UN deploys stabilizing forces. The two of them were somehow complementary. Da Costa also represented influential Brazil, which had invested heavily in peacekeeping in Haiti. The Brazilian general who led the peacekeepers, especially when it came to development, was another ally in this work. "We should do more to help the poor," he said to me the first time we met. "Too much time is wasted in meetings in Port-au-Prince and on protocol."

Early on, I told Annabi and da Costa that I'd been chosen for the job because of my knowledge of Haiti and of health care, food security, and education. I made it clear that I'd have little to contribute about peacekeeping, security, or Haitian party politics. (I had my doubts about the peacekeeping mission in Haiti, stemming from the events of 2004 and after.) It was a fraught topic and far afield from clinical medicine. The Special Envoy, Clinton, would be the leader and I, his deputy, would focus on what I knew best. On this first official trip, Annabi and da Costa listened carefully to my comments, trying to figure out where I fit into the complex UN structure. Sometimes I thought they were thinking, "Why on earth has an academic physician been chosen for a diplomatic role?" But no one ever said anything of the sort.

I also had the impression that some fraction of the UN leadership, which surely knew of my concerns about law-and-order approaches to security, was disappointed to hear my views. After all, security and local politics were the principal focus of UN peacekeeping missions. But others in the humanitarian-assistance machine seemed relieved when I emphasized human security. The food riots the previous year had led many UN officials to push for a shift in the focus on military peacekeeping toward development efforts, including providing basic services to the Haitian majority. Many Haitians noted the irony that this had long been the platform of the popular movement that arose in the mid-eighties. It was unclear, however, how widely the irony was appreciated within what was termed "the international community," which included not only the UN but representatives of many nations, international organizations, and nongovernmental groups. The United States had far and away the largest presence in Haiti, with a new ambassador and new leadership for USAID, its lead development agency.

This new, human-security-based approach had been long agreed upon but never really implemented. In espousing this approach—security will follow investments in basic social services and freedom from want—I was only trying to be honest. I'd long before concluded that jobs and such services, along with full political participation of the poor, were the best (and perhaps only) way to lessen violence and discord in the places we'd worked. But this was not an agenda I could push forward alone. The incoming UN development coordinator, Kim Bolduc, a Canadian born in Vietnam who had barely survived the destruction of UN headquarters in Iraq, shared this view. On a preliminary visit to Haiti, Bolduc had pushed to redirect the UN's focus toward sustainable and equitable development.

After letting the UN leadership know that I had Clinton's blessing to focus on health, education, and food security, even as we both promised to be cheerleaders for any and all decent (meaning propoor) development projects, I invited my new UN colleagues to visit our sites. "Come up to our hospitals and clinics," I suggested, "and you will see that basic services are what Haitians are asking for and can themselves, with accompaniment and support, provide. And President Clinton will help bring in private investors to support large projects and small ones, including those that help Haiti's farmers and artisans and market vendors." Saying this sort of thing wasn't innovative, but implementing it would have been—at least in Haiti. With Harvard's support, I began commuting between there, Haiti, and Rwanda. My new rank meant not only checking in with Mr. Annabi and others on each trip but also a great deal of time spent "interfacing with the international community." Listening to complaints was a big part of the job, and we heard from everyone: UN development experts seeking more resources to fund their projects rather than peacekeeping and military efforts; representatives of influential governments with bilateral development projects in Haiti; leaders of the Haitian government, who rightly deplored the scant support they received to monitor all (and implement many) of the health, education, and sanitation services; NGOs, large and small, which complained about the UN *and* the Haitian officials and took ill any critique of their efforts; and the business élite, who told us that government rules and regulations were not to their liking.

But if anyone had real cause for complaint, it was—and still is—the Haitian people themselves, so long excluded from any meaningful discussion of their fate.[21] To a list of grievances spanning at least two centuries, they added the inability of state and nonstate providers to ensure basic succor to those in great need, in spite of the large presence of humanitarians and NGOs. These sentiments—these complaints—have been the constant companions of almost everyone working in Haiti to deliver such services.

The failure to provide basic services—health care, education, water, sanitation—had reached a parlous state. In the fall of 2009, the Ministry of Education estimated that half of all school-age children were not in school, and that many of those who were in school attended what the Haitians call *lekol bolèt*—"lottery schools," so-called because, pedagogically, you take your chances there. The great majority of schools, maybe 90 percent, were private and relied on families' ability to pay tuition. President Clinton was convinced that if all children were in school and had at least one decent meal there, the stain of child servitude, referred to in Haiti as the *restavèk* system, would be dealt a serious blow.[22] The Haitians with whom we spoke agreed in principle, but finding the resources to make school fees, uniforms, books, and lunches available, and to improve the quality of education by training teachers, proved difficult. Although everyone seemed to agree on the diagnosis, and many on the treatment plan, failure to deliver led to another round of recrimination and blame. Similar discord was heard whether the topic was health care, access to potable water, clean energy, or ports and customs—the entire range of topics we were supposed to be addressing.

Practicing medicine in settings as different as Haiti and the urban United States taught me that scarcity (real and perceived) of resources was at the root of most of the discord. The team in the OSE—the Office of the Special Envoy—was committed to building back better in several senses. One was of course building or rebuilding infrastructure (from bridges to roads) and farmlands damaged by the storms. But we also had aspirations to build the development machinery back better. One of the books I gave to my new coworkers was a scathing indictment of development assistance, *Travesty in Haiti,* by anthropologist Tim Schwartz. I suspected it had won him few friends, but the book taught me a lot. His description of several abandoned windmills in the northwest could serve as a parable of foreign aid in Haiti:

> The wind generators stand like monuments atop a hill overlooking the city of Baie-de-Sol, the capital city of the province. They are the first thing one sees approaching the city, five majestic windmills, each one capable of producing fifty thousand kilowatts of energy. But they are useless, vandals having long ago ripped out their electrical guts. I had difficulty learning about them. No one could remember when they were installed. Government officials reported knowing nothing about them. . . . From missionaries I was able to learn that an unremembered foreign aid organization had installed the wind generators in the early 1990s, and that U.S. military personnel had tried to fix them during the occupation. That is all I got. But it was enough because it is the typical story regarding development all over Haiti: "it is broken, can't be fixed, and nobody knows anything else about it." And that was the whole point. To me the wind generators epito-

mized foreign aid. Their guts ripped out, never having functioned for longer than a *blan* [foreigner] sat watching and caring for them.[23]

We agreed that it was our duty to learn why foreign aid had failed, and to engage in goodwill efforts to improve it. Another of the duties of our small UN office (fewer than a dozen people, including volunteers) was to track pledges of development aid and see if they really ended up in Haiti. This process, which was directed by a hardworking and savvy young Australian on loan from UNICEF, Katherine Gilbert, marked the first time that one could check whether or not promised capital was moving. President Clinton also reached out to governments and agencies slow to keep their pledges, prodding diplomatically. These two interventions—a real-time window onto pledges and the courtly chivvying of the Special Envoy—led sometimes to more recriminations (including official letters of complaint from sovereign nations protesting that they had, in fact, fulfilled their pledges) but also started to speed up disbursement of some of the money. But this did not mean effective implementation, as Schwartz's windmills suggested.

Because many of the implementers were nongovernmental organizations, we also sought to develop a registry of NGOs working in Haiti. Nancy Dorsinville and Abbey Gardner, two longtime colleagues and friends who'd come with me to the UN, took on this project, promising to produce an online platform by the end of 2009. Although we found thousands of NGOs, we had no way to assess the quality or even the goals of their efforts. Sometimes we weren't sure organizations were still in existence. (Official records had not been updated in years.) Most importantly, despite the fact that the NGOs with the largest budgets (those funded by the United States and other bilateral and multilateral donors) were providing services for which the government was responsible, government officials had no way to monitor or coordinate their work.

We knew from experience that after the money arrived, if it did, issues of implementation would take over. Delivery of quality services and coordination of nonstate providers were the biggest challenges in health care efforts, certainly. For example, Partners In Health and

Zanmi Lasante had recently built the Ministry of Health a small community hospital, our tenth together, for only $700,000, and thereby created another two hundred permanent jobs. But such projects seemed too modest to those looking at the *big picture*, and critics—they were too numerous to count in all Haiti endeavors—could always dismiss any one project as either irrelevant or unsustainable.

Sometimes the *small picture* augured well for the bigger one, which invariably included, in development jargon, both implementation and integration of efforts across diverse sectors: social services, energy policy, governance, economic growth. It wasn't hard to point to regions needing improvement in all sectors—across Haiti but especially in isolated, rural areas. Part of my role as Deputy Special Envoy was to focus attention outside the "Republic of Port-au-Prince," where all development meetings took place. Again, this idea was hardly innovative—integrated rural development is one of the great clichés in such circles—but implementation itself was innovation. "GSD," as Clinton liked to say: get stuff done.

Some of the UN leadership in Haiti, along with a few friends of Clinton, visited central Haiti together in the fall of 2009. On one excursion to the town of Boucan Carré, isolated by a river that often flooded, we visited a rehabilitated public hospital covered with solar panels placed by locals working with Walt Ratterman. (He, along with the Solar Electric Light Fund, had solarized clinical facilities with us in Rwanda, Burundi, and Lesotho.) There was nowhere Ratterman wouldn't go to promote clean, renewable energy, and how he got those panels across the river was something I planned to ask him. He was all about GSD.

In Boucan Carré, one obstacle to getting stuff done was the challenge of getting there during the rainy season. We'd been talking about building a bridge there for years, but Partners In Health didn't have the expertise or resources to do so; the Haitian Ministry of Public Works was chronically starved of funds and expertise, too. In my UN role, I learned that the Brazilians had both military engineers and a robust bridge in a warehouse somewhere, and started importuning Mr. Annabi and the Brazilian force commander to help span the river at a place locals called *fonlanfè*—"hell's deep." Several people had died trying to ford the river, including two pregnant women the previous year, and we'd recently lost an ambulance there to a flash flood. With this coalition, I thought, we could surely build a proper bridge before the next rainy season. The Ministry of Public Works liked the idea, and so did the Brazilians, and so did Clinton. Denis O'Brien, an Irish cell phone magnate with deep affection for Haiti, said he'd pay for the labor and the little stretch of land necessary.

The people of Boucan Carré were also thrilled with the idea, as were the doctors and nurses there, including one of our protégés, Dr. Mario Pagenel, who had helped launch our efforts in Boucan Carré. Also pleased were all those who'd been stranded on the wrong side of the river when they needed the care we could offer in other, larger facilities. But getting the bridge up required a lot of paperwork, many meetings and calls, and then more paperwork. (One UN formality required that the Haitian government promise that no one involved in the project be harmed. The Brazilian general, as impatient with paperwork as anyone, scoffed at that stipulation, adding, with sarcasm, "I think we can take care of ourselves with the dangerous Haitians out there.") I pestered Mr. Annabi by phone and e-mail, begging him to make it happen; I begged the Haitian government, too. Each party (excepting O'Brien and the inhabitants of Boucan Carré) referred to certain forms that needed to be signed and approved. Just when we were starting to get discouraged about this fetishization of process, the Prime Minister (who also believed in the project) signed the last forms, Annabi gave the go-ahead, and a team of Brazilian engineers, a few Irish and American volunteers, and hundreds of Haitians pulled together to erect the bridge in a matter of days.

This remarkable project, as modest as it might seem to engineers, was a reminder that even patchwork coalitions could complete important, lifesaving work.[24] Ophelia Dahl described the bridge in a speech in the fall of 2009, a few days after it was completed:

> One of the areas in which we work is a commune called Boucan Carré, which has a clinic but is cut off for much of the year by a river, a river aptly named *fonlanfè* (or *fond d'enfer*—deep hell). This river has

swept away patients who were forced to try to cross it to get help; it
has gobbled up jeeps and an ambulance and even cattle being herded
across to get to market. Many who have worked there said we must
get a bridge. A bridge to cross deep hell to make sure that patients
have access to the road so that they don't bleed to death hoping that
the waters recede. You'll never get a proper bridge built in Haiti, said
many. You need heavy equipment and the coordination of the government. You won't cut through impenetrable red tape, you'll need resources and engineers and soil experts, and it'll never happen.

Six years ago, we started in earnest to bring together groups who
could help us, and we went down many a blind alley. We turned to
engineering firms here, and when they saw what would be involved,
they turned us down. But over time we found new partners: a cell
phone corporation, a foundation. We had an engineer from the U.S.
raise money and relocate to the village to move things forward. We
enlisted a general, the chief of the UN forces, the Haitian government,
and even President Clinton had a large role in bringing others into the
enterprise. Our colleagues in Haiti added this to their list of jobs:
Patrice [Névil], Louise [Ivers], Loune [Viaud], and many others. After
six years and many false starts, Haitians were employed to help with
the construction and, last week, we got word and pictures that the
bridge was finished. It is a strong and handsome structure made more
beautiful by its function; not just to provide access across the river
but to save lives and transform a community. Together we can build
extraordinary public-private partnerships and bring new people together to do whatever it takes to change the way the world works. Of
course the bridge is an obvious metaphor for what we do, but so are
the waters of hell. And I say if we can build a bridge over hell together, think what we can do for the mortal world.[25]

Getting that bridge up made me believe that our small UN office—
which was about nothing so much as building bridges—could get
stuff done and on a larger scale. It was modest as a project but potent
as a symbol, as were the glittering solar panels atop the Boucan Carré
hospital. I wanted others to see that such projects could be accomplished in rural Haiti.

Less than a month later, I crossed the bridge with one of Clinton's closest friends, Rolando Gonzalez-Bunster (who runs a large Latin American energy company and donated a big generator to the General Hospital right after the quake). We were again part of a large UN convoy and protected by UN security, which amused my Haitian coworkers. They'd welcomed me to Boucan Carré many times, but never with such an entourage. Thinking of patients lost to flash floods, and even of our ambulance, I crossed the river in what most would consider the correct way: safely, a dozen feet above the rushing water. As I held back tears, I told our first-time guests about the two women who'd died in childbirth stranded on the wrong side of the river. I was pretty sure they were unimpressed by the engineering—why the fuss over such a simple bridge?—but the Brazilian general and my coworkers, Haitian and American and Irish, understood why I was so moved.

But it was not to be a simple visit: as ever in Haiti, more drama awaited us. A few hundred meters past the bridge, on the rutted and muddy road to Boucan Carré, our convoy was blocked by an overturned UN truck that had scattered large sacks of food (none of it locally grown). We got out, planning to walk the rest of the way on foot, when some Haitian colleagues came to take us to the hospital. The main attraction for me was the fact that the hospital was by then almost entirely solar powered. Walt Ratterman wasn't there, but the director of his Solar Electric Light Fund explained the system to Clinton's friends and the UN visitors.

The hospital was busy. My Haitian colleagues (and a few students from Harvard Medical School) showed us the facility, which had been built by reclaiming an abandoned building, erected many years ago as part of a failed development project. Right next to the hospital was a bank run by Fonkoze, a Haitian microfinance group offering financial services to poor women. The guests were also shown an ingenious charcoal-briquette maker that used sugar cane waste rather than trees, and the beginnings of a tilapia hatchery we'd started near the bridge.[26] All I had to do was listen, but I couldn't help thinking about the promise of decent implementation and of the proper integration of efforts in health care, small businesses, pro-poor financial services, cleaner fuels, and better infrastructure. We were hoping that Rolando Gonzalez-Bunster and other guests would invest heavily in similar efforts across Haiti. It was a pretty impressive show and they said as much.

The overturned truck was still obstructing the road on the way back. As we walked around it, the head of UN security (guarding me, ostensibly) asked anxiously if we could find a doctor. "I'm a doctor," I replied with a mix of amusement and irritation: he was surrounded by medics, as Louise Ivers and David Walton were there, too. (My colleagues smirked a bit each time I was addressed as "sir" or "ambassador.") The UN employees pointed to a woman in labor on the side of the road, carried there by family members on a homemade stretcher; they were trying to reach the hospital in Boucan Carré on foot. Louise and I examined her as discreetly as we could: She was in arrested labor and needed immediate attention in a hospital where, if necessary, she could have a Cesarean section. She needed modern obstetrics.

We asked the head of UN security to take her not to Boucan Carré, but back over the bridge to the nearest Partners In Health affiliate—the hospital we'd just built for the Ministry of Health for $700,000. Thanks to the bridge, it was now only twenty-five minutes away. Off they went, with Dr. Walton in tow. We assured Rolando, whose birthday we celebrated over lunch in Mirebalais, that the baby would be born safely, attended by a nurse-midwife and an obstetrician. And two hours later, Walton joined us in Mirebalais with the good news: a healthy baby boy had been born into good care.[27] I gave silent thanks not only to the Haitian doctors and nurses but to Mr. Annabi and the engineers who built the bridge. Due to the partnership, the woman had been transported over deep hell to the safety of a proper hospital—and thus to a fate far different from that reserved for the two women and their unborn babies the previous year.

───

As 2009 drew to a close, there was a sense of progress elsewhere in Haiti, too. Some encouraging macro-economic indicators suggested a boost in agricultural productivity and the beginning of a recovery from the storms of 2008. Of course, there was brisk debate about priorities and an endless stream of criticism, but some endeavors seemed to be moving forward (though not on the scale of a Marshall Plan). Roads and bridges were in poor condition well before the hurricanes cut central Haiti off from the western coast the previous year, and several such infrastructure projects—deemed top development priorities by the government—had been launched.

Many of us also wanted to focus on complementary public works, with reforestation and watershed protection at the top of the list. Our UN team included two specialists in disaster risk reduction, one Swiss and one Cuban; in the second week of January, they set about planning a conference on implementation. Our standing joke was that the field of disaster risk reduction was "eminently technical" but that old-fashioned elbow grease was necessary for implementation. To this end, I begged them to spend more time in Haiti than in Geneva or New York.

Private investment in Haiti was not to be overlooked. It was for this reason that we'd taken Rolando and others to visit places such as Boucan Carré. But as physicians, we knew little about manufacturing, energy, or large-scale agriculture. To fill this gap, the Clinton Foundation seconded Greg Milne, an energetic and talented young lawyer, to the Office of the Special Envoy. Greg set to work with local businesses and institutions such as the Inter-American Development Bank to attract new investments and to "incubate" labor-intensive and environment-friendly enterprises. Denis O'Brien (who, in addition to helping us with the bridge, had also invested in schools throughout rural Haiti) brought scores of Irish investors to Haiti and allowed us to announce a new award for young women entrepreneurs. These awards were to be given out with the help of the Ministry of Women's Affairs—not just in Port-au-Prince but in each of Haiti's ten administrative departments. A hastily planned investors' conference in Port-au-Prince, headlined by Clinton, Préval, and Pierre-Louis, attracted people from across Latin America, the United States, and even Asia.[28] During the last months of 2009, it was difficult to find a hotel room in the capital. The biggest hotel, the Montana, was fully booked weeks in advance.

We weren't the only ones to sense progress. An article by a journalist knowledgeable about Haiti appeared in the Miami *Herald* on December 8:

> As my plane came in for a landing during a recent trip to Port-au-Prince, I was surprised to see five different planes from five different airlines on what used to be a deserted runway. Surprised to see that the traffic signals downtown, which rarely worked because of an electricity shortage, now run 24/7, not because there is more electricity—which there is—but because they are powered by solar panels. Even more amazing, drivers slow down for yellow lights and stop when they are red. Whether real or perceived, there is a sense of order on the streets. Such minor advances may seem insignificant in a country where monumental leaps are critical to its survival. But small steps, collectively, could be the magic formula for a poor, relatively uneducated population not predisposed to making drastic lifestyle changes imposed by the outside.[29]

Some didn't think this added up to much. The lack of any social safety net in health, education, and sanitation was clearly holding Haiti back. But it did seem possible, just then, to hope for progress. The city of Port-au-Prince was calm, and I let the UN know (diplomatically of course) that it was not necessary to provide me with so much security; I would be in Haiti often (including for the upcoming holidays with my family), and the bodyguards and motorcades seemed a waste of resources.

We hoped that Kim Bolduc, the new coordinator of nonsecurity-based UN activities in Haiti, would launch development projects like those she'd helped launch in Brazil, including conditional cash transfers for families in need. (The conditions on such transfers were that recipient families vaccinate and send their kids to school.) A similar program had helped millions of the poorest in Mexico and led to a national health insurance program.[30] And Bolduc was a veteran of some tough postings, including Iraq. She and I clicked, and our families rang in the New Year together in Port-au-Prince.

It would never have occurred to me that my new ally, badly injured in the explosion that killed seventeen UN staff in Iraq, would face such a violent affront to her survival only twelve days later.[31] Of the eight officials with whom we'd worked, seven, including Annabi and da Costa, would perish in the quake, as would Dr. Mario Pagenel and solar-power guru Walt Ratterman. Bolduc survived. So did the young specialist in disaster risk reduction, who had arrived in Port-au-Prince (to represent our office) two hours before the quake. One minute he was inside the UN headquarters and the next minute—the minute that mattered—he was not: he had stepped outside for better cell-phone reception.

# 3.

==

# JANUARY 12 AND
# THE AFTERMATH

*The matter of minutes,* the matter of time and place, was everything when the quake hit. Anyone in Haiti, or involved deeply with Haiti, can tell you exactly what they were doing at 4:53 P.M. on Tuesday, January 12, when a magnitude 7 earthquake ripped through the most heavily populated part of the country. I was in Miami, reading *The Best and the Brightest,* David Halberstam's cautionary tale about the United States' entanglement in Vietnam.[1] I had just spent Christmas and New Year's—a day the Haitians celebrate as Independence Day—in Haiti with my family. The century-old National Palace had been festooned with Christmas decorations. Nobody imagined that less than two weeks later, it would lie in ruins along with almost all of Haiti's federal buildings.

That morning, my family was preparing to leave for Rwanda, and I was ready to shut off my phone and read Halberstam's book. The problems we'd faced in Haiti the previous year had left me convinced that I needed to think harder about the tension between policy and praxis. Some of the implementation failures in Haiti were linked to a simple lack of follow-through, but others stemmed from misguided policies from Port-au-Prince and abroad. Although events in Vietnam during the sixties and seventies were distant, U.S. foreignpolicy misadventures there seemed relevant when thinking about the failure of aid in Haiti at the beginning of 2010. After my family had boarded their flight, I was planning to finish *The Best and the Brightest* uninterrupted.

But shortly before 6:00 P.M., I received a call from a Washington, D.C., area code. It was Cheryl Mills, Hillary Clinton's Chief of Staff and a friend who had made several trips to Haiti in the past few months. The new U.S. administration was aware of the difficult relations between the two oldest countries in the Western hemisphere, and Mills was one of those charged with improving them. She was taking the job seriously. Because Haiti is not seen by many in the U.S. foreign policy establishment as a region of strategic importance, and because it had been subject to erratic policy shifts under different administrations, I was grateful for Mills's interest. But I had no idea why she would be calling that evening.

"Are you and your family in Haiti?" she asked.

"No, we just left. I'm in Miami and they're en route to Rwanda. I won't be going back to Haiti until the week after next. Why?"

"Thank God you're safe," she said. "There's been an earthquake in Haiti. A big one."

"Where?"

"Looks like the epicenter wasn't too far from downtown Port-au-Prince."

This is what Haitians call "news that demands a chair." I was already sitting, but felt faint nonetheless. Port-au-Prince is the most fragile city I can think of: with a population of three million, it runs from mountaintops down steep hillsides to the harbor and waterfront slums. It is one of the most densely inhabited parts of the Caribbean and infamous for sloppy, makeshift, and almost entirely unregulated construction. In November 2008, a three-story school had collapsed without warning, killing almost a hundred students and injuring many more.[2] Mudslides occurred every year, sometimes consuming entire hillsides covered in houses and shacks. And the frequency of these incidents seemed to be accelerating with every rainy season, as the last of Haiti's forests were felled for charcoal, and as Port-au-Prince's crumbling infrastructure groaned under the weight of rapid urbanization and persistent poverty.

But an earthquake? A big one? This seemed unfair and statistically improbable. Could this happen after the hurricane season of 2008, when tropical storms Fay, Gustav, Hanna, and Ike had struck Haiti in only four weeks? It was impossible, just then, to take in another mental image of ruined infrastructure and injured and stranded people. And then, a second later, it hit me: What about our friends and family and coworkers in Port-au-Prince? We ran a dozen hospitals, and perhaps three times as many schools. Most of our patients and providers would be in Central and Artibonite Haiti, some hours outside Port-au-Prince, but all of them have family in what Haitians call "The City." And as on any weekday, many of our coworkers would be there. Hadn't I just asked a number of colleagues and friends to go there for meetings that day? Wasn't my brother-in-law there, along with three or four members of our small UN team?

"Paul, you there?" I realized that I was still holding a phone.

"Yes. But I have to get through to my coworkers and family."

Mills warned me that landlines were down, as were the cell towers that linked most Haitians, even the poor, through mobile phones. That alone was startling: how big an earthquake could take out both landlines and cell towers? But she invited me to join a conference call linking Port-au-Prince and Washington later that evening, and let me know that President Clinton would call shortly.

As soon as she hung up, I tried all the Haitian numbers on my cell phone. Nothing. I called my coworkers in Boston, including Ophelia Dahl, and learned that they'd had no more success getting through. The only word from Port-au-Prince came from Louise Ivers, who (as I later learned) had been in a meeting when the building cracked and fell around her. She got out one text message: "SOS. SOS."

Claire Pierre was, as chance would have it, in Boston. If anyone could get through to Haiti, it was Claire. She'd already reached her mother, who was alright and had promised to help connect me to Prime Minister Jean-Max Bellerive. (She didn't tell Claire that her childhood home had been flattened.)

I knew Bellerive pretty well. The previous October, when the Global Fund was considering cuts to their AIDS treatment programs in Haiti, Michèle Pierre-Louis agreed to help us attend to the Fund's concerns at a meeting later that year. The reason for the proposed cuts, as far as we could tell, was recurrent mismanagement at the central level of the program's administration since the departure of First Lady Mildred Aristide, the chair of Haiti's National AIDS Program until 2004. Although not involved at the central level, Partners In Health and Zanmi Lasante were among the largest implementers of Global Fund–supported programs, and our doctors and nurses and community health workers had patients who depended on these funds. We all wanted high-level government support, as we'd enjoyed under Aristide, in spite of the chronic central management problems.

Pierre-Louis, one of the early investors in such efforts, promised to help shepherd a unified response. But shortly before the meeting was due to take place, she was replaced by Jean-Max Bellerive, previously the Minister of Planning and External Cooperation.[3] The implementers (mostly health providers) insisted that the new government, now to be led by Bellerive, move the Global Fund grants higher up the official agenda. At a Christmas dinner hosted by Bellerive's sister, a few of us entreated Bellerive to reschedule the Global Fund meeting, and he agreed to help.

The date was set for January 12; the time, 4:00 P.M. Its significance was suggested by the attendees: the senior leadership of the Ministry of Health, including the Minister; leading AIDS researchers and care providers; AIDS activists and patients; and representatives of the French and U.S. development agencies. Loune Viaud and Nancy Dorsinville were representing Partners In Health and Zanmi Lasante, (and were among those I'd been calling repeatedly after hearing the news from Cheryl Mills). If I could talk to Bellerive, I could find out if my friends were okay—and also get his take on the dimensions of the quake before I spoke to Clinton.

Claire Pierre and her mother promised to keep trying Bellerive until they got through, and less than an hour after speaking to Mills, Claire's mother connected me to Bellerive by passing him her cell phone. I heard about every other word, but thought I got the gist: Yes, Bellerive had been at the AIDS meeting, and yes, my friends were unharmed. But much of the lower city lay in ruins, he said; "Downtown?" I asked. Yes—the palace and the ministries had been damaged or destroyed. Casualties would be high.

"Thousands?"

"Tens of thousands. Maybe more. We're in the dark. Tell President Clinton that we're going to need his friendship now more than ever. Port-au-Prince is ruined."

The restoration of telephone service was slow and spotty, but it was also responsible for many of the survival stories in the days following the quake. (Although the technology was introduced recently, Haitians from all stations of life seemed to have cell phones.) But most of the calls I received in the hours after the quake left me feeling helpless. A few were from survivors calling from under the rubble. (I wasn't always sure how they had obtained my number.) A couple of early calls came from friends who assumed I was still in Haiti. One was from an airport employee who rushed home to find his house destroyed and his seven-year-old son trapped under the rubble. The boy, Richardson, would perish, but not for three hours—and not without begging his parents and younger sister for a sip of water.

President Clinton did call that night; he asked me to come to New York. The next day, he would address an emergency UN session on Haiti. His Haitian counterpart, Haiti's Envoy to the UN office, was Leslie Voltaire, an architect and urban planner who had served in most of Haiti's democratically elected governments. Voltaire was already in New York. We'd been friends for two decades, and I knew that his duties as a diplomat were vying for space in his mind with the deep anxiety that gripped millions of other Haitians who lived abroad, or who, like Voltaire and Claire Pierre and my wife Didi, found themselves outside Haiti on January 12.

"Port-au-Prince is ruined." Bellerive's words rang through my head all night. We'd been speaking Creole, but the words mean pretty much the same thing in English, I thought. But I wasn't sure.

Did "ruined" mean damaged or destroyed? Did he mean that a certain part of the city was down? And was it true that other cities to the south had been damaged?

It wasn't easy to find out what was going on, even if by midnight the quake was the lead story on every television channel. Rumors about massive loss of life circulated widely on the Internet, but it was hard to credit them in the first hours. My mother and Jennie Block were with me, and together we packed our bags for New York. It was a relief to make an unplanned trip there, even if only to find out, more or less, what had happened.

We found President Clinton in a small room with a few members of his staff and with Ban Ki-moon, the UN Secretary-General. They were, in a sense, meeting to prepare their remarks. It was only fifteen hours after the quake, but they were probably working with better data than anyone else. We learned that some of the rumors were likely true: the temblor had leveled most Haitian federal buildings (soon we would know that it wasn't most but rather almost all) and the UN headquarters had collapsed completely. This last bit of news weighed heavily on those assembled in UN headquarters, though a heavier dread mantled the Haitians in the meeting. I still didn't have news of my wife's family, whom I hoped were safely in central Haiti. I still had little clue about my friends and coworkers, except for those who'd attended the same meeting as Bellerive.

The UN meeting was, of course, unscheduled, and I wasn't sure what role to play. Beyond my association with the Office of the Special Envoy (meaning President Clinton), few of those gathered knew how I fit into the puzzle any better than I did. Sitting in the small room, we heard Clinton and Ban Ki-moon agree that all energies needed to be focused on rescue and relief. This much was uncontroversial. But what else needed to be said? When Clinton asked that something be done to preserve the bodies of the Haitian dead so that they could be given proper burial, no one replied (although the theologian in the room was nodding vigorously).

The two leaders then left the room to deliver a grim set of public declarations at the official UN session. It was my job to sit behind President Clinton as his "plus one" (a term I'd never heard before

2009). He gave a brief statement that acknowledged the UN's losses but put the emphasis on the huge toll taken—we didn't have numbers, but it was clearly many thousands—on the Haitian government and civilian population. Pained but confident, Clinton struck a note respectful to the Haitians and apposite to the UN setting:

> Yes, Haiti is the poorest country in our hemisphere. Yes, 70 percent of the people or more live on $2 a day or less. Yes, they have had a long and tortured history. But they are good people. They are survivors. They are intelligent. They thrive in their diaspora communities. They desperately want to reclaim their country and give it a better future. And they need your help now. A lot of us at the UN, we believe in them. And a lot of us today are pretty low, because we know that some of our colleagues have died because they believed in Haiti. These people deserve a chance to bury their dead, to heal their wounded, to eat, to sleep, to begin to recover, and they can't do it just with government help alone.[4]

On January 13, Clinton's mix of idealism and pragmatism buoyed me. He had dealt with natural disasters before: he spearheaded recovery efforts for the 2004 tsunami and for Hurricane Katrina, and had called for more help for Haiti after the storms of 2008. Then, too, he'd pushed for immediate rescue and relief followed by a massive reconstruction response. But were these disasters of comparable magnitude? We had no idea, just then, but it couldn't hurt to have an experienced hand on deck.

This hope sustained me in the early hours before we had any sense of the body count. Good intel depended on reliable sources, and there were few of those on day two. When Clinton was asked whether estimates of one hundred thousand dead were off the mark, he responded, "They do seem high. If you think about the population of Port-au-Prince and the surrounding area, in excess of two million, one hundred thousand would be about 5 percent. What I am hoping is that, when they clear the rubble away, they will find that more people have survived these collapsing buildings than they think. We just don't know."[5]

Looking back, it's apparent that the rubble will take years to clear away and that the toll was far greater than feared. But on January 13, we didn't grasp the size of the disaster nor did we anticipate the magnitude of the relief efforts that would follow. Still, every report coming out of Haiti suggested that it was worse, far worse, than anything that had happened there before. Few Haitians were present at the UN meeting. Leslie Voltaire (also required to speak) was dazed, as I was. He still didn't know if his son was alive, and I still had no idea what had become of my in-laws, students, coworkers, and friends. Neither of us was sure that we were in the right place that day.

Thus began, well before the end of day two, the making of grim lists. In those first hours, Haitian families and their friends and colleagues kept lists, mental or otherwise, of those unaccounted for. The lists grew shorter with the hours, as searches and queries turned up the living and the dead. It was the living I wanted to help directly—that's why I felt out of place on the UN dais sitting behind President Clinton. At least Voltaire and the others were real diplomats. But what was I doing sitting in a meeting when medical needs were great? (Or was my ardent desire to show up in Haiti merely a symptom of some misguided personal quest for efficacy?)

Ill at ease listening to declarations in the UN general assembly, I knew I needed to get to Haiti immediately. There had to be a way, even though the airport had been damaged and was closed to all commercial traffic. Claire Pierre caught a train to New York to join me; she too wanted to return to Haiti, which was a great relief to me (and to her mother, who had spent the night after the quake on the lawn of the Prime Minister's office, along with hundreds of others). Voltaire wanted to go, too, and Clinton was ready to join us, he said, "as soon as I know I won't be in the way."

It took a dozen phone calls and Secretary Clinton's help, but by the end of the next day we boarded a small private jet headed for Haiti. On the plane was precisely the sort of team Dr. Alix Lassègue had requested: two orthopedic surgeons (a father-daughter team) and others able to take care of the critically injured, including a Haitian-American ICU doctor from New York. Flying to Port-au-

Prince from New York takes only three or four hours, but for about an hour, our plane circled the city. Smothered by near-total darkness, the only sources of light were small fires dotting the vast conurbation of Port-au-Prince.

I've lost track of the times I've flown into Haiti, sometimes during political violence and sometimes during disasters natural and unnatural. But I'd never arrived with a heavier heart than on that day. As soon as we opened the door, it hit us: a charnel-house stench filled the air of the windswept runway. I knew this smell but never imagined I would encounter it in an open space. Now it hung over the city like a filthy, clinging garment—the stench of a battlefield without the violence or din of war. Except for airplanes and helicopters, there was silence.

Loune Viaud and Nancy Dorsinville were there, as was the reporter Byron Pitts—he'd done a *60 Minutes* piece on our work in central Haiti and had become a friend. Pitts had flown to the Dominican Republic and hired a car to take him to Port-au-Prince. Although I felt entirely unprepared to speak on camera, Pitts was about the only journalist I was glad to see. We'd come with surgeons and medical supplies, and were headed for the General Hospital. Pitts and his team would meet us there, and I promised to sit down with him later that night. (It was already ten o'clock.) But first I went to the nearby UN logistics base, where my colleagues had cobbled together a makeshift field hospital under a tent and were attending to a number of survivors. I saw them—David Walton, Joia Mukherjee, and Louise Ivers—coming from rounds. David and Joia had flown to the Dominican Republic and come into Haiti by road, but Louise had been right in the middle of it all since the earthquake. She hadn't slept more than a few hours in the previous two days, and was signing out patients and duties to Haitian and American colleagues.

When the quake hit, Louise had been in a meeting about, of all things, food security and disaster preparedness. Ounsel Médé—pronounced "Mayday"—had driven her there, and a wall had fallen on the jeep, crushing the passenger side and taking out the windshield. Médé was uninjured but shaken. Louise found herself the only doctor amidst a sea of pain and suffering. But even the best doc-

tors are impotent without the tools of our trade. Her description of
the immediate aftermath says a lot about trying to provide care without proper equipment:

> The majority of injuries that I cared for in the first few hours and
> days of the tragedy were open fractures and crush injuries that re-
> quire antibiotics that we did not have and surgery that we could not
> perform. With the help of surgeons who had just arrived, forty-eight
> hours after I found him on the street where we had both escaped with
> our lives from cracking buildings, we amputated the arm of a young
> man on a table in the open air with no available anesthesia. Not to do
> so would have left him to die of gangrene.[6]

I didn't know these details when I landed but had a good sense by
then of what my colleagues had gone through. It was a relief to see
them—my protégés in the deepest sense of the word—and I em-
braced them all, especially Louise. Few words were spoken, but I
was flooded with gratitude for her presence. I could tell that she was
tired. But after eight years in Haiti, she was as committed to its people as a doctor could be.

I wanted to share the burden of caring for the patients streaming
into Haiti's crippled hospitals. Late that night, in two waves, we
made our way to Port-au-Prince's largest health care facility, where
Dr. Lassègue (and Byron Pitts and God knows what else) awaited us.
I still had little idea of what to expect, and wanted most of all to confer privately with two of my closest friends, Loune and Nancy. Now
we were together at last, alone in a jeep with Samuel, a driver we
knew well, and en route to the General Hospital.

We had been through rough times before: political strife, coups,
the loss of many friends and coworkers. (Loune and I had worked together for more than twenty years; she is one of the toughest people
I know.) Loune and Nancy tried talking, though not much came out.
They had both been in the Global Fund meeting along with Prime
Minister Bellerive and many of our colleagues. They didn't say much
about their experience because the building had not collapsed immediately upon them, and they knew how many others had not been so

lucky. But the ceiling had started to crack, and they heard another part of the building come tumbling down. Several voices cried out, and one of our friends fainted dead away, they said. But most in the crowded room did not panic; they gathered their affairs, helped their colleague to her feet, and filed into an open courtyard. Outside, a strange cloud of white dust picked up the late-afternoon light as Loune and Nancy moved to safer ground.

The street around them slowly filled with dazed people, many of them reaching for cell phones. As hundreds of thousands of people all tried at once to call friends and loved ones, overtaxed and damaged switching stations gave way. The city's residents were cut off from the world. The Prime Minister and other officials got a sense of what had happened—it took some minutes to understand it had been a quake, not a bomb—and sped off towards the city center. I'd gathered that much of the story from Bellerive shortly after the quake.

As we headed towards the General Hospital Loune and Nancy filled in some of the blanks about the first hours after the quake. In the busy neighborhood of Delmas, where the AIDS meeting had taken place, they could only guess the scope of the destruction. Power poles were skewed at strange angles or fallen, and a number of houses and commercial buildings, including some of the country's larger banks, had collapsed; other structures right next to them had not. It was rush hour, and confusion was welling, but many of Haiti's famously colorful tap-taps—the local equivalent of public transport—had pulled over as if their drivers awaited some harsher blow. Some cars and vehicles were crushed or damaged (like Médé's) by collapsed buildings and walls, but most stalled on Delmas's broad boulevard, as drivers tried to figure out what had happened.

Soon, confusion reigned. Something bad had happened; that was given and even expected in Haiti. But no one in Delmas or even in more heavily damaged parts of town knew how bad. As the news spread and as dusk fell, the city, then the nation, began keeping personal tallies. Loune and Nancy reassured me that my own relatives were alive and accounted for. But throughout the country, and then the diaspora, it was the week of grim lists.

Although I'd forgotten to ask, I later learned that at the top of Loune and Nancy's list were the almost fifty unaccompanied minors in the General Hospital: children with disabilities who had been born or treated in the hospital and whose parents had, before the quake, died or been unable to care for them. For more than two months, we'd been scouting neighborhoods north of the city for a safe haven where we could move them. But such matters take time, ample resources, and the blessing of the child-welfare system. We didn't want to bring the children to one of the many mediocre orphanages dotting the Haitian landscape; we wanted to find the right setting and the medical expertise these children needed. By January, Loune had found a few properties she thought might work as a home for special-needs kids of all ages, and she and Nancy and others had promised to take all the children into our care.

On the twelfth, as the sun set over the crippled city, the dimensions of the tragedy had not begun to sink in. But Loune and Nancy felt their first priority was checking on these children. As they made their way to the General Hospital, they saw, as everyone did, the wounded and the dead and the simply dazed. The way into the city center was obstructed by downed buildings and flattened vehicles and utility poles, but my friends pressed on. When they reached the hospital, they found chaos. Many employees not injured or killed had left their posts to search for family members; more and more casualties were arriving at the gates.

The dead were everywhere, but they discovered that not one of the handicapped children had been injured. (They were shifted to the "safe and accounted-for" list.) Staff moved the children into the open courtyard, where for two days they shared a crowded and foul space with the dead and wounded. The day before my arrival, Loune found safer lodging for them at an undamaged hospital run by a friend, a physician-priest. (Loune would later find a proper home for all of these children, whose number would grow to fifty-three.)

If Loune and Nancy recounted this part of the story as we headed to the hospital, it didn't register. What I do recall was that their accounts were interrupted by long silences. I didn't press them for details. Both were in anguish as we traveled through the ruined city they called home. It was my first look at it, and there was little to say. The headlights from our vehicle penetrated the darkness, which was complete save some scattered fires, thousands of candles, and the alien glow of helicopters of unknown provenance. Everywhere buildings spilled into the streets. Most commonly, concrete slabs—the buildings' floors—were pancaked down upon themselves, and it was from these buildings that the smell of death emanated. Some structures leaned over the streets, held in place at menacing angles by twisted steel.

We surveyed the wreckage while moving slowly through narrow openings. It was a transformed landscape, strewn with the ruins of some recognizable landmarks. We reached the densely populated area known as Bourdon. As a student in the eighties, I had spent many weekends with the Lafontants in a house on Martin Luther King Avenue, the main street from the airport to the center of town. To my left and right were scores of similar houses and also small businesses—many now stacks of floors with little more than a foot or two between them. At 5:00 P.M., businesses and homes and schools would have been full. Although we still had no idea of the death toll, it seemed unlikely that many would be pulled from this rubble alive.

Haiti is probably the only country in the world where a Martin Luther King Avenue runs into a John Brown Avenue, and we soon turned right on John Brown, down the hill towards the federal buildings. For twenty years, we'd traced this route to attend meetings at the Ministry of Health; now it led through empty streets lined by a new nightmare landscape. Could that really be the National Palace? The Ministry of Finance? The Cathedral? Even in the dark, it looked as if the heart of Port-au-Prince had been carpet bombed. People were already camped out in the broad open space in front of the palace, surrounding the famous statue of a marooned slave, broken fetters at his feet. Now his descendants were marooned under sheets pitched close by the symbol of Haiti's resistance to slavery.

The Ministry of Health was one of the first federal buildings on the street leading from the palace to the hospital. The heart of the nation's health system lay in a compact but messy pile of plaster, office furniture, and papers. Although I couldn't see much in the dark, I soon learned that not even a corner of the venerable building was standing.

We pulled up at last to the General Hospital. It looked the same as it had before the quake, and the gate was open. The rest of the neighborhood was clearly a mess. Echoing Dr. Lassègue, Loune and Nancy told me that the nursing school had been flattened, its students and faculty crushed. And once through the gates, we saw that like the neighborhoods and public spaces we'd just traversed, the once-familiar hospital campus was transformed. It was mostly dark: a few small generators were sputtering power into a couple of the main wards. Every open space on the campus was occupied by people who should've been inside the buildings, not outside. Even in the dark, we could make out people huddled around beds and cots and makeshift tents. Everywhere hung the same overwhelming stench that pervaded the entire city. I felt disoriented, and counted on Loune and Nancy to lead me to Lassègue, to the team I'd traveled with (none of them Haiti veterans except for the Haitian-American doctor who had trained there years ago), and to Byron Pitts, with whom I'd promised to sit and speak somewhere in this wreck and ruin.

In a disaster, shortages of personnel and supplies were to be expected. One didn't have to be an expert in disaster relief to know that. But the director of the hospital was there, as was the chief of nursing—even though it was after ten at night before we arrived. We found Dr. Lassègue and Marlaine Thompson tucked into a small office in the middle of the darkened complex, pouring over their own grim lists in the dim light—lists of what was needed but also lists of personnel unaccounted for. Outside the office, a handful of people were moving stacks of boxes and doing inventory; some of the tools of the trade, surgical and first-aid supplies, were coming in.

It was in this room, filled with stacked boxes of supplies, in the heart of a hospital that could not possibly provide the kind of care needed most—trauma care, much of it surgical—even if it had not been crippled by the quake, that I sat down with Pitts to discuss what was unfolding around us. I have little memory of our conversation, although one of Pitts's questions stayed with me: "Haiti was already in dire straits prior to the quake. Do you believe it's possible for it to recover?" I am paraphrasing here, because I've never had the courage to watch the piece through in one sitting, nor the reserve it would take to read the transcript of the interview and report.[7]

---

Although weary, Lassègue and Thompson were clearly happy to see us. We'd been last together a month before to cut the ribbon on a kitchen we'd helped build for the hospital. It was something we should have done years ago because our avowed philosophy—to make a preferential option for the poor—always led us back to dilapidated public institutions, whether in Haiti or elsewhere in Latin America or in Africa. After all, what institutions confer the right to health care? Not NGOs, universities, or patients and their families; not aid agencies or the UN. The government confers rights, and this was supposed to be the premier public hospital in the country. Our tardy and overmodest contribution to build a proper kitchen in the General Hospital was intended to help the hospital live up to its obligations. Feeding the patients was one such obligation, but as elsewhere in Haiti, patients' family members were expected to bring their meals to them. This practice had been extolled by some as community participation but had never been lauded by the poor, the sick, and the injured who found themselves in these institutions. (It reminded me of nothing so much as the fiction of community health "volunteers.")

If there had not been enough food for inpatients in Haiti's referral hospital a month before the earthquake, it wasn't hard to imagine what it would be like in its aftermath (in spite of the growing piles of medicines and supplies that served as the backdrop for my interview with Pitts). The hospital would also need food, fuel, and cash; it would need salary support. But very few of the Good Samaritans now pouring into Haiti were seeking to provide these basics. We wouldn't have been able to help much in those first days if family and friends, including a well-respected nun from Miami, hadn't given us thousands of dollars in cash to meet those needs.

Miami seemed like one obvious place to store other supplies we would need in the weeks ahead: medications, generators, anesthesia machines, water, tarps, portable ultrasound machines. (The lists went on and on.) Jennie Block's sister Laurie Nuell, a close friend of mine who lived there, helped organize such efforts. Before long, our teams in Miami and Boston had amassed hundreds of truckloads of supplies. The next issue was where to put them, and how to get them to Haiti. A New York–based supporter helped overcome this hurdle by donating a plane and a private airport hangar. (A number of our supporters in the business community, including Denis O'Brien and Rolando Gonzales-Bunster, also lent us planes.) Thanks to the logistical wizardry of the Partners In Health procurement team, which coordinated the entire process, private jets were soon flying in around the clock, picking up supplies and bringing them to Haiti. Laurie described it well:

We quickly had to learn the language of shipping—skids, pallets, tail numbers, flight trackers, slots, manifests, knowing which jets could hold which cargo. Calls to and from Boston occurred every couple of hours, from 7:00 A.M. to 2:00 A.M., detailing what supplies were needed, what plane was going to be in to pick them up. Calls went out all over Florida to procure the necessary items. My house became a makeshift depot with people delivering all kinds of supplies throughout the day. It quickly became apparent that Partners In Health was going to need more warehouse space, with a forklift and palletizing capability, and staff to run the operation. Within days, space was donated, and a staff person was on board. Phone calls began arriving from Haiti for personal requests too—staff needing clothes because they hadn't changed their clothes in weeks. Cots were needed so they didn't have to sleep on the rubble; tents were needed for shelter. Housing was being set up for staff, so everything was needed for that: blankets, towels, plates, cups, silverware, even a coffee maker. Every request, no matter how big or small, was fulfilled.

Many others made herculean efforts to help. But it was hard, even in the first days, to link the goodwill offers to the critical needs in Haiti because so much of what was needed and expected by medical volunteers was unavailable.[8] After decades of inattention and unwitting sabotage of Haiti's health system—too little foreign aid flowed to the public sector—there was suddenly a great deal of interest in helping Port-au-Prince's public hospitals. But helping is difficult in a broken and underfunded system. This is why many Good Samaritans simply erected their own MASH hospitals or worked in private facilities. Many lives were saved by such efforts, but what would happen when these Good Samaritans left, taking their temporary hospitals with them? What would happen if Haiti's for-profit hospitals continued to prove unable or unwilling to provide care for the destitute? Was there a way to help Haiti's dysfunctional health system function better in the long term?

The frustration of many volunteers and disaster relief experts was rooted in their inability to find a system capable of effectively using their resources and goodwill. "We were unprepared for what we saw in Haiti—the vast amount of human devastation, the complete lack of medical infrastructure, the lack of support from the Haitian medical community, the lack of organization on the ground," wrote three New York surgeons after a mission to the quake zone.[9] They first showed up at the General Hospital (where my colleagues had directed them) but felt that their efforts to help were futile: "This facility could not nearly accommodate our equipment nor our expertise to treat the volume of injuries we saw." A number of visiting medical teams felt similar frustrations well before they packed up and left. They had encountered, for the first time, the profound weakness of the underdeveloped public hospitals that should have been the frontline in the fight to save lives after the quake. From day one, friction grew between teams with much-needed skills and those, mostly Haitian, who had for years tried to keep such facilities from collapsing.

Most of this friction did not stem from cultural barriers. Some of the complaints came from Haitian-American professionals who spoke Creole and French just fine. (Many were happy to question, in these languages, the competence of their fellow Haitian professionals. It was a combustible mix, and a conversation to which non-Haitians contributed at their own peril.) These were, rather, *structural* problems. The urban public health delivery system, long weakened, was now all but destroyed. Beyond saving lives, medical practitioners faced a choice between giving up on the public system and seeking to rebuild it. It was for this reason we sought to direct expertise, skills, and goodwill toward the public-sector institutions still standing.

These frustrations were not new. In previous decades, we had encountered the same deficits and dysfunction while trying to provide health care to Haiti's poor. We learned early on about the friction between the diaspora and the Haitians we worked with—those who had never left. But such friction was not a given, nor did it prevent young Haitian-Americans from providing some of the best, most patient care in the days after the earthquake. I was lucky to count some of them as students. Natasha Archer, a young Haitian-American resident physician from Harvard, was one of the many volunteers based at the General Hospital. One night, after a long day of service, she wrote about the lifesaving work of a makeshift surgical team from Haiti, Boston, New York, and New Jersey. When a young girl presented with a rigid abdomen late one evening, and an x-ray suggested a perforated small intestine, she was immediately taken to the OR. The cause was likely typhoid. Natasha warned, correctly, that a lack of proper sanitation would lead to more such cases—and other waterborne illness.

I had reviewed the scant literature on typhoid in Haiti a decade before (it revealed the same high prevalence) and came to the same conclusion.[10] I'd issued the same warnings. A few years before the earthquake, Haiti was declared the most water-insecure country in the hemisphere.[11] After the temblor, sanitary conditions only magnified the threat of waterborne pathogens, including cholera—the most dreaded consequence of disaster and displacement. This was, again, what doctors termed an acute-on-chronic problem: one that should have been dealt with long ago, and one crying out for attention in the weeks after the quake. The good news was that, with proper surgical care, this girl's life could be saved, and it was.

Young doctors like Natasha were often the glue that held together people from what seemed like different worlds, people with the best of intentions.

––––––

The first week at the General Hospital was surreal and unsettling and sometimes inspiring. The campus was bursting with health professionals, many of them new to Haiti. All sought to provide care to the maimed and sick. Clashes occurred over matters grave and trivial—from arguments over control of space, personnel, and supplies to discord over where to park vehicles.

One nontrivial matter was providing salaries for the hospital staff. Many of those working were homeless and most had lost family; they were now surrounded by volunteers with skills much needed in Haiti, before and after the quake. The hospital needed not only these skills but also a living wage for those who could not afford to be volunteers. A few of the staff, bereaved and beleaguered, simply gave up. But most stuck with it, and more Haitian staff came back every day. If most had already returned, why was there still such demand for doctors and nurses? The answer, in large part, was that the hospital had never been properly staffed in the first place.

As the adrenaline wore off and the enormity of the catastrophe came into view, these structural problems of health care delivery also became apparent to the newly arrived volunteers. Despite the terrible suffering in this hospital and in others, there was something noble and inspiring in the spectacle of caregiving. Academic medical centers made a good showing: in the middle of the hubbub were surgeons and nurses and anesthesiologists from the University of Miami, Harvard, Dartmouth, Mt. Sinai, Duke, Montréal—to name just a few.[12] I saw scores of my former students and trainees, and countless colleagues. Many NGO and government-affiliated volunteers arrived soon after the earthquake. Chinese, Brazilian, and Israeli teams were there in as many hours as it takes to fly from Beijing, Rio, or Tel Aviv, respectively. There were rescue teams from fire departments and ambulance squads. And the Cubans, as ever, sent hundreds of specialists to join the hundreds already working in Haiti.

We saw more helpers from more countries during the wee'
January 12 than in the two decades previously. Most had ne
to Haiti before, but even groups with deep roots, such as I
Health, focused initially on bringing in surgical and re
There were so many relief workers that it became difficu
landing time at the Toussaint Louverture Airport. Alt!
cial air traffic to Haiti had ceased, humanitarian tr
could hear within miles of the airport; enormou'
jammed with supplies made a noise comm
Where once thirty flights would consti'
now sometimes a hundred flights in t!

Opening up the logjam required n
gistic capacity and patience. In
Haiti, we saw the messy side of
Countless stories were told of pai
stuck on the tarmac or in custom:
through. In the Partners In Health
teers—including board members an                        students—
learned new skills almost overnight, co               .traordinarily
effective teams of logisticians, visa exp             .u flight coordinators. The providers on the ground were gra..... even though few of
us saw with our own eyes the energy and time required to respond to
requests from the quake zone. Several of my former students rarely
left the Boston "war room." One, a Haitian-American named Luke
Messac, described it in the following terms:

> A motley crew quickly took up residence in a large, mostly barren
> room adjacent to Partners In Health's offices on Commonwealth Av-
> enue in Boston. The space came to be known as the "war room," in
> part, perhaps, because it recalled the spartan, kinetic office of a nas-
> cent political campaign. Our group included veteran logisticians, com-
> puter programmers, and program coordinators, former staff on leave
> from grad school and medical residencies, stalwart volunteers, and
> Haitian-American members of the Partners In Health family. A white-
> board at the front of the room tracked flights of cargo, medical volun-
> teers, and emergency evacuees going into and out of Haiti. Fueled by

the demands of the moment and generous offerings of pizza and coffee
from local eateries, our teams matched equipment orders and donations with precise lists of urgent needs prepared by Zanmi Lasante. Be-
use cargo planes and donated private jets departed and landed at
y time of day and night, the room was hardly ever empty during
week⁓ ⁓, the earthquake. The scale of the devastation
*d fo*uent reports from Haiti and the preternatural
*cuse*our stateside response—especially Partners
helia Dahl and Todd McCormack—helped

occurred at the Clinton Foundation,
hers pulled staff from regular activities
medicines and tents, and research every-
imbs to rubble crushers. In nearby Miami,
are      versities made earthquake relief a top prior-
as did in      n New York, Montréal, and many other cities.
The Office of      pecial Envoy was also working in overdrive.
(We'd just moved      of our unaccounted-for staff to the accounted-
for column of our own grim list.) The dozen or so staffers and volunteers camped out in our office—one that neither Clinton nor I had
visited since the day after the quake. They joined forces with Partners
In Health, the Clinton Foundation, the Haitian government, and other
new partners to move supplies and personnel to Haiti.

Even with supplies and personnel, the mortal dramas inside
Haiti's medical institutions—including those damaged and those
hastily confected—continued. People were still being brought in
from around and south of the city. A few survivors were still being
pulled from the rubble. A day after we'd been told to expect no more
survivors, a brother and sister were found under a collapsed building and brought to the General Hospital; people working there
cheered as they were carried in. Both survived after minor surgical
procedures.

The shortage of surgical capacity would be eased, we knew, by the
arrival of the USNS *Comfort*, a floating hospital with twelve operating rooms. As the first week of the aftermath drew to a close, plane-

loads of teams and supplies kept coming. It wasn't always clear where to send them. Not all the supplies and personnel were those needed, and the public health and disaster response authorities had been run ragged just trying to respond to offers of help. Efforts to coordinate all this goodwill emerged among UN-affiliates, big NGOs, and the beleaguered authorities. The first week was messy but not a total mess.

President Clinton made his first post-quake visit on day six and was anxious not to interrupt rescue and relief efforts with the protocol that attended visits from a former U.S. president. The UN Secretary-General had been in Haiti the day before, but I pushed President Clinton to make the trip to the General Hospital. We needed him to show up in part because we'd given him quite the shopping list: medicines we couldn't find at the General Hospital, dozens of generators, and a host of other supplies. We gave him all of forty-eight hours to complete the shopping, and Laura Graham and the staff at the Clinton Foundation had been asking for regular updates on what was needed.

Clinton was scheduled to arrive on the morning of January 18. I went to the airport with Prime Minister Bellerive rather than the UN team, but we were in the wrong place and missed the motorcade. (This was the sort of protocol error that would've driven Mr. Annabi mad. Clinton visited Haiti as a UN envoy, and it was our responsibility to welcome him and see him off.) I was pretty worked up over this error, having begged Clinton to come with supplies and to give moral support. His staff—a small and close-knit team—were expecting me to be on the tarmac to welcome them. In the chaos of the airport, even the country's prime minister couldn't get a straight answer about when the plane landed or where it was on the tarmac. Although the stench had lifted, the noise of the military cargo plane was still deafening, and Bellerive and I had to shout to hear each other. "You missed them," someone finally explained. "They're on their way to the General Hospital." We piled into Bellerive's jeep and headed through what Bellerive had aptly termed the "ruined city" towards the hospital. The traffic, humanitarian and otherwise, was already infernal.

Wearing a lime-green t-shirt, Bellerive looked tired—he had been logging twenty-hour days—but in good cheer. He was unfazed by our welcoming mishap. "Don't worry about it," he said. "We'll see Clinton at the hospital. He's not the sort of person to be irritated by us being at the wrong part of the airport when the control tower isn't functioning and phones aren't working well." Exactly right. Clinton wasn't at all that sort of person; he would be focused on rescue and relief. He was also likely to be thinking, already, about reconstruction. That would be the herculean task entrusted to Bellerive's government (or what was left of it) after the acute relief phase had passed. I didn't envy him a bit.

We tried to make small talk as the driver fought to catch up with the UN motorcade. But small talk was hard in the midst of such devastation. There was a certain fecklessness of collapse: you would see one intact building surrounded by crushed homes, huge piles of debris, and cracked walls at alarming angles. This unruly pattern of devastation would make both clearing and reconstruction difficult. As we drove by the fallen palace and then Bellerive's former office, laid low and with papers and filing cabinets cascading into the streets, I saw tears running down his face. We didn't speak again until we reached the hospital.

When we arrived, President Clinton was visiting patients and staff. (He was being led around by Mark Hyman, a doctor friend of his and the husband of the orthopedic surgeon with whom I'd flown to Haiti.) Dr. Lassègue was there, of course, but was doing more listening than talking. Bellerive waded through a crowd towards one of the makeshift postoperative "wards," where some children were recovering from surgery. Clinton had brought the surgical supplies and generators and anesthesia, as we'd asked. By then a dozen operating rooms were running, although the conditions were poor in the eyes of the visiting teams and the Haitians.

With President Clinton there, it was a double mob scene: there were scores of patients and families and relief workers but also a small horde of journalists and camera crews. This marked their first chance to ask Clinton questions directly. Still embarrassed about being late, I hung back, listening to his conversations with Haitian staff, American volunteers, and the press. One reporter asked what seemed the most pertinent question: "Have you, in your experience, ever seen anything as bad as this?" This was precisely the question I'd meant to ask him. He paused and then said, "I have seen many large natural disasters, in my country and in others. But never has there been one so concentrated in such a heavily populated part of a densely populated country, one that has devastated a capital city and with this much loss of life and infrastructure." Without pause, he added, "This is worse than what has happened before, but I'm confident that Haiti will recover and will build back better."

I never found out if this was reported exactly as he said it, but those three sentences finally put into context what I'd been struggling with, personally and professionally, since January 12. Was an inability to come to terms with the disaster's dimensions a reflection of a lack of imagination? For that matter, what *were* the dimensions of the disaster? Who was tallying the grim lists, and how accurate could they be? Did our powerlessness to save more lives—we all felt it—stem from incompetence or sluggishness in accepting offers of aid? (None had been spurned, as far as I knew, but deploying aid effectively was another story altogether.) Was there really hope of building back a destroyed city while survivors pitched "tents" made out of sheets and sometimes pieces of plastic or tin (donated tarpaulins had not yet arrived, nor had tents) between piles of rubble and in every other city space? We knew that hundreds of thousands had fled the city, but it seemed as crowded as ever, even in the worst-affected areas.

Clinton and Bellerive moved slowly through the hospital in a thicket of people. I was trailing them, trying to digest what Clinton had said. *Never in his experience had such a catastrophe struck the heart of such a densely populated capital city.* When a journalist asked me to comment, I couldn't get a word out in response. He was kindhearted enough to withdraw his microphone.

Clinton's words haunted me. I considered myself experienced in tough situations, but here was someone who had, for decades, dealt with flood and fire and quakes and every sort of misfortune, as public officials must. For eight years, he had done so as leader of a nation with a long history of responding to disasters beyond its borders. If Clinton hadn't seen anything like this, why was he confident that Haiti would claw its way back? I resolved to ask him when we were next alone.

It was a relief to move on to the next stop, even if only to think and breathe in the car. It was hot and crowded in the hospital, and the place still reeked. Some of the clinicians present, tired and irritable, didn't want to be disturbed. Small generators were adding to the general din; few places could have accommodated larger generators, had they been available, because the quake had scrambled the city's grid. (Rolando Gonzalez-Bunster, who had shipped the big generator overland from the Dominican Republic, was there that day with some of his Dominican friends, and Dr. Lassègue thanked him for his generosity.)

I was still lost in my own dark thoughts when Clinton's top aide pointed discreetly to a pile of bags on the ground in front of the pediatrics unit. "Some toys for the kids," he said, "from me and my wife." (The supplies on the plane had already been transferred to the appropriate officials.) With some pleasure I brought the bags into the ward, spilling them open in front of the tired nurses and children. All but the more heavily sedated kids looked on with excitement, triggering some of the few smiles I saw in days.

I left Haiti that night with President Clinton and had a chance to ask him why he was confident that Haiti could recover. His daughter was close by, but no one else was listening to our exchange. "Haitians have fought adversity for centuries. There's so much talent here, and perhaps they can turn this reversal into some new opportunities. And think about Rwanda." I did so all the way back to Florida and drew on this reflection in the days that followed.

---

After two days of rest (and restlessness), Louise Ivers and I found a ride back to Haiti on January 20 with a planeload of volunteers and supplies from the University of Miami. Who was going to coordinate them when they landed in Port-au-Prince? While waiting for hours in a small, unfamiliar airport while the plane was loaded with supplies, I asked Louise for help on an opinion piece that Claire Pierre and I had drafted for the Miami *Herald*. Finishing an op-ed was one way to kill time and to sharpen our thinking about the coordination of goodwill efforts pouring into Haiti as the enormous team of physicians and helpers loaded up.

Because the airport lounge was small and crowded, Louise finished it sitting in Jennie Block's car, which was idling in the parking lot:

> If any kind of chronology can be imposed on a disaster of this magnitude, we are moving into the next phase, where rescue and relief operations continue—miraculous rescues of those trapped are still occurring, with one young girl and her brother pulled from rubble the other day and now recovering at the largest urban hospital—and are complemented by slowly coordinated efforts to bring food, drink, shelter, and basic medical services to the millions affected by the quake.
>
> Some of the aid is starting to move, as repeat visits to the General Hospital of Port-au-Prince reveal: In the space of less than a week, the hospital, run by local staff, has been assisted by scores of surgical and medical volunteers and has moved from no functioning operating rooms to a dozen that are busy all day, every day, and throughout the night, too.
>
> This disaster has brought together goodwill and interest in Haiti such that for the first time in the country's history, there may soon be enough surgeons and trauma specialists. There are, of course, many kinds of trauma, and even those who escaped unscathed physically have lost friends and loved ones, to say nothing of material possessions.
>
> Across the country, as people continue to search for missing family members and friends, a kind of numbness is giving way to grief. Rescue workers and medical personnel and ad hoc logisticians, most of them Haitians, will need a break, as some of them have been working nonstop for over a week. One of our collaborators is still in the clothes in which she escaped with her life from her home.

To close the op-ed, we also took President Clinton's suggestion and started thinking about what lessons Rwanda's experience might offer Haiti. The tone may have been overly sharp:

> One potential model of recovery for Haiti is the nation of Rwanda. After the 1994 genocide, Rwanda was overwhelmed by the international helping class, which included, in addition to many people of good will, a flock of trauma vultures, consultants, and carpetbaggers. Under the strong leadership of the nascent government, including now-President Paul Kagame, leaders insisted that recovery and reconstruction aid be coordinated by the central and district governments. A number of nongovernmental organizations left Rwanda, but most would argue the decisions made then have helped to create a new model of collaboration between public and private actors, and contributed to Rwanda's remarkable post-genocide stability and growth.[13]

Louise looked rested, but we both knew that tough conversations were in order. The last time I'd seen her, five days before at the UN log base, we'd been enveloped by the stench. She had been through hell and now faced, along with all our colleagues, some difficult decisions. One of the biggest concerned the massive concentration of damage and injury in Port-au-Prince. Our medical work had always been based in rural areas outside the quake zone. It would have been easier, in some senses, to stay there. But, by 2010, Partners In Health/Zanmi Lasante had become the country's largest health provider; we worked closely with the Ministry of Health; we had support from the likes of President Clinton; the Obama administration had already declared earthquake relief a priority; and members of our Haitian staff were volunteering in the earthquake zone from rural sites and also from African posts. What did "business as usual" mean after all these changes?

Louise is as dedicated a physician as I've met and never one to shy away from a challenge. Because she'd been working in Haiti for eight years and was a key leader of Partners In Health's efforts, I knew she'd have clear ideas about the months and years ahead. Would we stay in the camps, and in the General Hospital? How could we train more doctors and nurses, now that the state medical and nursing schools were damaged or down? And what about the new hospital planned for Mirebalais since the storms of 2008—should it be a major teaching hospital or the smaller one we'd planned? (I'd already heard that Ministry officials were planning to ask for a large teaching hospital.) There were so many questions, such need for new ideas, that I didn't know where to begin. When we finally got on the plane, sitting next to each other en route back to Port-au-Prince, I asked Louise, simply enough, "Now what?"

"We'll figure it out," she replied. "We'll get our job done." She paused, and noted, more than once, "But I didn't sign up for earthquakes."

None of us did. None had been trained for such a shock to the body politic; none were prepared to manage, much less salve, such destruction, such a collapse of the systems, however inadequate, that struggled to keep people alive in a city of three million. Louise herself was an infectious disease expert and researcher and an excellent one at that. Now she was charged with leading our disaster relief efforts. None of us were prepared, but we were trying our best. Other self-described disaster experts had already informed us, gravely, that they were prepared. But privately, at least, we remained unconvinced. Now that the experts were there, would relief and recovery proceed rapidly enough for the millions—it was millions, we knew that much—in need of food and water and shelter? We were in uncharted territory and knew that a certain humility about diagnosis, prescription, and prognosis was surely warranted.

We landed in Port-au-Prince and were greeted by Loune, Claire, and Louise's driver, Médé; the vehicles were waiting for us right there on the crowded tarmac. We loaded Louise's kit and some supplies into a white Toyota jeep with a crumpled passenger side and sheets of plastic in place of windows. "It's kind of like the whole country," Médé remarked with good humor. "I've bandaged it up."

---

Claire and I headed back to the General Hospital, which still looked like an anthill poked by a stick. New tents had been pitched, and new tarps, too. (Many of the patients and some of the staff were still reluctant to go indoors.) Evan Lyon, Dr. Lassègue, and Miss Thompson ("Miss" is the Haitian word for nurse) were sitting in the same dark office where we'd left them. Casualties were still coming in, most as transfers from other institutions, but a few directly from the wreckage.

After an earthquake, there's only a limited amount of time to save those trapped under the rubble. And although the actual number of persons saved by the superhuman efforts of the rescuers tends to be small, some of those lucky, dusty, and dehydrated souls—like the siblings a few days earlier—were brought to the General Hospital (and other facilities), lifting the spirits of those working there. But in week two, we didn't expect many more of these "saves." Lassègue and Thompson (with Evan Lyon, Natasha Archer, and others at their side) spent most of their time on triage—a harsh and crucial part of emergency medicine. Most patients still needed surgical care; some were in renal failure; others needed advanced diagnostics unavailable at the General Hospital. Where should they go?

The arrival of the USNS *Comfort* a week and a day after the quake afforded one such site. So did certain MASH units (run by the University of Miami, the Israeli Defense Forces, and other groups) and the network of Partners In Health's affiliate hospitals to the north and west of the epicenter. (Surgical teams from U.S. academic medical centers had beefed up our critical care in Saint-Marc and elsewhere.) Central Haiti was also home to the venerable Schweitzer Hospital, founded seven decades ago by the Mellon family and still run by Mrs. Mellon's son. Louise, Claire, and I hadn't yet left the quake zone, but we knew from our friends that heroic efforts were ongoing elsewhere. One Dartmouth nephrologist, Brian Remillard, had already managed to get renal dialysis up and running in the town of Hinche (where it had never before been available), which heartened us and saved several young lives.

But even with these new assets in place and the floating hospital in the harbor, many patients needed care that was not available in Haiti. We could send some of them to Boston, Philadelphia, and Miami. Many went on their own to the Dominican Republic, but as we'd later learn, the care they received was not always good, nor was the welcome always warm. (Given the troubled history of these neighbors, most agreed that any post-quake assistance from the D.R. was a big step forward.)

The reason we could get critically injured Haitians to U.S. hospitals was always the same: personal connections with caregivers and hospitals, many of them Harvard affiliates. One new connection arose thanks to the efforts of my former assistant, Naomi Rosenberg, who was in her second year of medical school at Penn at the time of the quake. After hearing of swamped hospitals and clinics in Haiti, she became downright militant about these transnational transfers, spending her days sweet-talking hospital officials and professors (all inclined to help), working with Partners In Health and Homeland Security on paperwork, and coming to Haiti to accompany patients back to the States. On the day that newspapers announced the end of such transfers (because, absurdly, of fears of "saturating" U.S. facilities), she traveled with two more earthquake victims from Port-au-Prince to Philadelphia—an exception noted in several national papers.[14] Within a month, Naomi had set up a home for these patients and family members, and she decided to take the rest of the year off from medical school to tend to their needs. (She details this experience in her essay "Those Who Survived" in this book.)

Those of us in Haiti felt pretty sure that anyone who ended up in a U.S. hospital would be okay. We were less sure about people who remained in Haiti, except the ones who received care in the giant hospital ship a half mile offshore in the Bay of Port-au-Prince.

Even transfers to the *Comfort* required close follow-up. In Chapter 1, I wrote of a young man in respiratory distress whom I'd come across in the General Hospital, and of our efforts to stabilize him through the night until a helicopter could airlift him to the *Comfort*. When I reached the General Hospital the following morning, I asked our "resident physicians" (Drs. Natasha Archer and Phuoc Van Le, who were, with formidable composure, juggling tasks ranging from providing direct care to coordinating volunteers to transferring patients) about the fate of the gasping young man. (I had scant hope.)

They were sure he'd been intubated and transferred to the *Comfort* but had heard nothing after that. This was unusual because the ship's staff was meticulous about follow-up. He was alive, barely, when we left the hospital that night. Some of our coworkers had heard that he had died, but three residents weren't sure.

The young man therefore remained on my grim list as unaccounted for. His parents began sending out bulletins on the radio, asking if anyone had seen their son. This was unnecessary (he hadn't gone missing somewhere radio listeners would visit) but to be expected. They wanted to know he was alive or to have, at least, proof of death. Through a mutual friend, Father Fritz, I promised the young man's parents that I would look for him on the *Comfort* while checking on some other patients we'd transferred there. Phuoc had been on board several times, and told me that the commanding officers would be glad to receive us. The medical staff on board had some infectious disease patients they wanted me to evaluate and perhaps help move to one of our facilities. The ship also had patients who'd received surgical care, but needed to be transferred where they could receive longer-term postoperative care and rehabilitation. Might they go to Cange?

The coordination of such services was slowly improving, but such questions remained unanswered for most of the gravely injured. Many would require prostheses and rehabilitation; some were paralyzed and unlikely to walk again. Many of the younger victims would require long-term nursing care, but adequate facilities simply didn't exist in Haiti. Families struggled alone with such burdens. Haiti's handicapped citizens had never had the kind of disability rights nor resources they deserved.

The *Comfort* is a converted oil tanker, huge and ungainly. But it lived up to its name. The only ways to get there were by boat or helicopter, and we were due to meet a regular transport boat down at the docks. Before the quake, I'd given a talk at the U.S. Naval Academy about the potential significance of a mission like the *Comfort*. Now that the ship was in the Port-au-Prince harbor, I wanted to see it but feared wasting staff time. Rescue-and-relief teams were still focusing all energies on saving lives.

Phuoc was waiting for Claire and me at the rundown docks just south of the city center. (The city's largest docks had been heavily damaged.) This deserted spot was the loading site for *Comfort* personnel—a mix of civilians (some colleagues from Harvard hospitals), merchant marines, and members of the Navy. Most had volunteered for the assignment.

As we headed across choppy waters towards the giant ship, Claire and I started reviewing what we hoped to accomplish: we would thank the people taking our referrals, as is customary in medicine; we would check on a few patients, as we'd promised colleagues and patients' family members in central Haiti; we would see if we could help the on-board staff transfer patients needing skilled nursing care or rehab services on land (so the overbooked ship could take on new surgical patients); we would review some of their infectious disease cases, as requested; and we would look for the thirty-four-year-old question mark looming large in my mind. This would require, we feared, a trip to the on-board morgue.

We reached the ship in about twenty minutes and walked up a gangplank to a large hole in the hull—the front door for those coming by sea. (It was clear from the noise overhead that the front door via chopper was on a top deck many levels above us.) By this time, the on-board staff was familiar with Partners In Health because we'd been coordinating patient transport from the General Hospital and elsewhere. As we signed in, a senior Navy medical specialist from Jacksonville, Florida, greeted us. (We later became friends and eventually lured him and other *Comfort* staff to visit our facilities in central Haiti to see some of the people they'd saved.) Soon, we were getting the grand tour.

The ship was vast. We hiked up a few levels to our first stop, the emergency room. It wasn't crowded, although we'd heard that the ship was as full as it had ever been since being recommissioned as the *Comfort* almost twenty-five years previously. On a loudspeaker overhead we heard a page for Dr. Mill Etienne, a young Haitian-American Navy physician who had gone to college with Natasha. As a Creole-speaking neurologist, he was no doubt being pulled in many directions during his stay in Haitian waters.

We didn't have time, on this first trip, to meet all the goals we'd discussed on the transport boat. But we did see a number of patients—all in good hands—and conferred with those seeking to transfer stable patients back to facilities on land. We also got a good sense of the *Comfort's* quality: it was, truly, an American hospital—not as fancy as Harvard hospitals, perhaps, but clean and efficient and spacious.

I was wondering how to suggest visiting the morgue when one of the commanding officers pulled us aside and offered to take us there. Everything on board ran by protocol, even the morgue. The attendants were expecting us. They'd been told about the patient we were looking for and had already run through a list of potentials—people in our patient's age range who had arrived early in the transfer mêlée. An officer advised me that there might be no need to go into the morgue. First he would show me images on a computer, and then, if still necessary, I could examine the unidentified bodies.

The second image on the screen was my friend's son, in a black body bag. Only his face was visible, but it was him, and I said so. "We are so sorry for your loss," said the officer. It was formulaic, and I knew he'd been trained to say it, but I was grateful nevertheless for the civility and compassion that I will always associate with the ship. I was also grateful that I could count on Father Fritz to break the news to the young man's parents. Another name had just moved from one grim list to another.

The math was becoming clearer, and the grimmest list of all was growing. Sober estimates a week or two after the quake were that more than two hundred thousand had perished. This figure included at least a quarter of Haiti's civil servants. (Almost all federal buildings had collapsed.) I wasn't sure how such numbers were generated, but I suspected the tally would continue to grow.

So, too, would the tally of the displaced and homeless. Each day more spontaneous settlements appeared in the few remaining open spaces in Port-au-Prince. Some estimates pegged the number of displaced at close to a million; we later learned that these were too low. Without water, sanitation, and food, the camp dwellers would be in trouble. As President Clinton had predicted, shelter would prove the hardest nut to crack; epidemics of waterborne disease and gender-based violence were growing concerns.

These challenges—housing, water, and sanitation, but also gender-based violence—were questions of recovery and reconstruction, not rescue and relief. I'd made a pledge to focus on building back better, so a few days later, I headed back to the airport, at Clinton's request, to help prepare for a donor conference in support of Haiti's reconstruction. Although the previous ten days had been grueling, working with patients and their caregivers seemed somehow less daunting than an international meeting. But medical care was not going to rebuild Haiti. The meeting was in Canada, so I started looking for a warm coat.

---

"Donor conference" wasn't, I soon learned, the correct term for the gathering in Montréal on January 25. It was rather a "ministerial conference" to prepare for a donor's conference on Haiti's reconstruction. It was a meeting about a meeting. Recovery would require billions of dollars in capital, and one didn't have to be a trained economist to see that those billions weren't going to come from within Haiti. So I was to join Jean-Max Bellerive, Gabriel Verret (a Haitian economic advisor), Edmond Mulet (Special Representative of the UN Secretary-General), and Gilles Rivard (Canadian Ambassador to Haiti) on a small jet bound for Ottawa. Canada was one of the largest per capita donors to Haiti, and Quebec and Haiti have particularly strong ties. Michäelle Jean, then Canada's Governor-General, is of Haitian descent. I knew her slightly and was hoping to see her and some other Haitian friends when we reached Montréal.

In Port-au-Prince's damaged airport, still redolent of a morgue, I ran into Marie-Laurence Lassègue, the Minister of Culture and Communication and the wife of Dr. Alix Lassègue. Like Leslie Voltaire, she'd held a number of cabinet posts in post-Duvalier Haiti. We'd known each other for years and had, before the quake, discussed making a joint trip to Rwanda. The deafening racket of arriving and departing aircraft made it hard to catch up. I managed to ask her, as I

had asked other surviving civil servants, whether there was anything we could do to help. She said she could use a satellite phone.
In disbelief, I handed her one a colleague had given me a few days
before. (I hadn't even used it.) That the Minister of Culture and Communication still needed a satellite phone two weeks after the quake
spoke to the basic deficits paralyzing Haiti's government. She was
probably accustomed to attending meetings about meetings, and
wished us well.

As the Canadian jet lifted off the runway, I tried to suppress the
sense that I was abandoning quake victims in need of emergency
medical care and colleagues trying to provide it. Most of the passen-
gers on the plane hadn't slept much since the quake and were nursing their own private thoughts or soon asleep. Before long, we flew
over Haiti's northern coast, and I saw a giant tourist cruise ship resting in the turquoise waters. I'd written disparagingly about the
tourist industry twenty years before.[15] But after the quake, the
ship—and the undamaged northern reaches of Haiti—looked serene
and somehow hopeful.

The plane made a brief stop in Turks and Caicos to refuel. Several
people at the tiny airport there were collating diapers, clothes, and
other relief materials for Haiti. Bellerive, especially, was moved by
this modest gesture. Across the world, people were thinking about
his country. There were other stirring examples: Partners In Health's
teams in rural Rwanda sent 10 percent of their salaries to their colleagues in Haiti; they also hosted, along with Didi and our oldest
daughter, Catherine, a series of fundraisers in Kigali; colleagues in
Lesotho raised $20,000 in two weeks; colleagues from Peru helped
out on the difficult border between Haiti and the Dominican Republic; some of my closest friends and many of my former students were
camped out in the Boston war room; the New York businessman
who'd lent us a warehouse in Miami had continued his support.
Spontaneous expressions of solidarity like these might go unnoticed
in professional development circles, but they were encouraging to
consider en route to a meeting about long-term reconstruction.

We stepped off the plane to some diplomatic rigmarole and a bit-
ing cold. A Canadian official handed me a coat and scarf, and the

delegation packed into a series of town cars bound for a meeting in Ottawa. I wasn't needed at that meeting and headed directly to Montréal. Images of the flattened city left behind invaded my mind's eye as I looked out over the frozen landscape.

My colleagues from the UN met me in Montréal with briefing documents, a change of clothes, and yet another coat. The Canadian foreign ministry hosted a dinner at the hotel attended by delegates from perhaps twenty countries—another sign that the eyes of the world were on Haiti.

I had an early breakfast with Bernard Kouchner, the French Foreign Minister and also a physician and cofounder of Médecins Sans Frontières. We'd met in the 1990s, when he was France's health minister and I was looking for help improving tuberculosis care in Russian prisons. We hadn't always agreed about Haiti, but that morning we did. We talked about health care financing and the need for an insurance system to protect the poor.[16] Kouchner also supported integrating NGOs within Haiti's public sector. (As noted, experiences in Haiti and Rwanda had convinced me that this was a necessary step if we were serious about building robust and sovereign health systems with local partners.) I described the disarray at the General Hospital and asked whether France might help rebuild it. Such an effort would require a good deal of capital, partners, and patience, but it was infrastructure projects like this that would help Haiti recover and create jobs.

An hour later, Kouchner and I joined dozens of others at a round table. People were jockeying, quite literally, for a seat at that table, and the big players were the big donors: wealthy nations, multilateral development banks, UN agencies, the odd international NGO. At this point, two weeks after the quake, more than $1 billion had been sent for immediate relief. But this conference sought to test the waters about longer-term reconstruction aid: would donors be willing to make significant and long-term pledges to help rebuild Haiti? The United States, Canada, Japan, Spain, Brazil, the European Union, the Inter-American Development Bank, the World Bank, and others were represented by their leadership. In addition to Secretary Clinton and Minister Kouchner, there were a dozen other foreign ministers, as well as high-level functionaries from Italy and Japan. The cast seemed promising.[17]

Stephen Harper, Prime Minister of Canada, opened the meeting with a call for long-term support for reconstruction: "an initial ten-year commitment is essential," he insisted. This emerged as the conference's encouraging (if vague) "take-home message," as my medical students would say. A ten-year commitment sounded good, especially if resources pledged on March 31—the date chosen for the donors' conference in New York—were used more effectively than they had been in the past. Most present seemed willing to acknowledge, at least behind closed doors, that the aid machinery itself was flawed and that Haiti had been particularly vulnerable to these flaws. Almost none of the billion dollars already spent on rescue and relief went to the public sector. Although this was understandable for acute relief efforts—after all, government employees and infrastructure had been dealt a rude blow, and it was difficult to move resources through broken conduits—it was not a good formula for reconstruction. Those present were, after all, representatives of their own countries' public sectors; they must have understood the implications of relying on contractors and NGOs.

The delegates, who had all read stories about poor aid coordination, agreed that the Haitian government needed to lead the charge. Hillary Clinton put it succinctly: "The government of Haiti must and will be in the lead. We cannot any longer in the twenty-first century be making decisions for people and their futures without listening and without giving them the opportunity to be as involved and make as many decisions as possible."[18] The people who we needed to listen to were not in that room, of course. The only Haitians there had flown up on the Canadian jet with me or were members of Canada's large diaspora. Finding a way to include Haitians from all social strata in discussions about Haiti's future was clearly going to be a bone of contention in the coming year.

The participants also seemed to agree that rebuilding would take not only time but also a lot more money, although the numbers were still all over the map. The grim lists were still growing—by late January, estimates of loss of life reached up to a quarter of a million—

and few, it turned out, knew how to assess the value of a destroyed capital city. The Haitian government, at least privately, had estimated that at least $3 billion would be required to rebuild Port-au-Prince. That sounded like a lot at the time, but it turned out to be too little to rebuild the city, much less build it back better. And so there was surface consensus on one more point: aid would be most effective if a rigorous needs assessment were conducted before the big donor meeting. This, it seems, was the reason for the meeting about the meeting. Secretary Clinton explained: "We're trying to do this in the correct order. Sometimes people have pledging conferences and pledge money, and they don't have any idea what they're going to do with it. We actually think it's a novel idea to do the needs assessment first and then the planning and then the pledging."[19]

Few disagreed. Perhaps no one did. This sentiment would crystallize into the Post-Disaster Needs Assessment, to be led by the Haitian government in collaboration with the UN, the Inter-American Development Bank, the Economic Commission for Latin America and the Caribbean, the World Bank, and the European Commission. The needs assessment would lay the groundwork for the New York donor conference, with the hope of generating a large pool of dedicated reconstruction funding.[20]

On the surface there was nothing but consensus, but there was an undercurrent of dissensus. Publicly, some raised doubts about the ability of the Haitian government and its implementation partners to absorb the large influx of capital necessary for reconstruction—a lack of "absorptive capacity." Privately, there was much talk of corruption and inefficiencies of all sorts.[21]

Although the purpose of the meeting was to promote reconstruction and growth, Prime Minister Bellerive seemed anxious. The half-dozen of us who'd just come from Haiti knew that the disaster was still unfolding and that the acute needs of the Haitian people were immense. Several times Bellerive steered the discussion back to the immediate needs: the wounded in need of medical care, children without food and clean water, families without even a tarpaulin for shelter. Haitian president René Préval, who had already taken a public shellacking for failing to move more quickly to meet the immediate needs of the victims, had sent a written memo calling for two hundred thousand family-sized tents and one-and-a-half million food rations.[22] Some gathered in Montréal found it odd that Préval would issue a written plea to an international donor body before formally addressing his own country; others criticized him for passivity or incompetence. But the Haitian authorities felt trapped, as did so many of the rest of us, between immediate needs and interventions that might bear fruit in the long term.

The Haitian government was in a tough spot. It was struggling to run the country from a small police station. On the afternoon of January 12, Préval had avoided being crushed in his own home because, moments before, he had carried his infant granddaughter outside for a breath of fresh air. Sitting in Montréal, at a meeting about a meeting, it was impossible not to think about both the grim lists and the burdens of leadership in general. Why, I thought, would people fight for these jobs—president, prime minister, secretary of state—especially when resources seemed always in short supply? Governing Haiti was a pretty thankless job, and sometimes a lethal one. Préval faced acute disasters on top of chronic problems—from joblessness to dirty water, from homelessness to deforestation, from hunger to crumbling schools—that would have given any head of state nightmares.[23]

Perhaps the question of reconstruction was best addressed outside of the quake zone, removed a bit from its nightmares. Harper's and Clinton's commitment to a Haitian-led reconstruction effort was reassuring, but which Haitians? Those gathered in Montréal seemed to have the interests of the Haitian people at heart, but they also had only a vague and summary knowledge of the country, its leaders, and its challenges. As noted, few Haitians were present: two high-ranking government officials and a handful of Haitian-Canadians, some of whom hadn't lived in Haiti in decades. I thought about how difficult it was, in such meetings, to "echo and amplify" the voices of the rural Haitians we'd worked with for almost thirty years: members of women's groups, church groups, peasant cooperatives, and other Haitian organizations too small to be included in any international meeting, much less a gathering of ministers. How might we bring in their perspectives? Neither those squatting in crowded tent camps nor their families in the countryside had been invited to this meeting or any other outside Haiti—and to precious few within it. Although it's easy to make such critiques, the logistical challenges of incorporating the views of Haiti's most vulnerable citizens were sobering. The rural poor don't have passports and visas, much less the money for a plane ticket to Canada. Realizing inclusivity in a class-divided society with a large and far-flung diaspora would be no easy task. After the conference closed, I called Nancy Dorsinville. As an advocate for the poor from a relatively privileged background, she was familiar with people on both ends of the spectrum. For years, she'd helped me understand (and span) these worlds—they had seemed like separate worlds to me—and now I confessed my anxieties about attending a meeting so far away, geographically and socially, from our colleagues and patients in Haiti.

Our discussions hatched the idea for a project called Voices of the Voiceless. We would interview mothers, *ti machann* (market women), farmers, fishermen, factory workers, the unemployed, and others often excluded from such discussions; we would ask them about reconstruction, about what they considered the greatest priorities and most urgent needs. This was no original idea. Many development projects claimed "community participation" and engagement with "civil society." But in Haiti and other parts of Latin America, these buzzwords usually refer to institutions run by the relatively privileged and based in capital cities: NGOs, funded human rights groups, and mainstream political associations to name a few. The urban poor, the displaced, and the *moun andeyò*—the "people outside" (outside Port-au-Prince)—had little to do with such institutions. Nancy agreed that to plumb their opinions we would need help, especially if we wanted to pull something together before the big donor conference. Who would be able to span such diverse worlds?

Michèle Montas, a journalist and defender of the rights of the poor, sprang to mind. She and her husband Jean Dominique ran Radio Haiti-Inter for three decades, pushing an ambitious (and thus

dangerous) social and political agenda that called for genuine democratic participation in Haiti's government. Michèle and Jean had
trained young journalists to interview peasants, coffee farmers,
youth groups, the urban poor, and others effectively barred from
the public sphere. Radio Haiti-Inter was the first radio show to
broadcast in Creole, the lingua franca, in addition to French.
Michèle and Jean played a big part in the fight against the Duvalier
dictatorships and against the repressive coup-backed régimes of the
late eighties. Back then, I listened to their show every day. Jean
Dominique's deep voice is still a vivid memory, speaking, for example, of "Haïti, la belle prisonnière de l'armée" ("Haiti, the beautiful
prisoner of the army"). He was assassinated in 2000 in downtown
Port-au-Prince.[24]

After Jean's death, Michèle became Ban Ki-moon's spokesperson at
the UN and helped launch the Office of the Special Envoy. She still
worked with the UN but had returned to Haiti after the quake.
When Nancy and I floated our idea, she agreed not only to lead the
effort but to present the project's findings at the donor conference in
March. Under her direction, Voices of the Voiceless took root, funded
by friends and coworkers. (We tried to obtain funding from the UN
but encountered red tape and protocol; we decided it would be
quicker to do it ourselves.)

I carried down dozens of tape recorders, and before long a small
team of Haitian interviewers fanned out across the country to survey
the opinions of the rural poor about reconstruction. It would have
been easy for an effort like this to be sidelined and never completed.
But Michèle and others involved wouldn't let this happen. They
would have something to present by the time the larger donor group
gathered in New York and the real pledge-making began. The donor's
conference suddenly seemed right around the corner.

That same night, Régine Chassagne and Win Butler, the husband-
wife force behind the band Arcade Fire, met me for dinner. Régine's
parents fled Haiti in the 1970s, and she'd been born and raised in
Montréal. She wrote a stirring piece for the Irish Times called "I let
out a cry" about what the quake meant to the diaspora. I quote it at
length:

Somewhere in my heart, it's the end of the world. These days, nothing is funny. I am mourning people I know. People I don't know. People who are still trapped under rubble and won't be rescued in time. I can't help it. Everybody I talk to says the same thing: time has stopped. Simultaneously, time is at work. Sneakily passing through the cracks, taking the lives of survivors away, one by one. Diaspora overloads the satellites. Calling families, friends of families, family friends. Did you know about George et Mireille? Have you heard about Alix, Michaelle etc, etc? But I know that my personal anguish is small compared to the overwhelming reality of what is going on down there. When it happened I was at home in Montréal, safe and cosy, surfing the internet, half randomly, like millions of westerners. Breaking news: 7.0 earthquake hits Haiti near Port-au-Prince. Such emotion came over me. My breath stopped. My heart sank and went straight into panic mode. I knew right away that the whole city is in no way built to resist this kind of assault and that this meant that thousands were under rubble. I saw it straight away. I ran downstairs and turned on the television. It was true. Tears came rushing right to my eyes and I let out a cry, as if I had just heard that everybody I love had died. The reality, unfortunately, is much worse.[25]

Régine and her bandmates had been loyal supporters of Partners In Health for a number of years. After traveling to Haiti together after the storms of 2008, they pledged a substantial fraction of their concert and album earnings to our work. They were also about to launch, along with fellow Haitian-Canadian Dominique Anglade (who lost both of her parents, the Georges and Mireille mentioned in Régine's essay, in the quake), an NGO that would offer poor families in central Haiti access to credit and basic services such as health care and primary education.[26] After the ministerial meeting, it was good to discuss grassroots efforts—even though we knew them to be necessary and worthy and still insufficient after the quake. Reconstruction would require billions of dollars and a new way of deploying them in Haiti. That's why my next stop was Washington, D.C., where I was scheduled to address the Senate Foreign Relations Committee.

Régine drove me to the Montréal airport the next day. Having spent the morning preparing remarks for the Senate, I bought a few magazines and papers to read en route to Dulles. Each of them featured Haiti on the cover. One of the dailies ran a story about a young Canadian man who, wanting to help out in Haiti, flew to the Dominican Republic and drove west to Port-au-Prince without much in the way of cash—or anything other than his goodwill. Before long, he ran out of money, and the Canadian embassy had to help send him home. It was meant as a lesson about the importance of planning and the shortcomings of goodwill alone.[27] But it could stand as a parable for foreign aid, except that not all aid has been as honorable in intent. That would be a point to make diplomatically in the Senate hearing.

I met a colleague, Cassia Holstein (who later agreed to help co-edit this book along with Abbey Gardner), at Dulles, where we sat in a coffee shop and watched the State of the Union. President Obama moved through a list of domestic grievances, as was his job, but we were pretty certain he'd turn soon to Haiti. (Ophelia Dahl had been invited to the formalities by the Speaker of the House.) A crowd of airport staff, many of them émigrés from disrupted regions in the Horn of Africa, had also gathered to listen to the President's remarks. It was hard not to wonder if humanitarian aid and development strategies and donor conferences had helped much in their corner of the world. Scanning the coffee shop filled with people displaced by forces beyond their control, I wondered how often their thoughts turned back to distant cities and villages.

Obama did indeed bring up the earthquake. He reaffirmed the United States' commitment to help Haiti: "As we have for over sixty years, America takes these actions because our destiny is connected to those beyond our shores. But we also do it because it is right. That's why, as we meet here tonight, over ten thousand Americans are working with many nations to help the people of Haiti recover and rebuild."[28] Ten thousand Americans, and probably as many more from other countries (there were almost a thousand in the Cuban medical brigade alone)—it was easy to forget just how substantial the relief effort had been.

But it was important also to make sure that the purveyors of relief added up to at least the sum of our parts. That's why we were headed to the Senate Foreign Relations Committee. It wasn't the first time I'd testified there. In 2003, I'd called for an end to the de facto sanctions of development aid to the government of Haiti.[29] At the time, influential American institutions were effectively blocking four loans to Haiti from the Inter-American Development Bank—for primary health care, education, potable water, and road improvement—because they didn't condone the outcome of Haiti's 2000 elections, which brought left-leaning Aristide back to power. At least, that's what I believed.[30] The stated reason for our unstated freeze of assistance to the Haitian government was dissatisfaction with the process of parliamentary elections.

Political views aside, any doctor working in Haiti during these years had reason to object to manipulation of development assistance that slowed credit approval for major water and health care projects. The Haitian government, with a national budget smaller than that of a single Harvard teaching hospital, could not clean up water supplies or revitalize its health system without access to credit. Although our own work was independent of such aid, we were tired of seeing waterborne diseases and other easily preventable conditions afflict our patients. A few years passed before we got wind of this state of affairs and started writing op-eds (one of them with Jeff Sachs, who was equally appalled[31]). The loans were still blocked at the time of the 2003 hearing; my testimony made it crystal clear that I viewed the situation as little more than manipulation of development assistance for political reasons. It took all the guts I had to make these points in Washington.

I'd also made a more general point in my 2003 testimony: it wasn't a good idea to funnel foreign assistance exclusively through NGOs and private contractors. Without real and sustained commitments to strengthening the public sector—including its capacity to monitor and coordinate services offered by NGOs—who would make sure development funds were being used efficiently? During the same years as the aid embargo, international trade policies cut Haitian farmers off at the knees, accelerating vicious cycles of urban migration and deforestation. These twin epidemics of urbanization and ecological decline set the stage for food insecurity, vulnerability to heavy rains and storms, massive overcrowding, and shoddy construction in Port-au-Prince. (The quake would, of course, reveal the anatomy of such weaknesses in high relief.) I hadn't seen much point in mincing words. Although my 2003 comments were met with civility, I wondered if such candor were the best way to unfreeze the development projects (the reason I had come). I wasn't sure I'd be invited back.

This time, in 2010, the invitation had come from Senator John Kerry, the father of one of my medical protégées and coworkers. He would be chairing the hearing. I knew Kerry cared about Haiti, and he set the tone for the session: "The task before us remains far from over. . . . We need to use this humanitarian crisis to begin reversing the poverty and human degradation that plagued Haiti before this catastrophe. . . . We need to help Haitians build a sustainable foundation—physical, social, economic—for a stronger and more stable society. This is a chance for Haitians to reimagine their country as they rebuild it."[32]

As any fan of Haitian art knew, the Haitian imagination was rife with utopian visions. And even more were emerging after the quake. Rebuilding would require new vision to move away from a system of foreign assistance that rewarded private contractors richly even when outcomes were not those promised or desired. It was my goal that day to be critical and constructive about humanitarian aid—to reassure the committee that relief efforts to date had saved lives and assuaged suffering (and truly they did both) but also to suggest that Haitians would need a different kind of development assistance to build back better. A new set of ground rules for foreign aid was needed. Saying all this in front of the Senate felt like walking a tightrope. One way to broach the subject was to focus on the shift from relief to reconstruction, which everyone agreed was necessary.

This transition was upon us even two weeks after the quake. Ongoing relief efforts, focused on addressing the initial wave of devastation after the earthquake, were turning to a new set of concerns.

Building safe schools and safe hospitals, even makeshift ones, were obvious needs, and installing storm-resistant housing was a priority with the rainy season approaching. Likewise, the planting season demanded fertilizer, seeds, and tools. Hastily cobbled together camps—Port-au-Prince alone had hundreds of them—were at risk of outbreaks of cholera and other waterborne diseases; camp residents needed more tents, tarpaulins, and latrines (or composting toilets). The Haitian government had hoped to avoid huge camps, which are difficult to manage, but these were precisely what came to fill every open space in the capital. In my 2010 testimony, I told those gathered in the Senate Office Building how humbling it was to see ambitious recovery efforts move slowly, in large part because of delivery challenges that predated the quake. Recovery faced acute-on-chronic problems.

If past were prologue, Haitians themselves would be blamed if such problems were not addressed. But many factors, within Haitian borders and without, had weakened Haiti's institutions and made its people so vulnerable to the quake. The foreign aid apparatus, for one, kept too much overhead for its operations and relied too heavily on international NGOs and contractors. This was another acute-on-chronic problem. Even before the quake, there were more NGOs per capita in Haiti than in any other country around the world, save India. The "Republic of NGOs" came about in part out of need (the government certainly could not provide adequate services for its citizens) but also because of U.S. laws, including the Foreign Assistance Act of 1961 "and later revisions," which prevented direct investment in the public sector.[33] It was an outmoded way of doing business, I argued. Post-quake Haiti needed many of the foreign contractors and NGOs because its implementation capacity had long been weakened. But Haiti also needed new approaches to foreign assistance that might create good jobs for Haitians and reduce Haiti's dependence on aid.

In Washington, where attention spans are short, it also seemed prudent to remind those present that, over the past three decades, U.S. aid policies had seesawed between the permissive and the punitive. Neither the international community nor the United States had provided credible, long-term, financial investment in Haiti. We needed to revisit these policies. Forgiving Haiti's crippling debts was an easy place to start.[34]

This argument would have been out of place in the quake zone, where the daily business of survival reigned. But as recovery followed relief, we needed to think beyond mere survival and about job creation, local business development, watershed protection, alternative energies, and access to quality health care and education. Goals such as these could orient strategic choices for the self-described friends of Haiti. For example, cash transfers to women, who hold the purse strings in many Haitian families, would have a significant and salutary effect, as would investments in girls' education.[35]

My chief point that day echoed Senator Kerry's: the quake offered a chance to do reconstruction right. We needed to construct hurricane-resistant houses, build communities around clean water sources, and reforest the terrain to protect from erosion and to nurture the fertility of the land. Above all, the quake offered a chance to push job creation as a recovery strategy. It was a strange irony, I noted, that supporters of economic assistance to Haiti were then obliged to shill for "cash for work" programs—the quaint notion that people should be paid for their labor. It was absurd to argue that voluntarism and food-for-work programs would create sustainable jobs or meaningful development. With more just ground rules, the process of reconstruction itself could stimulate enough jobs to help get the Haitian economy back on its feet.

That, in any case, was my argument and conclusion: "If even half of the pledges made in Montréal or other such meetings are linked tightly to local job creation, it is possible to imagine a Haiti building back better with fewer of the social tensions that inevitably arise as half a million homeless people are integrated into new communities."[36]

In spite of its errors—no formal pledges had been made in Montréal, except the pledge to meet again at the end of March—the testimony was well received, which was a relief. But beyond relief, my strongest sentiment was déjà-vu: I'd made many of these same points in the same room less than seven years before.

Such testimony becomes part of the public record, so I later looked up my 2003 remarks. One of the conclusions was eerily familiar: "Haiti needs and deserves a Marshall Plan." Also from 2003: "Rebuilding Haiti will require resources. The Haitians have a saying: you can't get blood from a rock. Massive amounts of capital need to flow into Haiti in order to stay the humanitarian crises I've described. But this capital cannot go only to groups like ours—to NGOs or 'faith-based organizations.' We're proud of our work in central Haiti, but that's where we live and work: in a circumscribed bit of central Haiti. Only the Haitian government has both national reach and a mandate to serve the Haitian poor."[37] These repetitions are underlined here not to suggest some prescience or consistency, but rather to highlight the persistent pathology of inaction—or worse—spanning previous decades of development assistance and foreign aid to Haiti.

The presentations were scripted, but exchanges with senators and the global peanut gallery (such hearings are broadcast live on C-SPAN) were not. After the two other presenters (James Dobbins of the RAND Corporation and Dr. Rony François, former Secretary of Florida's Department of Health) had delivered their remarks, Senator Kerry guided the discussion. He first asked about food shortages. In the short term, it was hard to think of an alternative to the World Food Program's logistically robust food distributions. But almost none of the food it procured was locally grown. I was proud to be able to offer an example of local production: vitamin-enriched peanut butter had proven a miraculous treatment for childhood malnutrition while also creating jobs and stimulating local agriculture (simply by purchasing locally grown peanuts). It wasn't nuclear physics. Such investments could help diminish hunger, support local farmers, and build food-processing capacity in rural Haiti.[38]

Senator Ben Cardin of Maryland asked an important question: How might we learn from past mistakes in aid delivery? Most of those present wanted to correct the inefficiencies in the aid system. People in the audience, seated behind me, passed notes to me in the hopes that I might underscore important points. One such note was affixed to a news report from that morning, which announced that the Haitian government had received significantly less than 1 percent of U.S. relief aid since the quake.[39] Later we would learn that it was not only U.S. aid that bypassed the government: an estimated 0.3 percent of all Haitian quake relief went to the public sector.[40] In fact, more went to the government of the Dominican Republic than to Haiti's government. The lion's share of every U.S. dollar spent on earthquake relief went to the U.S. military's efforts, which included search and rescue and the logistic support needed, as we had learned, to save lives.[41] But the military leadership we'd met in Haiti would be the first to say that relief is not the same as recovery.

Although it wasn't clear how best to make the leap from relief to recovery, I returned to Haiti torn between optimism (the goodwill in Montréal and in Washington felt real) and pessimism (we'd been saying the same things for well over a decade). One thing was certain: there was little knowledge, in Washington, of Haitian history or of the close links between the two oldest republics in the hemisphere. Most Haitians I've met argue that it's impossible to know the history of either country without knowing that of the other.[42] But the powerful could afford not to know.

I hoped that a new infrastructure of transparency might grease the aid machinery's skids and improve performance on all sides. Colleagues in our tiny UN office were already tracking aid pledges and publishing disbursement rates (mostly shortfalls) online. It was our shared hope that this platform—the infrastructure in question—would help Haiti build back better and move us beyond rudimentary declarations of support to a focus on delivery. Otherwise, why have meetings a thousand miles away from those needing water, sanitation, medical care, solid homes, and decent jobs?

These were the questions on my mind when I headed back to Haiti after the Montréal meeting and the Senate testimony. Thirty days after the quake, we were once again preparing to receive President Clinton, who was coaching us on the transition to reconstruction. Claire Pierre had been working closely with the Minister of Health, Dr. Alex Larsen, who encouraged us to focus on rebuilding health infrastructure. In one meeting, he asked us to rethink the hospital we'd been planning to build in Mirebalais since before the quake. "You need to set your sights higher," he said. "The hospital needs to be a place where you can train young doctors and nurses, and also allied health professionals—the people who run labs and pharmacies—and community health workers. It needs to be bigger, many times bigger, than what we agreed upon." He planned to say as much to President Clinton, who would return to Haiti on February 11.

We were working with Clinton's team and the Office of the Special Envoy to plan this next visit. I suggested that Clinton should visit the Haitian Group for the Study of Kaposi's Sarcoma and Opportunistic Infections (GHESKIO), a Cornell-affiliated NGO led by Dr. Bill Pape. Pape had been one of four physicians invited to the White House when, in 2003, the Bush administration contemplated the launch of its AIDS program. (The President's Emergency Plan for AIDS Relief, or PEPFAR, as it would be called, would prove to be the most ambitious global health program of the preceding decade.) I was there too, and had worked with Pape for almost twenty-five years. After the quake, he also began pressing me to focus on the health sector—not because we were physicians but because improving access to health care was, like improving education and sanitation, something everyone could agree on.

Pape's suggestion was fine by me. I wanted to focus on health to drown out the mounting clamor about everything from land tenure to urban planning. The challenges of rebuilding a single hospital were daunting enough; coordinating diverse interests to help the Haitians rebuild a health system would require energy and time and resources. Clinton knew I felt overwhelmed by our broad brief. He knew I felt out of place when it came to discussing rebuilding industry and roads and civil society, and that I wished to work in the arena I knew best.

During President Clinton's visit to GHESKIO, both Pape and Larsen suggested to him that my energies be focused on the health sector. Clinton made a joke of it: "Farmer, did you pay them to say this?" A moment later, an American nurse brought us an infant with a congenital heart defect. "This child needs surgery at once," she said to the

President, who took the baby in his hands. He turned to me and said, "Okay, Paul, make sure this boy gets the care he needs. Can you do that?" I nodded. That was something I knew how to do.

We'd received patients like this boy, named Héros, for years at our facilities in central Haiti. Most were cared for in Cange, but some ended up, as he later did, in Harvard's affiliate hospitals. Héros needed open-heart surgery (if less urgently than averred), a procedure that wasn't yet possible in Haiti. That was one of the reasons we were taking the Minister of Health's recommendations about Mirebalais seriously: Haiti needed at least one state-of-the-art hospital. In the interim, there was the hospital in Cange—far from state-of-the-art but still a decent place to practice medicine. I was anxious to return. It was one month after the quake, and I still didn't feel as if I'd been home.

Returning to Cange would lessen my persistent anxiety regarding friends and others still unaccounted for—an anxiety all of us shared. Most had found their way onto grim lists: dead, injured, safe. But for weeks, some few remained unaccounted for, and families kept on hoping against hope. Little by little, and often late at night, I whittled my own list: my brother-in-law injured; a number of colleagues dead; most of my nearest and dearest safe. Nonetheless, I counted close to fifty colleagues and friends who had lost their lives in the space of a minute.

My colleagues and patients, almost all of them Haitian, were safe because the network of hospitals and clinics we'd built up over the years was well outside the quake zone. I wanted to get back to Cange, although I wasn't much needed there: my coworkers had their hands full since day two when the first waves of injured survivors began arriving from the capital. They had sent many doctors and nurses to help out in the burgeoning camps in Port-au-Prince. (Haitian physicians working with Partners In Health in rural Rwanda, Malawi, Lesotho, and Burundi also returned to the capital to pitch in.) But in the chaos of the broken city, I thought more and more about getting back to Cange, if only for a couple of days, to see friends and family. My sister-in-law, a nurse-anesthetist in Cange, was in the OR almost around-the-clock, but I knew we'd find time to catch up.

I was also anxious to see Father Fritz and Yolande "Mamito" Lafontant, the elderly couple who had been like surrogate parents to me since 1983. Although their house was damaged and their daughter's home destroyed, they'd survived the quake because they too were in central Haiti. Many of their friends were not so fortunate. Their lives beyond Cange had been focused on Haiti's Episcopal Church, which had been battered by the quake: Saint Trinity Cathedral, with its famous murals, had been leveled, as had the diocesan offices and the convent. The bishop's wife was badly injured and had taken refuge in Cange; she needed to get to the *Comfort* and perhaps, my colleagues thought, to the United States. I hoped to be helpful on that score. It was a relief to make rounds in a hospital that was clean and orderly and busy. Mostly, however, I wanted to spend a night in my own house.

The drive to Cange used to take well over three hours, even though it's less than fifty miles from Port-au-Prince. The road had recently been repaved, and had cut the time, and the jolts and aches, in half. I convinced Claire Pierre to go with me. We hadn't yet left the quake zone, and had seen few neighborhoods, or even vistas, without fallen buildings and debris. But the wreckage became less frequent as we drove north, disappearing altogether a few miles outside the city.

What didn't disappear were the spontaneous settlements. By the beginning of February, they stretched into the empty plain—almost a desert in the dry season—between the city and the mountain chain separating it from the Central Plateau. Some of these camps boasted proper tents; others were crafted mostly of tarps, plastic, and tin; none were very orderly. Alongside the road leading across the plain were groups of people carrying tools and materials to build more camps. With no trees or water, but many cacti, this wide-open space looked more like a bit of arid west Texas than a tropical island. It was hard to imagine how anyone encamped there would get by for even a few days. And more refugees were coming, we'd heard.

We traveled over the first mountain range and into the lower Central Plateau, which had more trees. There too we saw the beginnings of new settlements— "IDP camps" in UN argot because they were peopled by internally displaced persons—and wondered if those pitching them were originally from these parts or simply seeking refuge from the chaos and aftershocks of the city. We didn't stop in Mirebalais, the lower plateau's chief town, although we'd promised to meet with the mayor about our plans to rebuild their hospital—a project spearheaded by Dr. David Walton and a Boston contractor, Jim Ansara, who had been in Haiti on and off since the quake. If we were to proceed in keeping with the wishes of local and national authorities, we needed to go back to the drawing board on the proposed hospital, because some of our partners—the Health Ministry, the medical and nursing schools, and the General Hospital—were in shambles or ruins. Although David and Jim had asked me to stop by the proposed construction site, I was too anxious to get home. We reached Cange by late afternoon.

Although it seemed like an oasis then, Cange had once been a treeless squatter settlement: an internally displaced persons camp established after the valley was flooded by a huge hydroelectric dam.[43] When I first saw it, in 1983, it was a mix of tin- and thatched-roof huts and lean-tos and had almost nothing in the way of cement buildings. The place could've used a few tarps. Father Fritz had built a school and chapel there, and together with others, we'd built a clinic that, over a decade, would be transformed into a hospital. (Specialty clinics, a blood bank, operating rooms, and staff dormitories were added piecemeal.) The school became a magnet school, and the chapel enlarged into a church that could seat almost a thousand. Trees planted in the eighties had taken root, and the hilltop and valley below were now forested. Most people who visited, and even many who lived and worked there, had forgotten that Cange had been nothing more than a squalid refugee camp less than thirty years ago.

Although it was a far cry from the Harvard teaching hospitals, and poorly designed compared to what we were planning in Mirebalais, the hospital in Cange had become a medical Mecca in Haiti over the years. Free or heavily subventioned care and a good pharmacy and labs drew more patients and then more staff, which drew still more patients. The hospital and clinics became the de facto providers of last resort for afflictions too numerous to count.

After the quake, it was only to be expected that Cange would be a refuge for the injured and a docking station for those seeking to help them. When Claire and I arrived, the campus was overrun. There were ambulances and vehicles and a throng of people around the church (although it was Saturday), and a huge crowd encamped around the hospital. People were lying on mats and sheets near the clinics. Nurses and doctors and all manner of helpers in surgical scrubs were moving between the church and the hospital and the central warehouse.

Although the campus was mobbed with patients and providers, it was the most orderly scene Claire and I had witnessed since the quake. Before we went to pay our respects to Father Fritz and Mamito, we wove through the crowd in front of the church. After stepping aside for two men carrying a woman on a stretcher, we went inside and I caught my breath: the entire church had become a post-op ward. The pews were gone, and from lintel to altar lay row upon row of mattresses. Above the altar, a black Christ (a beautiful batik from Uganda) presided over a scene of expert mercy: there were casts and external fixators and suction dressings on almost all the patients.

Expert mercy is what the wounded needed and seemed to be receiving. Unlike the scene at the General Hospital, the ersatz post-op ward was clean and smelled it. There was no groaning or weeping, in part because of adequate analgesia; the only noise came from patients and family members praying or singing and from hushed clinical conversations as doctors and nurses—mostly Haitian, but some from the United States and Ireland, Louise's home country—tended to the patients. It was, somehow, uplifting, and we hadn't yet set foot in the hospital or clinics. An internist-pediatrician from the Brigham, Koji Nakashima, came by to welcome us back. He looked exhausted but told us that almost everyone lying there would make it.

Our mental health team, led by Father Eddy Eustache, Dr. Giuseppe (Bepi) Raviola, and Cate Oswald, were busy treating countless cases of acute mental distress, most of which went unaddressed in those first weeks. Like all of our teams, they needed reinforcements, and soon got to work training and recruiting new caregivers: before long, their ranks had grown from three psychologists to seventeen, from twenty social workers (and assistants) to fifty.[44] They were also working closely with the Haitian health ministry to help strengthen national mental health delivery and training systems. But not all mental health needs were clinical: in the weeks after January 12, Father Eddy and others led memorial services at Cange and other ZL sites; these were among the only moments dedicated for reflecting on the past month and remembering loved ones lost. In February, Bepi and Father Eddy and Cate knew all too well that their work was just beginning: mental illness associated with the temblor and its aftermath would persist for years to come.

It was soothing to be in Cange and to see Mamito and Fritz and all of our coworkers; it was soothing to see something orderly and clean and almost calm. The hospital was more than full, the ORs had not been closed since the quake, and the church wasn't the only facility transformed into a post-op ward.

It was an uplifting sight, but there had been heavy losses. Our team mourned friends, colleagues, and family members. Fritz and Mamito had just buried their son-in-law, who had a heart attack right after the quake. We lost interns in medicine and social work. We lost colleagues such as Dr. Mario Pagenel, an eccentric young family-practice doctor who worked in Boucan Carré and in other Zanmi Lasante sites, always insisting that we maintain a "self-critical dialogue" through academic presentations and discussions. On the afternoon of the earthquake, he'd been hard at work on one such presentation when his home collapsed upon him. We never found proof of his death in the rubble where his house had once stood.

Many coworkers lost family. Samahel, a tireless and resourceful pharmacist, lost his parents, his brother, and all but one of his children. In an e-mail, he wrote that the only thing keeping him going was that his wife and infant son had survived. One nurse, Naomie

Marcelin, rushed home from Cange to Port-au-Prince, where she found that her sister and niece had been crushed as a church fell apart around them. Like many of our team whose families were torn apart by the quake, she returned to work the next day. Naomie told one journalist who was visiting Cange, "Yes, I lost my sister and niece. I told myself I can't have them back. So if I can help sick people get better, that is exactly what my sister would want me to do. I'm helping other people stay alive. That is my strength."[45]

Many had shown the same strength, and it was good to see them in Cange. One was a student of mine, Thierry Pauyo, who was born in Montréal to Haitian parents. During his first year at Harvard Medical School, Thierry told me that his dream was to work as a surgeon in Haiti, a place he had never visited but regarded, somehow, as home. As a senior medical student, he got his wish: Thierry lived in central Haiti during the latter half of 2009, learning new skills while improving the quality of surgical care. He stayed with his aunt and uncle in Port-au-Prince on weekends, at long last meeting and befriending the rest of his extended family. On January 12, eight of his cousins became orphans. He brought them all to Cange for the time being.

Thierry had been in the OR nonstop since the quake, but he asked me to see a patient with him that night—a woman with a massive soft-tissue defect. "Half her thigh is gone," said Thierry. "The bone is exposed." This turned out to be a friend who I'd been hoping to transfer to the *Comfort*. She was woozy from pain meds but managed a few words. As we removed her dressings to examine the wound— it was clean—Thierry also spoke of his own loss and new responsibility. His chief concern, he said, was getting his cousins to Montréal, where his parents could take them in. And then, he added, his next order of business would be to return to Haiti to get back to work. The patient smiled at him and said, "Dr. Paul, what a nice boy he is. And what a good doctor." We transferred her to the *Comfort* the next day, and Thierry stayed on in Cange. She seemed more worried about Thierry than about her own mangled leg. Such was my student's first taste of his homeland.[46]

Returning to Cange was a relief in part because I got to move some of my friends and coworkers from one part of the grim ledger to another. The lists were often changing, and not all the injured and maimed would survive. But Cange reminded me that many would survive and that the Haitian people have long been resilient in the face of tribulation.

It was important for all of us to remember the saves and recoveries. On another night in central Haiti, in another hospital, an elderly man grabbed my arm and said: "Haiti is finished." Two younger Haitians, a doctor whose family home in Petit-Goâve was turned to rubble and a former patient who was enrolled in nursing school at the time of the quake, overheard the comment. "No," they both said. *"Ayiti p'ap peri"* ("Haiti will never be finished").

We were in Lascahobas, and the evening was mild and starlit, as if a million miles from the quake zone. But the quake had come to Lascahobas. My former patient, Natacha, and the young physician, Christophe Milien, were reminders that no one in Haiti was untouched by the quake: both were now homeless, as were their families. Dr. Christophe asked me to see another patient who represented the sorrow and burden of Haiti's chronic social problems. Roseleine was not a trauma patient, not in the sense of so many we'd seen in the past month. Dr. Christophe mentioned that she was a teenager with severe tuberculosis. "Both lungs are badly damaged," he said, "and she's emaciated." The young doctor, an obstetrician who had been running the community hospital there, paused a bit and added, "I think she's very depressed. She's an orphan."

Natacha perked right up when she heard this. Since the quake, she'd been living in a tent with other Partners In Health volunteers, pitching in however she could. "This sounds like a job for me," she said with her usual confidence. She had survived her own teenage trauma: not only tuberculosis, but drug-resistant tuberculosis. Back in the nineties, she'd been the youngest patient in the tuberculosis referral center in Cange—the only place in the entire country, back then, that provided treatment for tuberculosis' drug-resistant forms. In the course of that year, Natacha went from being skeletal and depressed and coughing up blood to being one of our best-loved patients. Everyone cheered when she returned to high school and cheered again when she decided to pursue nursing studies. If Natacha was confident she could help Roseleine, she spoke not as a nursing student but as a survivor. "I will know how to cheer her up," she said. She was living proof that Haiti would never be finished.

Roseleine was as Dr. Christophe diagnosed: gaunt and depressed. Her chest film was as bad as he'd said, but even worse was what doctors term her "social history." Roseleine was indeed an orphan, but also a *restavèk*—a child servant who had been abused for years and hadn't even started school. She wept as she recounted her travails, which had worsened when she got sick. The day before the quake, the family for whom she toiled kicked her out, and she'd been wandering the streets since, looking for help, coughing and gasping for air. It was a terrible story but not wholly unfamiliar to me or my former patient. Natacha assured Roseleine that she'd recovered from the same affliction when she was a teen. Roseleine's eyes were fixed resolutely on the floor without any signs of hope. But the two doctors present shared Natacha's optimism: we were pretty sure we could cure Roseleine's lung disease and her malnutrition. We left her alone with Natacha to talk about her other acute needs—and her emotional ones, too.

Haiti would never be finished if it continued to count as citizens people like Dr. Christophe and our indefatigable, if homeless, student nurse, Natacha. We met patients as inspiring and confident as the caregivers, and some of the patients became caregivers themselves.

The stories of two survivors, Shelove and Carmen, who reached the hospital in Cange after sustaining severe injuries during the quake, are a case in point. Shelove was born in Boucan Carré, the same isolated town that had required a veritable international coalition to build a bridge connecting it to the rest of the Central Plateau. But like so many young people from rural Haiti—Shelove was twenty-five on the eve of the quake—she saw no future in the dwindling agricultural sector in which her parents toiled, so she went off to school in Port-au-Prince. She leavened her studies with hard work, attending school by day and moonlighting as a waitress.

On January 12, Shelove was in her aunt's apartment—on the third floor of a six-story building—along with her sister and a half-dozen aunts and cousins. When the three floors of shoddy cement construction overhead rained down on them, Shelove, more fortunate than most, was buried in the debris, her left leg crushed. "The house was just shaking and shaking," she recounted, "and soon I was falling down with the wall. And then I had a big block of cement on my legs. When I touched it, I knew my leg was crushed . . . I thought that I would never walk again."[47] Two cousins, nine and eighteen, perished in the rubble; the survivors sustained severe injuries.

Shelove managed to crawl into the street, caked in fine powder from the wreckage—the telltale mark of many in Port-au-Prince that afternoon. She soon passed out. After lying there for two days, alongside others maimed by the quake and now without food or water, an aid worker from Médecins Sans Frontières found her and bandaged her leg. This emergency care *in situ* wasn't much help, since Shelove needed surgery and any physician would have known what procedure was needed—amputation. As chance would have it, a Haitian priest on his way to central Haiti loaded Shelove into his truck and delivered her to the doorstep of the hospital in Cange. Our surgical team recommended amputating immediately, before her crushed limb became gangrenous. She remembered little of that discussion and nothing of the procedure itself.

When Shelove awoke, her left leg ended at the knee. She remembered thinking that she would be in a wheelchair for the rest of her life, if she was lucky enough to obtain one. As was the case for many quake victims, salvaging her leg had never been much of an option. Even after amputation, she required more "revisions"—two more trips to the OR. The post-op pain was nothing compared to what she experienced for two days under the rubble, and in Cange she'd found herself among dozens of strangers similarly afflicted. Shelove recovered rapidly and with a zeal that buoyed fellow patients as well as doctors and rehabilitation workers in the post-op ward (in a dim storage room on the first floor, under the ORs). When I walked into that room during my first hour in Cange, she lit up the place with her smile, even before we reassured her that she would walk again.

Carmen, also from the Central Plateau, lost both legs to the quake. "I was sitting near a big wall," she recalled in a matter-of-fact voice, "and the wall fell down on my legs. My legs were crushed. I went to the General Hospital and was referred to the Mirebalais hospital. They removed both of my legs."

Both Shelove and Carmen recovered thanks to the work of surgeons and nurses and people like Koji Nakashima and a physical therapist from Miami, Carmen Romero. Fitted for prostheses at a nearby hospital, Shelove learned how to stand, and then, less than six months after the quake, to walk. For most of Haitian history, losing a limb, especially a leg, was a sure ticket to beggar status; disability begets pauperism among those working in agriculture.[48] Carmen was one of the first amputees to take steps, in her case on bilateral prostheses. And Shelove was among those inspired by Carmen's determination to learn to live fully in spite of her disability: "When Carmen arrived, she just put the prostheses on and she stood up! And I had this brace on my other leg, so I couldn't stand up. She asked, 'you aren't going to push yourself to stand up? Okay, just stay that way!' She was showing off playing soccer. And this encouraged me to try harder. Even when my leg was hurting, I tried to walk."[49]

Not all patients who had surgeries fared so well. Some never got the prostheses and wheelchairs and rehabilitation care needed to live normal lives again, and exceedingly few have been able to find work. It was in part anxiety about such fates that fueled widespread resistance to certain surgical interventions such as amputation. One could find, in the first months after the quake, online articles about hasty amputations, for example, "Surgeon Seeks to Prevent 'Unnecessary Amputations' in Haiti's Earthquake Zone."[50] A sound caution, perhaps, but there were scores of survivors who could have done better—or survived longer—with an amputation. Many of the patients we saw in the first week after the quake, Shelove and Carmen among them, knew almost immediately that they needed amputation but had trouble getting medical attention. A few more days, and both would have died of gangrene or sepsis.

That said, amputation was a hard procedure to recommend, especially when, as was often the case, the patients were children or young adults. This anxiety accounts for some of the delays, and it was fully shared by the physicians, especially when we knew patients personally. One such patient was Sanley, the daughter of a friend from Cange. I'd know her since she was born nineteen years ago. She'd been on my grim list, in the injured category, since her older brother told me she'd gone back to Cange for care. "She hurt her right foot, but it's not too bad." This meant she slipped off my unaccounted-for list; she'd be in good hands. But his diagnosis was off the mark: the teams there found multiple fractures in her ankle and heel and reluctantly recommended amputation. Her family, dismayed by this treatment plan, took her over the border to a hospital in the Dominican Republic. But they feared she was a low priority there, in wards crowded with Dominican and Haitian patients. She traveled back to Cange, in blazing pain and without analgesia, and was seen by a plastic surgeon from the Brigham, a physician I'd worked with for years. Like her family, I wanted to hear that her leg might be saved. "A limb-sparing procedure might just be possible," Chris Sampson said cautiously. "But it would need to be done at the Brigham and in several stages. It might not work, but given her age, it might be worth a shot."

So we made plans to get her to Boston. Sanley, a girl of sunny disposition who'd been living a nightmare month of pain and fear of losing her limb, smiled for the first time in a long time: she was going to Boston, where medical miracles were routine. By the time this decision had been made, the Partners In Health team had become expert at medical evacuations, and she was soon en route to the Brigham. I spoke with her by phone on the bumpy ride from Cange to Port-au-Prince. She'd had pain meds and was sunny again, sure she'd be fixed by the Harvard doctors. "Thank you so much," she repeated over and over.

But it was not to be. A half-dozen radiologists and as many surgeons reviewed her case, arguing every angle. Amputation was the consensus. None of us felt bad about having taken so long to reach the decision, and I was deeply grateful to Dr. Sampson, who treated her as if she were his daughter or mine. Sanley's mother asked me to break this news to her. It was terribly painful; Sanley was sobbing in her room while her mother wept silently outside. Sampson reminded me then that one of the surgical residents, a former student of ours, had undergone an above-the-knee amputation as a child and subsequently became a competitive skier. Most people who worked with her—she stood long hours in the OR—had no idea that she was an amputee. I asked her to speak with Sanley. These conversations helped her, as did the prospect of being free from incessant pain. After the procedure, which occurred fully six weeks after the quake, the worst of her pain soon subsided; all her problems had emanated from her crushed right foot. Within a week or so, Sanley turned back into herself and began planning her future, which she regarded as more promising than ever.

As February drew to a close, many of us realized that we'd been working for six weeks without a day off, without a moment to think or pray, without a chance to take stock of what so many had endured or been spared by luck or fate. As noted, Father Eddy was among those counseling us all to slow down and take stock of our losses. The quake had killed so many, had maimed so many, and had disrupted families and friendships. The caregivers were worn down; we hadn't seen our children. (My own nephews had joined Didi and our children in Rwanda, an ocean away, and, although unharmed, were sundered from their parents for months.) For six weeks, it was all earthquake, all the time, and we were the lucky ones: more than a million people were living under tents and tarps. As March approached, tempers began to flare and even those blessed with sunny dispositions were tired or frustrated or anxious. Some of those working hardest felt unappreciated. We needed to pause and reflect, but also to celebrate something.

But what might we celebrate? We settled on a long-planned graduation ceremony. From the beginning, we knew that service delivery would never be enough. How could we improve the quality of these services and also proffer them to more people in rural Haiti and elsewhere? Training had to figure in our strategy. A group of Harvard physicians, including Jim Kim and Joia Mukherjee, were working with our Haitian and African colleagues to codify a training program in "global health delivery." The stars in that firmament were the Haitian doctors who had led programs across Haiti and parts of Africa in the preceding decade, and we wanted to acknowledge their work and studies in public health and program implementation with a sort of diploma in global health delivery. We had planned the ceremony for late January but of course had to postpone it. But on February 27, representatives of Harvard Medical School (two deans), the Brigham and Women's Hospital (the new president and her predecessor), the Haitian Health Ministry (including the Minister), Partners In Health (Ophelia Dahl and many others), and the Clinton Foundation gathered in Cange for a moving graduation ceremony that included patient testimonies and speeches in English and French. (Claire Pierre, David Walton, and I took turns translating, since it was heavy going, emotionally.) It was the first celebratory moment since the quake, and celebrate we did—although one diploma was awarded posthumously, to Mario Pagenel.[51]

There were other happy reunions, too. My mentor Howard Hiatt, who had served for a decade as dean of the Harvard School of Public Health and had since dedicated himself to global health and Partners In Health, described one such reunion—between some of our patients in Cange and visiting USNS *Comfort* staff. In truth, we had almost kidnapped these doctors, including Lieutenant Commander Dr. Jeffrey Stancil. (We'd promised to have them back on board that night, which was patently impossible.) They went along with the ruse and were happy to see some of the patients they'd cared for, as Dr. Hiatt wrote:

> We invited several of the crew from the *Comfort* to come with us on our visit to the Partners In Health hospital in Cange. As we walked into one of the wards recently set up in a neighboring church, the faces of many patients noticeably lit up as they saw the Navy uni-

forms. One patient, who, among other injuries, had lost an eye in the collapse of a building, recognized Lt. Commander Todd Gleeson, the doctor who had treated her on the *Comfort*. Her mattress was on the floor, and as she struggled to rise, he knelt down beside her, and she wrapped him in a bear hug that lasted for several minutes. Her joy at seeing him was apparent, as was his emotion upon seeing her. This scene was repeated more than once during our visit, and according to the *Comfort* crew it is common when they visit the hospitals on land to which their patients have been discharged . . . The *Comfort* and its crew represented hope for Haiti, yes—but hope also for the United States.

Celebrations remained rare in Haiti, and March brought mounting anxiety as all those involved in relief efforts began thinking in earnest about reconstruction. It took me weeks to finish reading *The Best and the Brightest*. I'd been meaning to read it for years and had pinched it from a friend's bookshelf. It's about not only Vietnam but also the ways in which the fog of war and undue confidence in the trappings of power can lead, and did lead, to disaster. For me, it was also about people affiliated with academic institutions and the choices they made decades ago. Two months after the quake, as we took stock of the damage, assessed rescue and relief efforts, and considered what might happen in the coming months and years of reconstruction, I finally finished Halberstam's book.

Reading and reflection led some of us to record our experiences. This was surely part of my job as a professor, and it was about that time that I decided to write this book. The earthquake and our responses to it posed anew questions I'd struggled with while spanning the uneven worlds between Harvard and Haiti. Broadly, how could we diminish the growing inequalities in the world, which lead to, or (for those shy about claims of causality) are associated with, so much death, disability, and social instability? More specifically, just how "natural" a disaster was the one that struck Haiti on January 12? What made Haiti peculiarly vulnerable to the quake, as it was vulnerable to the storms of 2004 and 2008? How much of this vulnerability was social, rather than natural, and caused by bad policies, foreign and homegrown? What is the role of massive development agencies, and their contractors, in rebuilding whole cities and towns? What are the proper roles for the thousands of nongovernmental agencies that give Haiti its equivocal nickname, "the Republic of NGOs?"

These are old questions, both in Haiti and without, that often generate self-serving (and sometimes contradictory) responses and acrimonious debate. Even when the topic is seemingly innocuous—providing health care to the Haitian poor should be pretty uncontroversial—there is a great deal of discord and heat. Given the acrimony and discord, and the life-and-death power struggles to which anyone working in Haiti in recent decades has been witness, it's tempting to focus on immediate clinical questions. In the quake's aftermath, most doctors did just that. But what are the appropriate roles for doctors when responding to disasters, natural and unnatural? We're there to bind wounds, stanch bleeding, and treat those already injured, certainly. But does the physician also have a special obligation to think broadly about etiology, diagnosis, and treatment? Finally, as a physician-educator, what is the role of the American research university, one of the most direct channels into the halls of power (as described by Halberstam), in addressing the great social problems of our time? (The quake in Haiti surely ranked as one such problem.) In a social field littered with humanitarian groups, NGOs, and UN peacekeepers, we needed to rethink the ways in which we might draw on academic medical centers and on universities in general.

These questions were forced on us every day. They brought back the experiences of individuals and families, neighborhoods and cities, the injured and the whole, the caregivers who sought to tend to broken bones and crushed limbs. Grim lists were always step one in any analysis of the quake.

Step two, a month or two after the quake, was to take stock. As they say in medicine, you have to do the physical exam yourself: to palpate and percuss and listen to the patient. A thorough examination, whether termed a "post-disaster needs assessment" or some-

thing else, must progress rapidly and be linked to quantitative assessments, however imperfect. (Data were still hard to come by—at
least hard data—and we knew that even the official numbers one
sees in reports and news stories are a product of guesswork.) When
four storms hit Haiti in the fall of 2008, Haiti's GDP was said to have
dropped by 15 percent.[52] Then what was the cost, in every sense, of
the quake? Although it was still early to lay out the economic costs
of the earthquake, it would be far greater than those of the storms.
Estimates of the body count still varied. By March, as the donors'
conference approached, some said 220,000 dead; others more and
others less. By late March, we knew that a third of Haiti's population
had been affected directly, and this meant that most Haitians would
be affected as the displaced sought safer places to live. An estimated
25,000 nonresidential buildings had collapsed and, even worse,
some 225,000 or more homes. Some reports claimed that close to 40
percent of all federal employees were injured or killed and 28 out of
29 government ministries leveled.[53] Again, the numbers were all over
the map. Another assessment noted that about half of all public-sector health facilities in Port-au-Prince collapsed or were deemed unsafe; some 14 percent of Ministry of Health employees died, and
two-thirds lost their homes.[54]

And injured was not the same as killed, as the experiences of Shelove and Carmen and Sanley suggest. The extent of inner-city damage, along with the inability of the local and international authorities
to move swiftly to address the shelter crisis, was the reason why
crammed and unsanitary informal settlements, almost one thousand
of them a month after the quake, had blossomed across the city and
to the south; they spread north as people sought safe shelter. Haiti,
already food-insecure and vulnerable to flash floods (because of deforestation), might have to feed an estimated two million displaced
people with a mix of locally grown and imported food. The rainy
season would arrive by April or May, then hurricane season after
that.

What was the status of the health system after the quake? The
kinds of problems we encountered at the General Hospital existed

throughout the country, even far from the quake zone. Before the quake, only 5 percent of the government's budget went to the health ministry—Rwanda's commitment was more than twice that—and consequently, stock-outs of key medications and supplies were the rule, public-sector staff were poorly paid, clinic hours were short, and health indicators were some of the worst in the hemisphere. The quake had clearly worsened a bad situation: the post-quake influx of medical aid saved lives but didn't do much to help the public sector recover.[55]

In clinical medicine, questions like these are answered by seeking the best available data, often from the lab or other diagnostic studies or the patient's history. The events of January 12 and after are best approached by understanding Haiti's remarkable and troubled history, to which we now turn.

# 4.

## A HISTORY OF THE PRESENT ILLNESS

*One month after the earthquake,* the wrack and ruin in Haiti was still more or less unchanged. This was, in a sense, a paradox: countless people were looking for work just as billions dollars of aid were pouring into Haiti and huge amounts of work needed to be done. Why were so many still unemployed? In clinical medicine, the evaluation of every patient follows a certain logic. Physicians working in Haiti used this logic every day, not only when caring for individual patients, but when contemplating the enormity of the problems facing the country.

By some macro indicators, Haiti had made slow improvements the year before the quake. Agricultural outputs had increased; infrastructure projects were underway; foreign investment began to trickle into Haiti. However, short-lived gains did little to address the country's deep-rooted social and economic problems: shoddy housing, bare hillsides and overfished waters, scarce access to clean water and modern sanitation, an undesirable business environment, cash-strapped health and school systems, high structural unemployment, frequent political upheaval. On top of these longstanding problems came the worst natural disaster to befall the region in centuries: an "acute-on-chronic" event.

A month later, there was little evidence to suggest that the tsunami of goodwill that crashed over Haiti after the quake could effectively address such layered afflictions. Whether one looked at job creation, health, education, potable water, or safe and affordable housing, similar conclusions could be drawn. First, great weakness in the public sector made it difficult to deliver even basic services at a significant scale; second, not enough of the pledged earthquake relief reached those in need through mechanisms that might address this central weakness. In other words, existing development and reconstruction machinery did little to mitigate Haiti's acute-on-chronic problems in spite of many good intentions and extraordinary generosity. Might responding to the acute needs of people displaced and injured by the earthquake afford us a chance to address the underlying chronic conditions that had rendered them so vulnerable in the first place? To answer this question, we need to know the history of the present illness.

Haiti, an independent nation for more than two centuries, has the worst health indices in the Western hemisphere. Whether we look at malnutrition, maternal mortality, or life expectancy at birth, Haiti is an outlier in the region—not just in comparison with the United States or Canada but also with the more modest economies of Jamaica, Cuba, and the Dominican Republic. Such outlier status looms large in any discussion of Haiti's future health and economic development. (Haitians are not surprisingly tired of their homeland being labeled "the poorest country in the Western hemisphere.") But few agree about the causes of Haiti's present condition. Simple stories of corruption or ungovernability (although real problems) do little to explain the chronic nature of such problems, nor can we invoke the crutch of cultural difference to explain the challenges before Haiti.

To be credible, and to yield workable recommendations for building Haiti back better, to use Clinton's optimistic phrase, analysis of Haiti's current woes must be historically deep and geographically broad. Such an approach may also provide some inoculation against the old and pernicious tendency to blame solely Haitians—and Haitian culture—for their misfortunes. This default logic relies on the erasure of history.[1] For many who arrived in Haiti immediately after the quake, history began the moment they got off the plane. But Haitians from all classes will tell visitors that to understand Haiti's problems, you need to understand its history. As Mark Danner has written:

> Whether they can read or not, Haiti's people walk in history, and live in politics. They are independent, proud, fiercely aware of their own singularity. What distinguishes them is a tradition of heroism and a conviction that they are and will remain something distinct, apart— something you can hear in the Creole spoken in the countryside, or the voodoo practiced there, traces of the Africa that the first generation of revolutionaries brought with them on the middle passage.[2]

Haiti's history has been recounted before in a literature of mixed quality. This includes a Haitian bibliography that is quite robust, considering the low literacy rates since independence. In the nineteenth century, Haiti contributed more books per capita than any other country in Latin America. From the end of the revolution in 1803 to the withdrawal of U.S. Marines in 1934, after a nineteen-year occupation, Haitian élites wrote tome after tome in impeccable French about the country's glories and travails.[3] Although books in Haitian Creole, the lingua franca, remain rare, Haitians from all classes seem to agree about the nation's beginnings: the colonial experience and the fight against slavery constitute the template of modern Haiti.

---

The story starts at the close of the fifteenth century. Haiti was the site of Europe's first New World settlement after one of Columbus's three ships foundered off the northern coast of Haiti in 1492. The island's native Taíno population, numbering at least in the hundreds of thousands (some demographers say millions),[4] was mostly wiped out within a century of the Columbian exchange by assault from pathogens ranging from slavery to smallpox. When a 1697 treaty ceded the western third of Hispaniola (Columbus's name for the island called *Ayiti* by its doomed inhabitants) to France, not a single

Taíno remained alive. For those who say Haiti's history is written in blood, this is the first chapter.

The second chapter is equally brutal. Although the Spanish began importing slaves from Africa in the first decades of the sixteenth century, it was the French who moved the slave trade into high gear: by the mid-eighteenth century, Haiti was the Americas' chief port of call for slavers. By 1540 some thirty thousand in chains had reached Haiti's shores.[5] Saint-Domingue—the name given to the French colony on Hispaniola from 1659 until it became the independent nation of Haiti in 1804—became the world's leading exporter of coffee, sugar, and other tropical produce. It brought in more income for the French, noted Moreau de St-Méry (the chief French chronicler of the era), than all their other colonial possessions combined.[6] Moreau de St-Méry's two-volume treatise wasn't able to completely sanitize the horrors and excesses of the period. But it was the Haitian slaves who would later write the most damning accounts:

> Have they not hung up men with heads downward, drowned them in sacks, crucified them on planks, buried them alive, crushed them in mortars? Have they not forced them to eat shit? And, after having flayed them with the lash, have they not cast them alive to be devoured by worms, or onto anthills, or lashed them to stakes in the swamp to be devoured by mosquitoes? Have they not thrown them into boiling cauldrons of cane syrup?[7]

Revolts were frequent everywhere chattel slavery was practiced. But none had succeeded in ending slavery, much less founding a nation in which slaves would become citizens. In Haiti, the numbers were heavily skewed in favor of the slaves, who accounted for 85 percent of the colony's population by the time of the French revolution.[8] A major uprising in 1791 laid waste to many of the plantations and fields in the north and soon coalesced into a full-scale revolution led by former slaves such as Toussaint Louverture. European armies from all the great powers of the era (and the newborn republic to the north) proved no match for those organized by Louverture. But the slave leader was soon kidnapped in a parley with the French, later dying in a French prison, probably of tuberculosis.

Such treachery only stiffened the resolve of the Haitians, now under the leadership of the fiery Jean-Jacques Dessalines, who vowed
to fight for as long as it took to found an independent nation. It
would be the epic battle of the era. In 1801, Napoleon sent his
brother-in-law, Captain-General Leclerc, to retake the colony. Leclerc
sailed at the head one of the largest armadas ever to set forth for the
New World; his more than forty thousand troops included not only
French soldiers but also German, Polish, Swiss, and Dutch mercenar-
ies. But the European troops fared poorly against the guerilla tactics
of the Haitians, as General Leclerc, who later died there (of yellow
fever), was to learn. In one of his last letters home, Leclerc wrote that
the only remaining tactic was to "destroy all the negroes in the hills,
men and women, sparing only children under twelve, destroy half of
those living in the plains, and leave behind not a single man of color
who has worn a uniform—without this the colony will never have
peace."[9] Dessalines and his irregulars routed the French and their
conscripts by November of 1803. On January 1, 1804, Dessalines declared Haiti a sovereign nation, the first (and only) one born of a
slave revolt. "I have given the French cannibals blood for blood," he
said. "I have avenged America."[10]

The end of slavery in Haiti caused ripples throughout the Americas, from Venezuela to the United States and back to Europe, where
plantation slavery had been spawned. Many have observed that most
modern human rights movements trace their origins to the fight to
end the slave trade and slavery itself. Britons proudly claim that this
fight began in their own country, when Thomas Clarkson, William
Wilberforce, and others used moral suasion and legal and political
means to end the British slave trade.[11] But the first decisive blow
against slavery was struck in Saint-Domingue in 1791, culminating
in the defeat of Napoleon's vast army in the hills and plains of his
soon-to-be former colony. For those who doubt the grand aspirations
of the victorious slaves—to establish an independent republic free
from slavery—we have only to consult the historical record. The dis-
covery, in late March 2010, of the only surviving copy of Haiti's 1804

Declaration of Independence in the British National Archives leaves no doubt: Haiti's military leaders used rights language unstintingly. These are Dessalines words:

> And you, a people so long without good fortune, witness to the oath we take, remember that I counted on your constancy and courage when I threw myself into the career of liberty to fight the despotism and tyranny you had struggled against for 14 years. Remember that I sacrificed everything to rally to your defense; family, children, fortune, and now I am rich only with your liberty; my name has become a horror to all those who want slavery. Despots and tyrants curse the day that I was born. If ever you refused or grumbled while receiving those laws that the spirit guarding your fate dictates to me for your own good, you would deserve the fate of an ungrateful people. But I reject that awful idea; you will sustain the liberty that you cherish and support the leader who commands you. Therefore vow before me to live free and independent, and to prefer death to anything that will try to place you back in chains. Swear, finally, to pursue forever the traitors and enemies of your independence.[12]

If the prize was great, the price paid for it by the Haitians was steep. Dessalines was killed in a power struggle a few years after he penned these stirring words; his former masters orchestrated an economic and diplomatic embargo, the first of many, against the troubled young nation. Hemmed in by the Caribbean's slave colonies and, to the north, by the only other independent nation in the Americas (which also practiced slavery), the nascent republic was born into a hostile world. Senator Robert Hayne of South Carolina summed up the United States' stance toward Haiti in 1824: "Our policy with regard to Hayti [sic] is plain. We can never acknowledge her independence. . . . The peace and safety of a large portion of our union forbids us even to discuss [it]."[13] Many U.S. statesmen continued calling Haitians "rebel slaves," and the government refused to recognize Haiti's existence until President Lincoln did so in 1862.

It can be reasonably said that no one helped the Haitians on the road to independence, and that many forces, the deliberate policies of their neighbors among them, stymied their growth as a nation. France, as might be expected, was a particularly sore loser—and influential with its allies in the region, especially the United States. Absurdly, the French demanded reparations, and not just for the losses of French plantations but for the losses of their slaves, too. Desperate for trading partners and international recognition, Haitian leaders agreed, in 1825, to pay France 150 million germinal francs.[14] Never before or since has a poor but victorious nation indemnified the rich and defeated in this manner. For more than a century, well into the 1950s, the Haitians paid this debt.

Many adverse events ensued: coups, invasions, military occupations, dictatorships, epidemics. Let me quote Danner's recent essay once more because it sums up the effects of these national beginnings on the course of Haitian politics:

> The new nation, its fields burned, its plantation manors pillaged, its towns devastated by apocalyptic war, was crushed by the burden of these astronomical reparations, payments that, in one form or another, strangled its economy for more than a century. It was in this dark aftermath of war, in the shadow of isolation and contempt, that Haiti's peculiar political system took shape, mirroring in distorted form, like a wax model placed too close to the fire, the slave society of colonial times.[15]

Diverse claims of causality are now made to explain Haiti's poverty and inequality. But the nagging sense that Haiti had paid dearly for achieving, however briefly, the goals of liberty, fraternity, and equality for all is the most commonly heard explanation in Haiti. "We're still paying the price for defeating the architects of slavery," a young Haitian recently told me, and most others would likely agree. The French debt looms large in internal discussions but is scarcely remembered beyond Haiti's borders.[16] How much money went from the former slave colony to one of the richest countries in the world is debated, of course, as is the significance of this transfer to the parlous state of modern Haiti. One scholarly history, written in 1953 by the Haitian anthropologist Jean Price-Mars, blames the local élites for accepting the 1825 agreement: "From a country whose expenditures and receipts were, until then, balanced, the incompetence and frivolity of the men in power had made a nation burdened with debts and entangled in a web of impossible financial obligations."[17]

Regardless of how blame is doled out, Haiti was not, as some have said, cut off from the world in the nineteenth century. The fledgling republic actively supported the anticolonial project in the Americas, helping to bankroll and supply Simón Bolívar, for example. Its economy, though moving away from its slave-labor roots, was still wedged in the tight and unequal embrace of international commerce. The country had been redivided into smaller holdings on which peasant farmers continued to grow—in addition to food for their families and local markets—coffee, cotton, and sugar for export.

During these first decades after independence, a tiny élite began consolidating control over the busy ports in the capital. Recurrent palace coups, often with foreign sponsorship, fueled the centralization of power in Port-au-Prince. The British, Americans, and Germans traded briskly with the Haitians, even though they had no formal diplomatic relationship. The subaltern status that led to the disastrous treaty of 1825 continued to shape trade arrangements favorable to the *blan,* as Haitians now termed the world beyond their shores. From the late nineteenth century on, the United States kept gunboats in or near Haitian waters. In 1915, after yet another internal coup, we sent in the Marines.

The nineteen-year U.S. occupation of Haiti—like the French debt, remembered by all within Haiti and few without—was justified in the usual manner, with a host of contradictory claims. Just as the "peace and safety of our shores" was the early nineteenth-century reason for refusing to recognize Haiti's sovereignty, so was early twentieth-century Haiti's mayhem held to be infectious. But President Wilson may have put it more honestly when he said, "control of the customs houses constituted the essence of the whole affair."[18] U.S. banks took over Haiti's treasury. The Marines also disbanded the army, the last, tattered remnant of the revolutionary army, long bereft of a non-Haitian enemy.

The new rulers cobbled together by the Marines would also lack for nondomestic targets: foreign occupation engendered local dissidence and fierce resistance. By 1919, when the United States was distracted by the closing chapters of the war in Europe, simmering resentment boiled over and rebellion erupted throughout the country. The violence was fiercest in rural regions, where forced labor had been used to build roads and other public works. Thousands were killed as the Marines and their newly formed Haitian constabulary sought to suppress the rebellion. Haitian historians (such as Roger Gaillard) estimate that 15,000 were killed or seriously injured, and internal U.S. reports put the numbers in the thousands, too.[19] Such news disturbed pacifist groups in the United States, which brought attention to the U.S.–Haitian conflict, if only after the rebellion had been suppressed. For example, Emily Greene Balch, a writer and peace advocate, repeatedly called for an end to the occupation of Haiti.[20] (She won the Nobel Peace Prize for these and other efforts some years later.) The affair stained the reputation of the Marine Corps, even according to its internal assessments.[21] On October 14, 1920, the *New York Times* noted an in-house investigation conducted by Brigadier General George Barnett, former Commandant General of the Marine Corps, who concluded that 3,250 "natives" had been killed:

> On 2 September, 1919 [General Barnett] wrote a confidential letter to Colonel John H. Russell, commanding the Marine forces in Haiti, bringing to the latter's attention evidence that "practically indiscriminate killings of natives had gone on for some time," and calling for a thorough investigation. . . . "I think," General Barnett wrote to Colonel Russell, "this is the most startling thing of its kind that has ever taken place in the Marine Corps, and I don't want anything of the kind to happen again."[22]

Rebellion aside, Haiti, along with much of the Caribbean basin, was firmly in the U.S. sphere of influence by the 1930s. Naked force was no stranger to many of the small island republics surrounding Haiti, including the Dominican Republic (to the east) and Cuba (to the west). Most Americans knew little of these matters: there wasn't much appetite, during the Depression, for such foreign adventures. Although President Roosevelt was no isolationist, he too favored ending the occupation. (During his campaign, Roosevelt had once boasted of learning a thing or two about government by writing Haiti's constitution.[23]) In 1934, Roosevelt made his second trip to Haitian waters to announce the withdrawal of U.S. troops. (He was the first and only U.S. president to visit northern Haiti until Bill Clinton did so just before the quake.)

The U.S. government had little intention of leaving a power vacuum in Haiti. As local factions struggled to control the state, and as another world war was brewing in Europe and Asia, U.S. leadership cast its lot firmly with the military and economic élite. This pattern was repeated throughout the Caribbean and Latin America, where military-civilian élites were rapidly assuming greater power and an increasing share of scarce resources. Throughout the region, participatory democracy broke down; elections served as charades to showcase power and boost meager legitimacy; and puppet régimes and military dictatorships became the rule.

Thus did the U.S.-trained army and a small number of families hold the upper hand in Haiti until 1957, when François Duvalier was "selected" (as Haitians say) president in fraudulent elections. Duvalier ("Papa Doc") built up his own militia and began using terror liberally to tighten his control over the country. Wave after wave of refugees, including professionals and other élites, left Haiti for safer shores. Graham Greene pilloried Papa Doc in *The Comedians*; Duvalier, idly banning the book, vowed to remain in office until the end of his days.[24] He did just that, naming his nineteen-year-old son, Jean-Claude ("Baby Doc"), as his successor before he died in 1971. Baby Doc held onto power until 1986, when the Duvaliers left Haiti for gilded exile in France.

There was much talk, in 1986, of bringing the Duvaliers to justice—or at least trying to recover some of the millions they'd looted from public coffers. It was a heady time, one chronicled by Jean Dominique and Michèle Montas on Radio Haiti-Inter, and others also seeking to introduce the country's first free press. Broadcasts and broadsheets reached more and more Haitians, and the word "democracy" could be heard across the country. A new constitution was drafted, one that declared Creole the national language and banned Duvalierists from office. It was a period of restless hope.

It was also a violent interregnum, in which the military and economic élite again vied for power.[25] Frequent clashes between pro-democracy demonstrators and the military claimed many lives. Most demonstrations were organized by young people in the city, but rural farmers also began taking arms against unjust social arrangements and pressing for land reform. In the city and countryside, some of the most outspoken community organizers were Catholic clergy influenced by liberation theology. One was Father Jean-Marie Vincent, who worked with peasant farmers in the northwest. The notion of basic social and economic rights for the poor—the right to land, jobs, and basic services—resonated with those so long denied them but was anathema to regional landowners, to some in the military, and to many of the wealthy. During the late eighties, violence broke out not only in Port-au-Prince but anywhere land reform, literacy campaigns, or political enfranchisement were discussed openly.

Such discord—essentially class conflict—took the country by storm. Military and paramilitary forces, many of them holdovers from the old order, often fired on demonstrators pushing for change. The most infamous attacks targeted progressive church leaders, including Father Jean-Bertrand Aristide, a Salesian priest who rose to prominence because of his fiery sermons and his work with youth groups and the poor, and because he and his followers were persecuted by the military and parts of the Catholic hierarchy. In one lethal episode, hundreds of peasant farmers were killed in the northwest and Father Vincent narrowly escaped with his life.

Repression did little to stop the popular movement, which hadn't yet organized under one particular banner but was coalescing around the rights long denied to the majority: political and civil rights and also (perhaps more boldly) social and economic rights. The chief order of business was to organize proper democratic elections. In 1987, an attempt to hold elections ended in a polling station massacre, and the military—implicated in the killing—stepped in and declared martial law. It was during these years that Jean Dominique's rich baritone voice declared Haiti *la belle prisonnière de l'armée*. And it was during these years that Aristide survived several assassination attempts, which only increased the numbers and devotion of his followers.

Genuinely democratic elections seemed unlikely to occur under the army's patronage, but that's just what army leadership promised a few months after the abortive 1987 poll. Numerous accounts—in French and in English, partisan and less so—cover these years after the fall of the Duvalier family dictatorship. One of the best comes from Amy Wilentz, who was present for much of this violence and chronicled the rise of the popular movement. She offered the following assessment of the 1988 elections organized under martial law:

> The January election had been one big joke. Manigat's voters were given rum and money; "campaign" workers doled out dollars to voters from the back of a big black car outside Cité Soleil. A foreign journalist, a white man, was paid five dollars to vote for Manigat. The voters, ragtag groups in most places, toured the towns by tap-tap, voting—and then voting again.[26]

Wilentz might have witnessed one of the last gasps of the old order when she survived the sack of Saint-Jean Bosco church on September 11, 1988. A group of hired assassins set fire to the church while Father Aristide was saying mass. Aristide (and my future coworker and friend, Loune Viaud) survived; at least a dozen did not.[27]

The attack on Saint-Jean Bosco was among the darkest chapters of the period and surely one of the great crimes against the democracy movement (and the Church) in Haiti. It was, alas, soon eclipsed by other crimes and more political violence, as great numbers of Haitians continued to push for free and fair elections. But the military leadership held firm, in spite of growing pressure from the international community. There was meeting after meeting, commission after commission, inquiry after inquiry, and a handful of interim governments in Haiti before enough players agreed that elections and democratic rule—in keeping with the new constitution—were the only way out of this quagmire.

How to hold elections in such a fevered environment wasn't clear, but Father Aristide's candidacy led to a stampede of last-minute voter registration. The ballot was set for December 16, 1990. Having weathered the 1987 election-day killings in Haiti, I knew I ought to stay out of Port-au-Prince that day. But with so many international observers and such infectious enthusiasm amongst my friends, I wanted to see it with my own eyes.[28]

Although there were a dozen candidates, Aristide won 67 percent of the vote; he had cast his lot with the poor majority and they had cast theirs with him. But the army and many of Haiti's wealthy families remained, by and large, staunchly opposed to the young priest and his dangerous ideas (the ones he'd been preaching in his parish). Sure enough, another military coup—one of the bloodiest—toppled Aristide only seven months after his inauguration. If the previous four years had been difficult, it was hard to find words to describe the months after September 1991. Tens of thousands fled, by land and by sea. Aristide was sheltered in Caracas. Thousands more found no shelter at all.

More than five years after the fall of Duvalierism, Haiti had another military government. But most Haitians refused to be governed by unelected military officials or their civilian backers. The slums and poor neighborhoods from which Aristide drew his support fought back, the economy continued its downward spiral, and the army wasn't able to govern effectively, even with liberal use of force. Such repression fueled further waves of migration, and the "refugee crisis" was much discussed during the U.S. presidential elections in 1992. (Restoration of Haitian democracy made its way into the Clinton-Gore platform.) But there was foot dragging on all sides, especially from the Haitian high command. Aristide himself had decamped from Caracas to Georgetown, D.C., to participate in these discussions. It was not until 1994, when President Clinton intervened to restore constitutional democracy, that Aristide returned to his homeland.

Not a shot was fired during this "immaculate invasion," to quote one account of the period.[29] But guns and bullets were on people's minds because these—not the ballot box—had always been the instruments of régime change in Haiti. How best to end this sorry cycle was much discussed in Haiti. Aristide proposed demobilizing the Haitian army, which since its creation by the U.S. Marines had never known a non-Haitian enemy. President Oscar Arias of Costa Rica endorsed this suggestion. (His country was one of the few in Central America without a standing army and also one of the few free from recurrent coups d'état.) Arias was in Haiti in 1995 when Aristide became the first Haitian president to hand over the reins of power to another elected civilian, agronomist René Préval, who had served as Aristide's Prime Minister in 1991. The hand-off was surely an achievement of note, and Arias, by then a Nobel laureate, wrote an op-ed saying as much: "Aristide happily noted that the only members of the army still on the government payroll were twenty marching band musicians."[30]

Behind the scenes, though, power struggles continued, involving the usual players in the Haitian political class, the diaspora, the business élite, foreign embassies, and international institutions. Everyone seemed to have a prescription for Haiti, which limped along—deforestation continued apace, and erosion further threatened crop yields—until Préval also won a record: he became the first Haitian president to serve his complete term and pass the reins to the next elected president. He was replaced by none other than Aristide, who this time had won more than 90 percent of the vote. Would the former priest become the second Haitian president to serve out his term and move Haiti towards a constitutional democracy in which orderly transfer of power was the rule rather than the exception?

Bitter disputes about what happened next characterize almost all commentaries on the period.[31] But some things are clear: although Aristide could easily win the popular vote, he had not endeared himself to the wealthy, nor to some members of the second Bush administration. (That the newly elected U.S. President's father had held the same office during the previous military coup against Aristide was a topic of much commentary in Haiti.) It is also clear that the agenda of the popular movement—a just partition of wealth and improved access to basic social services—had deep-seated opposition. Some of its detractors could be found among the local beneficiaries of the old order; some were still influenced by Cold War mentalities. A handful of doughty conservatives counseled the new U.S. administration to obstruct capital outlays, including credit and development assistance, to populist, left-leaning régimes. This might not have mattered much in Cuba or Venezuela, but Washington's policies had, as usual, loud echoes in Haiti. As noted, the United States and others sought to slow direct assistance to the Haitian government because they disapproved of recent election cycles. How much influence these policies had on other countries is unclear, but they seem to have guided the hand of certain countries (such as France and Canada) and development agencies; U.S. assistance, certainly, went to NGOs instead of the public sector.

How cash-poor was Haiti's government? In 2002, governing a population of almost ten million, its budget wasn't much bigger than that of the city of Cambridge, Massachusetts (with a population of one hundred thousand); neither amounted to a quarter of the budget of the Harvard hospital in which I trained. Without resources, it was impossible for public providers to provide much of anything; many professionals went to work for NGOs, which did not have a mandate to serve all citizens; others left the country altogether. Public health and public education faltered, as did other services of special importance to the poor—such as access to safe drinking water. Choking off assistance for development and basic service delivery ended up choking off oxygen to the government. But that had been the intention all along: to discipline or dislodge the Aristide administration.

Although U.S. assistance didn't flow to the public sector, it did flow, some of it to civil society groups that opposed the Aristide administration. A handful of wealthy families also helped finance these groups. At the other end of the spectrum, urban slums were becoming ever more factionalized into gangs, some of them heavily armed. Young gang members, called *Chimè*, were blamed for much of the urban disorder. Madison Smartt Bell, the novelist, wrote an affecting essay in *Harper's* about these troubled times. Here's what he said about the *Chimè*:

> One word usually means many things in Haiti, and . . . the word *Chimè* carried me toward a deeper meaning. Before that term was coined, Haitian delinquent youths were called *malélevé* ("ill brought up") or, still more tellingly, *sansmaman* ("the motherless ones"). They were people who'd somehow reached adulthood without the nurture of the traditional *lakou*—communities that the combined forces of poverty and globalization had been shattering here for the last few decades. That was what made them so dangerous. The *Chimè* were indeed chimeras; ill fortune left them as unrealized shadows. With better luck they might have been human beings, but they weren't. These were the people Aristide had originally been out to salvage; "*Tout moun sé moun*" was his earliest motto ("Every man is a man").[32]

*Tout moun se moun* really means "every person is a person," and it was the favored motto of the poor, who continued to support their champion even as others, including many civil society groups, defected. The toll taken by the unacknowledged aid embargo was steep—a fact that was much commented upon in Haiti, even as it was denied by those who'd slowed their aid. As mysterious "rebels" (many of them demobilized soldiers from the Haitian army) massed on the Dominican border, Aristide was roundly condemned by officialdom for having the cheek to bring up the distasteful subject of the French debt. The Haitian president asked the French government to repay the money France had extorted from Haiti in the nineteenth century, and was only too happy to let them know how much 150 million germinal francs were worth in 2003 terms: with interest, $21 billion.

It was another violent interregnum. In central Haiti, our medical teams did their best to care for victims of border raids. These included, in the space of a few months: a judge, a vice mayor, several police officers, and security guards at the hydroelectric dam. Most were shot dead. The "rebels" also kidnapped Dr. Wesler Lambert, a protégé and colleague, and four nurses interviewing for a job with

Zanmi Lasante. Dr. Lambert was driving an ambulance—clearly marked as such—and when released asked only that it be returned, along with the medicines he'd been transporting. We never got them back.

Entire books (containing many discrepant claims) have been written about this violent period, and more will surely follow.[33] But some facts were incontestable: there would be no repeat of the 2000 transfer of power from one elected president to the next. In February, 2004, Aristide and his Haitian-American wife, the lawyer who had chaired the national AIDS commission, were spirited away to the Central African Republic, itself governed by a military man who had installed himself in a recent coup. U.S. and French diplomats insisted the Aristides had been taken to a country of their choosing; but the destination, a lawless place neither he nor his wife had ever visited before, seemed to support the president's claim that they'd been kidnapped.[34] American officials, including Donald Rumsfeld and Colin Powell, dismissed this claim as absurd, and denied any U.S. involvement. As Amy Wilentz noted in the *Nation*:

> What happened in Haiti was a coup d'état, and it's almost funny to hear Donald Rumsfeld, Colin Powell, and Scott McClellan call that claim "absurd" and "nonsense." The coup didn't come in one fell strike, which in fact camouflaged it for a time; we're used to a coup being a coup—which means a cut or blow in French—something sudden. But the coup against Aristide, and by extension against the Haitian people, was prolonged, a chronic coup. It began when Aristide was first elected at the end of 1990 and continued right up until he was hustled aboard a plane and flown to what he was told would be a place of his choice but that turned out to be the former homeland of fabled killer and diamond collector Jean-Bedel Bokassa, a country where, according to the CIA country report available on the web, a ten-year elected civilian government was recently replaced by a military coup d'état.[35]

Regardless of the disputes over Aristide's departure, the régime that replaced him didn't really take. The U.S.-selected caretaker government was unpopular, unrest continued to grow, and Port-au-Prince became the kidnapping capital of the world in spite of a large UN peacekeeper presence. Local police forces were weak or corrupt—a pale reflection of what they should have been—as were the public health, public education, and judicial systems. Haiti again proved difficult to govern without elections.

The next two years weren't much better. The leader of the UN peacekeeping forces, a Brazilian general, took his own life in the Montana Hotel. Another UN diplomat, Jean-Marie Guehenno, compared the plight of Haiti to that of Darfur. "Haitians in Cap Haïtien," he noted, "are in a worse situation than some of the [internally displaced persons] I saw in Darfur."[36] In terms of security in its broadest sense—freedom from want and freedom from attack—Haiti was in bad shape. No member of its interim government had been elected; the elected president was in exile (first in the Central African Republic, then in Jamaica, and finally in South Africa); armed "rebels" moved freely throughout the country; the Prime Minister and other government officials had been jailed without due process; and there were persistent shortages of food and fuel and other basic necessities. It was hard to imagine that those who had supported the latest coup would be satisfied with such an outcome. It certainly made delivering basic health services difficult.

As the months dragged on, as people accustomed themselves to the UN peacekeeper presence, myths and mystifications about Aristide's departure were in no short supply. But as in the preceding decade, the appetite for constitutional rule and an end to de facto governance was great. In 2006, Haitian voters again elected René Préval, whose second term would be fraught with problems not entirely under his control. In 2008, an international flare in food and fuel prices caused riots and a vote of no confidence in his prime minister. His next choice, Michèle Pierre-Louis, was not approved by the parliament for months, which meant, essentially, that any bold development policies would be difficult to implement. And any hope of reversing Haiti's ecological disaster, accelerated by deforestation, needed bold policies. Every rainy season brought landslides, floods, and deaths. The 2008 hurricane season was, as noted, the worst on record.

This, then, is the short version of what physicians call the history of the present illness. During the twentieth century, Haiti had survived a foreign occupation (followed by various régimes of short duration, none properly elected), a twenty-nine-year-long family dictatorship with scant interest in long-term development, a series of military-civilian juntas, brief democratic rule, more coups, and the slow sundering of a once united popular movement. In the decade or so preceding January 12, 2010, Haiti was deforested and fragile but was not peopled by the same zombified populace (to use the local term) who suffered in seeming silence under the Duvaliers. A large portion of the current population was born after 1986, the year the dictatorship crumbled. Its people were strong and proud, but its government and institutions were weak and largely unable to deliver the basic services for which the population clamored.

The earthquake was another reminder of the weakness of Haiti's public institutions and the vulnerability of its population without any kind of social safety net. Into the breach have come humanitarian groups, NGOs, development experts, missionaries, and many others, but whether such goodwill can be converted into substantial reconstruction projects that grow the Haitian economy, mend its infrastructure, strengthen its health, education, and sanitation systems, and furnish its government and institutions with sovereignty and resources remains to be seen.

# 5.

## INTO THE CAMPS

*A*ppreciating the historical roots of Haiti's chronic problems did not make solving them easy, as was clear before the quake. And it would be hard to rank Haiti's post-quake problems in order of importance. But it was increasingly clear that living conditions in the spontaneous settlements that stretched across the city and to other affected areas would be near the top of the list.

Although my coworkers from Partners In Health and Zanmi Lasante were providing medical services in four of the camps, I hadn't spent much time at these sites. It was tempting to assume that others with more expertise in such matters were helping Haitian authorities address this new crisis of homelessness. A number of large institutions with experience in such settings—including the International Organization for Migration, the UN Office for the Coordination of Humanitarian Affairs (OCHA), and Red Cross affiliates—were charged with tending to the displaced, and the UN had pulled together a "shelter cluster" to coordinate responses to the knotty problem of shelter. In retrospect, I had a naïve view on how long these tent cities would be around before people would find their way to safer temporary shelters or repaired homes. How temporary was temporary? During a visit to one of those camps, Chelsea Clinton shocked me by noting that, on average, displaced persons in Africa spend well over a decade in such "temporary" settlements.[1]

As it became clear that displaced Haitians would fill Port-au-Prince's interstices and public spaces, from soccer pitches to public parks to churchyards, the shelter experts in humanitarian disasters devised dozens of plans. But plans didn't always, or often, lead to implementation. Hundreds of thousands lacked adequate housing—many were living under bedsheets jerry-rigged as roofs—as well as food, water, and medical care. Although the Haitian government had suggested building numerous small camps instead of a few large ones—because security and sanitation worsened with increasing sprawl—the majority of those *anbatant* ("under the tents") lived cheek-to-jowl in large encampments. By mid-February, more than one million people were living in almost a thousand such camps.

It's not that we weren't thinking about the shelter problem from the beginning: it was impossible to walk for more than a few minutes in Port-au-Prince without seeing spontaneous settlements. A few days after the quake, before we'd even heard the term shelter cluster, I met several Partners In Health and Zanmi Lasante colleagues for an impromptu meeting about our urban strategy. We debated for hours in the UN logistics base. Should we be providing medical services in the rapidly forming camps, or were the experts on the case? And what about adding staff in the city to complement our teams already working there?

These were weighty decisions that would, we knew, affect our work for years to come. Setting up tent clinics would require additional staff, some of whom we could surely recruit from among camp residents. But even well-staffed clinics couldn't do much without medications, equipment, food, water, sanitation—and we had none of those things in urban Haiti. In the same heated meeting, my colleagues asked simply, "What is our obligation to the camps and to the General Hospital?" Loune Viaud, who had spoken very little, gave a shrug as if to say, "What choice do we have?" She was pretty sure we could set up decent clinics and recruit staff rapidly. The other Haitians there also seemed confident about our capacity for growth in

Port-au-Prince. The more reluctant staff feared we wouldn't do a good enough job; all of us knew camp conditions were brutal. One of the most experienced doctors put it this way: "I went into one of the camps and, although I hate to say it, almost lost all hope." Thinking as UN Deputy Special Envoy, I couldn't ignore the camps on the grounds that they were "outside our catchment area," as public health professionals are wont to say. And although I respected the shelter experts, no group had as much experience implementing projects in Haiti as Loune and our Zanmi Lasante teams did. I was relieved when consensus emerged that we would try to help out in the camps.

The spontaneous settlements were dispiriting in large measure because of the execrable living conditions. Many of those providing services within the camps also felt dispirited; by mid-February, some humanitarians were already speaking of failure. Wasn't it a failure that the vast humanitarian machine could not move the internally displaced to higher ground before the rains started? Couldn't they at least make sure camp residents had enough to eat and drink?

In mid-February, I visited Parc Jean-Marie Vincent, one of the largest camps in Port-au-Prince. (The actor Sean Penn and his group had set up shop in the only larger camp, sitting precariously on what was once the Pétionville Golf Club.) The park was named after Father Jean-Marie Vincent, the Haitian priest, who was martyred in 1994 for helping to organize the poor in Haiti's parched northwest. Father Vincent had launched literacy projects and a bank for poor people (an anticipation of the microcredit movement) before being gunned down on the steps of his own rectory. I'd known him personally, and wondered what he would've thought about the park-turned-camp bearing his name. It wouldn't have shamed him, I felt sure. These were, at least, his kind of people.

One of the many fine people we'd met (and hired) was Dr. Dubique Kobel, a young Haitian physician trained in Cuba who had recently returned to live and work in the poor Port-au-Prince neighborhood where he'd grown up. His wife, Nadège (also a doctor), had given birth to a baby girl mere months before the quake leveled their neighborhood. The Drs. Kobel took the baby, who was unharmed, and sought shelter in the tent city being hastily erected in Parc Jean-

Marie Vincent from all sorts of ersatz construction materials. Few tents were available, but the Kobels eventually found one and pitched it on a stretch of cement. (The park had been made in part out of an abandoned runway.) The Kobels's new home was a few hundred yards from where they'd lived before the quake. Along with new colleagues from Zanmi Lasante and Partners In Health, they soon found themselves delivering medical care to a population the size of a medium-sized city.

Dr. Dubique guided me through the camp. It was a stunning scene: on that day, he estimated that about forty-eight thousand souls were packed into the tiny space. But Dr. Dubique was upbeat, glad to have medications, basic lab capacity, and some experienced colleagues from central Haiti, including one of my favorite protégés, Dr. Anany Prosper. (In spite of the setting, there were some happy reunions that day.) Anany had helped launch a clinic in a town called Petite Rivière de l'Artibonite and had recently assumed similar duties in Parc Jean-Marie Vincent and three other spontaneous settlements.

Some progress had been made: regular clinical services (delivered, alas, in sweltering tents); the slow transformation of shelters from dun-colored to blue as cardboard and sheets were replaced by turquoise plastic sheeting; a couple of new tent schools; some minor improvements in lighting. (The pitch darkness into which the camp was plunged each night increased the risk of sexual violence and other crime.) But there didn't seem to be more than a few score latrines, and the entire place was hot and dank. How long could the good morale among doctors and nurses last in these conditions? Surely the shelter experts were working on these challenges?

Shelter experts were, in fact, also unhappy with the pace and quality of the services offered to the displaced. Although Parc Jean-Marie Vincent was bigger than most camps, it was in other senses par for the course. Dr. Dubique underscored the need for scaled-up provision of food, water, and shelter—the same services we tried to afford our patients in rural Haiti. He also pushed for more investment in security to make the camps safe for women and children. But it was clear, as Dr. Dubique took me through the camp, that resources and expertise were insufficient to meet all these needs.

The day after the quake, hours after President Clinton's speech at UN headquarters, I'd met with John Holmes, the head of OCHA. He seemed like a reasonable and experienced professional. Perhaps I should seek his counsel about security, water, sanitation, and alternatives to tarps and plywood and tin? Holmes directed me to internally displaced persons experts in the shelter cluster. My colleagues from Partners In Health (including Louise Ivers) had already consulted them, and were finding that the U.S. military and a missionary group, Operation Blessing, were more reliable partners when it came to working in the park.

What exactly was the cluster system? The UN's cluster strategy divided labor into discrete areas according to its lead agencies: the WHO (World Health Organization) was charged with coordinating medical aid; the World Food Program, with food aid; and UNICEF, with attending to children's needs. As the weeks passed, swelling settlements and crowded hospitals revealed a wide gap between the existing humanitarian capacity and the unmet needs of Haitians affected by the quake. The cluster system needed reform. Dissatisfaction with aid delivery was abundant and not only within the camps. An internal memo written by John Holmes himself was leaked to the press on February 17. I include it here, with gratitude for his candor:

> Exactly one month after the earthquake, I visited Haiti to measure progress in the humanitarian operation and to gain a better understanding of the challenges we continue to face as a community in our efforts to support the national authorities in their emergency response. It is clear that, thanks to the collective efforts of so many people and organizations, we have achieved a great deal. However, it is also clear that there remain major unmet humanitarian needs, particularly in critical areas such as shelter, other NFIs [non-food items], and sanitation.
>
> With the rainy season looming, these unmet needs are taking on additional urgency, not least from the health and protection points of view, and given the potential consequences in terms of both politics and security of large demonstrations in some sensitive places.

If I read him right, Holmes wasn't sure that the A team was on the job; nor did he think that enough resources were reaching the most urgent projects. Holmes continued:

Part of the problem relates to our overall operational capacity. I fear we have simply not yet injected the necessary resources in some areas in terms of capacity to implement practical programmes and deliver on the ground. The magnitude and complexity of the disaster are such that all major organisations need to deploy their most experienced disaster response staff and to make sure they are procuring, delivering and distributing what is needed as quickly as possible. This is a major test for all of us and we cannot afford to fail. So I ask you all to take a fresh hard look at what you are able to do in the key areas, and pursue a much more aggressive approach to meeting the needs.

Regarding coordination, I was disappointed to find that despite my calls for the Global Cluster Lead Agencies to strengthen their cluster coordination capacity on the ground, very little progress has been made in this critical area. In most of the twelve clusters established, cluster coordinators continue to struggle without the capacity required to coordinate efficiently the large number of partners involved in the operation. One month into the response, only a few clusters have fully dedicated cluster coordinators, information management focal points and technical support capacity, all of which are basic requirements for the efficient management of a large scale emergency operation. This lack of capacity has meant that several clusters have yet to establish a concise overview of needs and develop coherent response plans, strategies and gap analyses. This is beginning to show and is leading others to doubt our ability to deliver.

Among the many lessons already identified from this disaster is the need for robust cluster coordination teams with adequate seniority to take charge of cluster coordination at the outset of the response. To place one person as a cluster coordinator is simply inadequate and falls critically short of what Global Cluster Lead Agencies have committed to.

We cannot, however, wait for the next emergency for these lessons to be learned. There is an urgent need to boost significantly capacity

on the ground, to improve coordination, strategic planning and provision of aid. Good coordination between clusters and within each
cluster is needed not only to channel the contributions of UN agencies, the Red Cross/Red Crescent Movement, IOM [International Organization for Migration] and NGOs, but also: (1) to ensure close
coordination with the efforts of national authorities; (2) to channel
the contributions of the private sector; and (3) to make maximum use
of the logistical support and other assistance provided by the military. OCHA stands ready to assist and can provide further support
and advice, when needed.

I would therefore like to repeat my request to Global Cluster Lead
Agencies to boost their cluster coordination teams immediately, and
to provide sustained coordination capacity on the ground. I would
also like to request NGOs to look at ways of strengthening their own
capacity on the ground and to consider contributing personnel to
support cluster coordination efforts.

The scale of the devastation in Haiti has overwhelmed everyone. Despite the untiring efforts of so many people, we are still struggling to
provide enough basic assistance in some vital areas to Haitians affected
by the earthquake, many of whom remain in life-threatening situations.
We can scale our efforts up further and we must do so urgently.[2]

Holmes identified a number of perennial challenges facing humanitarian groups—from poor coordination to the gaps in the delivery
pipeline. For a top UN official to express such disappointment was
news only because it was leaked. But how could he avoid drawing
such conclusions after visiting the camps? Some of those working in
Haiti took umbrage that a senior official had said their work wasn't
good enough. But the Haitians were even more vocal and forthright
in their complaints: this work *wasn't* good enough by any stretch of
the imagination. A walk through the camps was all it took to reach
this same conclusion. Some working in the cluster system were self-
aware enough to make mocking t-shirts. A few weeks after the quake,
I saw one young humanitarian in Léogâne sporting a shirt with "I survived the shelter cluster" printed on the front. If the leak helped
spark a self-critical dialogue among the many aid purveyors in and
outside Port-au-Prince, it was surely helpful.

At the time the memo was leaked, OCHA estimated that 40 percent of displaced persons in Haiti were still without any form of transitional shelter. That meant at least four hundred thousand people, and perhaps many more, still lacked a safe and dry place to sleep over a month after the earthquake in spite of the massive humanitarian presence. Press articles published during this spike in aid critiques pointed to the airport bottleneck—more than one thousand relief planes were backlogged—and to stories of containers full of supplies detained in ports and customs areas by extortionary fees or simple incompetence. It was not the brightest moment in the history of humanitarian aid, which already had a long and checkered history.

Much more could be (and was) said about the imperfections of the aid machinery and about the sorry history of development and humanitarian aid in Haiti before and after the quake. But Holmes's memo did not solve the problems in the camps; no memo or declaration or editorial could. Camp conditions improved at a snail's pace, and reports of gender-based violence increased.

At night, it was easy to see why the camps were fetid: girls and women, especially, were afraid to walk to the latrines because they'd heard stories of others being raped there. Such stories surfaced even in camps that had organized women's patrols with fluorescent t-shirts and whistles to accompany girls to the latrines. (We'd helped set this up in one camp.) Why didn't this system work? All we got in response to that question were shrugs. Some humanitarians also suffered from a sort of attention-deficit disorder. One NGO installed lights in a settlement only to take them away again when their tour of duty was up. A study conducted by Louise Ivers and her senior aide, Kim Cullen (another quake survivor), found that, three months after the quake, in Parc Jean-Marie Vincent, more than 40 percent of camp dwellers thought camp conditions were too dangerous for children and women to get water at night. Another 7.4 percent reported having already been attacked.[3] This camp was, by comparison to most others, well-managed.

The settlements continued to grow during the summer months, and so too did the social pathologies. Didi made her first trip to post-quake Haiti in the summer, and spoke with women and girls who had been abused in the camps and also with a Zanmi Lasante social worker there. She posted the following, linking the lack of basic sanitation to gender-based violence seen at all the camps:

> Sexual assault and rape were common in pre-earthquake Haiti—hence some of our own ethnographic studies of "forced sex" in rural Haiti—but the social structures of family and neighborhood networks provided some protection for Haiti's women and girls. The collapse of this social infrastructure on January 12 brought with it a destruction of the physical and social safeguards against violence, leaving women and girls completely vulnerable to sexual violence. Many girls spoke of being raped. As vulnerable as Virginie [one girl living in Parc Jean-Marie Vincent] is within her family's "shelter," she and other girls are at even greater risk when they venture to the bathroom—little more than a crude dark closet with a hole in the ground where they squat in darkness. Latrines are far away. Numerous girls described being followed and attacked on the way to the toilets. While armed police may patrol some camps in the day, and citizen brigades have formed in some camps to help escort women and girls to latrines and cooking areas at dark, armed men continue to prey upon them.[4]

It was clear by the start of the rainy season that the problems in the camps, including the lack of safe and affordable housing, would not be addressed effectively in the short term. Groups with long-term commitments to Haiti would be stuck working on behalf of those sequestered in the camps, and their responsibilities would increase as short-term relief groups prepared to leave (even as the camps continued to grow in size and number). I thought of an experience I'd had in 2008 when visiting a dusty refugee camp in a rural district of Malawi not far from where we were building a hospital. Although that camp had dwindled in size, we'd been asked to help rehabilitate its clinic. I ran into a couple of young people, who were surprised when I greeted them in their native language, Kinyarwanda. They'd been living there, they said, since the Rwandan genocide—which had occurred fourteen years before.

# 6.

## FROM RELIEF TO RECONSTRUCTION
### *(Building Back Better?)*

*Two months after the quake,* Haiti was still struggling to transition from disaster relief to reconstruction. There were still many acute needs: injured and sick people needing medical attention, children without food and water, families living in burgeoning tent cities who needed safer shelter. As in February, many of us split our time between assisting with direct relief and trying to resume whatever it was we were doing when the quake hit.

As we struggled to recapture a sense of normalcy, continuing tragedies kept pulling us back to the making of grim lists. Most such tragedies occurred in Haiti, but no one was really spared. One of our hardest working members of the Office of the Special Envoy, Aaron Charlop-Powers, lost his mother (whom I'd known as a Partners In Health supporter) in a bike accident in New York on March 17. Everyone in the UN offices stopped work and tried to let Aaron and his grieving family know that we were there with them. But, as with Haiti, it seemed too little and too late.

President Clinton and his staff were gearing up for the March 31 donors' conference. I wouldn't have to speak at the conference,

which was a relief for reasons ranging from stage fright to epistemo-
logical anxiety (how could we be sure about the numbers?). As his
deputy, I would be responsible for questions about medicine and
health, but could refer questions about other aspects of recovery to
the Special Envoy himself. Clinton wasn't shy about discussing any
of Haiti's dilemmas, including structural problems with deep historical roots; nor did he mince words about our country's role in worsening Haiti's plight, unwittingly or otherwise. A few weeks after my
Senate testimony, the former president was in the same room giving
his. He offered a brave mea culpa about the role of U.S. food imports
in undermining Haitian agriculture. He could have blamed the Foreign Assistance Act of 1961 or ecological decline or the inferior productivity of Haitian farmers, or any old thing, as politicians often do.
But here is what he said to the Senate Foreign Relations Committee
on March 10:

> Since 1981, the United States has followed a policy, until the last year
> or so when we started rethinking it, that we rich countries that pro-
> duce a lot of food should sell it to poor countries and relieve them of
> the burden of producing their own food, so, thank goodness, they
> can leap directly into the industrial era. It has not worked. It may
> have been good for some of my farmers in Arkansas, but it has not
> worked. It was a mistake. It was a mistake that I was a party to. I am
> not pointing the finger at anybody. I did that. I have to live every day
> with the consequences of the lost capacity to produce a rice crop in
> Haiti to feed those people, because of what I did. Nobody else.[1]

This sort of candor meant a lot to me and to many others; it helped
start a conversation about needed reforms to the machinery of foreign assistance and global trade.

I next left Haiti with Claire Pierre and Garry Conille for a March 15
conference in the Dominican Republic. This was yet another meeting
about a meeting, but one in which the broad outlines of the upcoming pledging conference were to come into view. Flying from Haiti
into the more developed Dominican Republic was always startling,
but the differences—economic, ecological, infrastructural—between

these two countries, sharing a single landmass and once inhabited by a single people, had never been more jarring than after the quake. The border visibly instantiated the divergence between the two countries' fates: where the Haitian side was stripped bare of trees after decades of unchecked deforestation for charcoal production, the Dominican side retained a healthy forest cover. (I'd recently learned that bakeries, laundromats, and household cooking fires were three of the largest consumers of charcoal in Haiti.) Infrastructure and construction quality were noticeably more robust after crossing the border. One could not help but wonder how much less damage there would have been—and how many fewer lives lost—had the earthquake struck a few hundred miles east (though no one would ever wish such a fate upon any country or people).

The three-day meeting in Santo Domingo aimed to help the Haitian government develop its national reconstruction plan and to coordinate donor activity leading up to the March 31 conference in New York. This meeting was, after Montréal, the second public step in the process of aligning the goodwill of the international community to help rebuild Haiti and one of the last steps before a more scripted agenda was set for New York. Without much to contribute, I listened and watched, often disquieted, as foreign ministers, international organization representatives, and disaster relief experts improvised in what often felt like political theater. Different players—some powerful, some less so—tried to get a word in edgewise, taking turns sitting and standing in a dance that seemed to reassert an unspoken hierarchy of power and prestige. The more interesting conversations occurred *dans les coulisses*—"in the hallways"—where it was possible to be frank and find those who were deeply committed to Haiti.

Some participants had experience rebuilding cities and regions after disasters natural and unnatural. Most relevant, perhaps, were the teams who'd worked in Indonesia after the 2004 tsunami as part of the Multi Donor Fund for Aceh and Nias (two of the hardest-hit provinces). They shared experience of disaster-resistant construction, resettlement of refugees, and the resolution of property disputes—all challenges Haiti was already facing and ones that would only grow in importance on the long road to reconstruction.

A number of Haitians expressed—not impolitely—doubts about the relevance of such examples and overly prescriptive advice. Prime Minister Jean-Max Bellerive said, *dans les coulisses,* "Look, I don't want my country to look like the Dominican Republic or Indonesia or some other place. We're searching for a genuinely Haitian way of rebuilding." Haitians from "civil society" were already grumbling that they weren't getting much of a say in the recovery process. But they'd been invited to Santo Domingo, which is more than most of our patients in central Haiti could say. We hoped, of course, that Michèle Montas's testimony (based on the Voices of the Voiceless project) would help fill this gap at the March 31 donors' conference, which by the end of the Santo Domingo meeting had been titled, "Towards a New Future for Haiti."

Attendance at the preparatory meetings—in Montréal and Santo Domingo—suggested that significant commitments would be made. It did not mean, however, that all promises would be kept, nor did it mean that resources would be deployed fairly or wisely. The New York convocation was slated to be much larger than the previous meetings, drawing representatives from an estimated 150 member states and international institutions. It remained to be seen whether having so many participants would mean much to the people cobbling a life together in Port-au-Prince, but it would have been worse than cynical not to give it a try.

Past experience tempered naïve optimism. Meetings like these were common coin after natural disasters. We'd witnessed the flimsiness of aid promises since the Washington, D.C., International Donors' Conference in April of 2009, a meeting to generate support after the 2008 storms rocked Haiti, leaving Gonaïves under water and causing billions of dollars worth of damages.[2] During that meeting, labeled "A New Paradigm," Ban Ki-moon and others spoke of a "new juncture" and pledged long-term support for Haiti. (Some of the new was redolent of the old, including the idea of turning Haiti into the "Taiwan of the Caribbean."[3]) In any case, not enough came of the financial pledges made in Washington: of $402 million promised for the Haitian government's Economic Recovery Program, only about $61 million, or 15 percent of the pledges, was disbursed.[4] And, to risk repetition, of the money that did reach Haiti, little went to the public sector.[5] (Isn't the government an important player when trying to rebuild a country or prepare for future storms?) Donor conferences, it seemed, needed to be "built back better," too.

Jean-Max Bellerive was slated to introduce the Action Plan for National Recovery and Development of Haiti, which drew on the Post Disaster Needs Assessment launched in Montréal. The action plan and the needs assessment were drafted by the government of Haiti in collaboration with foreign technical assistance (a clutch of consultants, some working pro bono and others seconded from various agencies); they sought to lay out a vision for reconstruction and identify funding gaps. These documents drew on a wellspring of development and recovery initiatives proposed by previous Haitian governments after upheavals (such as the 2004 coup) and disasters (such as the 2008 hurricanes).[6] The new action plan introduced a number of schemes to build back better, from political restructuring to massive housing plans to scaling up an ambitious education agenda. There was a profusion of plans, but little in the way of implementation.

Was this giant March meeting to yield more of the same? Sometimes it seemed that the quake had changed everything, but as the history of chronic problems revealed, much had not changed. Uneven development, the gap between rich and poor, the ongoing exclusion of most of the latter, the unseemly quest for control of the frail apparatus of the state, the ecological crisis, the reliance on fractured foreign aid, and the privatization of basic services (when they were available at all)—all were longstanding problems worsened by the quake. It was tempting, at times, to give an ivory-tower shrug of inevitability and assume that it was all too hard to improve, much less to fix. The donors' conference would be bigger, but surely it could also do better. Garry, Claire, and I were physicians, and we were there to give reconstruction our best good-faith effort, knowing full well that we would fall short of our aspirations and those of the Haitian people. But we had to try.

And so on we went, organizing and cajoling and seeking to make New York not just bigger but better. The Office of the Special Envoy team had been working around the clock, as had President Clinton and his staff, official teams from the hosts (the UN and the U.S. government), and many Haitians who had worked on the needs assessment and action plan.

The conference was held on the second floor of the General Assembly Building of the United Nations. Security was tight at the UN and across New York because so many dignitaries were flying in for the meeting. The morning consisted of welcomes and introductions; all speakers underlined the need for long-term financial support for Haiti's reconstruction (as they'd done in Montréal). Ban Ki-moon spoke, then Hillary Clinton, then René Préval. The Haitian president thanked those present for helping Haiti, but also noted that his government had received little support from the international response to date—a paltry $23 million of the $1.35 billion disbursed for immediate earthquake relief.[7]

My job was to sit behind Clinton, along with Laura Graham, and to brief him on the "civil society" session he would be chairing. He knew my views—that although the session brought in perspectives from certain NGOs, certain parts of the Haitian diaspora, and certain private sector groups, no poor people were present. During the plenary session, Michèle Montas would summarize the views recorded by the "Voices of the Voiceless" team. Because we couldn't hear directly from those most affected by Haiti's social and economic fragility, Michèle's testimony was the part of the conference that mattered most to me.

Michèle knew the rural and urban poor as some of the sharpest critics of Haitian society and politics and the development enterprise. Her statement, not much more than ten minutes long, presented their suggestions about rebuilding Haiti. Although her elegant contribution to this book introduces the Voices of the Voiceless project in more detail, I'd like to underscore how her words, echoing this, challenged a number of assumptions about Haiti that persisted among those gathered in New York. In contrast to reports of Haitians passively accepting handouts in refugee camps, these interviews revealed that leaving the camps was a priority for almost everyone surveyed. Camp dwellers desired nothing more than to return to their homes—some of them little more than heaps of rubble—or to rejoin family in the countryside. Interviews far from the quake zone were also instructive. Rural farmers interviewed were adamant that Haiti needed to rebuild its agricultural base before it could reap the benefits of local and international trade; mothers and fathers demanded adequate food for their children and their neighbors' children; many stressed the importance of aid independence and sovereignty after reconstruction was underway. During the few short minutes that Michèle spoke, I wondered if some new paradigms of foreign assistance and economic development might come out of all this.

Clinton's optimism and Michèle's testimony set a tone of hopeful pragmatism for the afternoon, when the pledging sessions took place. As in Montréal and Santo Domingo, the meeting had its share of posturing and grand promises. But for the most part, the concern and willingness to help expressed by foreign ministers, international organization representatives, and other delegates seemed genuine (as political theater often does). When Venezuela and the United States began vying for the biggest pledge, it seemed best to applaud politely. Even those from nations with divergent interests handled themselves with a certain comity. And the numbers—the amount pledged—kept going up.

A stunning $9.9 billion of reconstruction pledges were made on March 31.[8] The funds were earmarked not just for rebuilding but for rebuilding better: $5.3 billion for the near term (2010–2011), $4.6 billion for the long term. Venezuela and its allies emerged as the largest contributors, pledging more than $2 billion; the European Union collectively pledged $1.6 billion; the United States pledged $1.15 billion.[9] It was an impressive show. "Today it has been demonstrated," concluded Préval, "that the international community will continue to support Haiti in the long term."[10] Hillary Clinton noted in closing that after the Asian tsunami, some 80 countries pitched in with humanitarian relief, while about 20 pledged reconstruction assistance; in Haiti the numbers were more than 140 and 50, respectively.[11] Ban Ki-moon was similarly optimistic: "As we move from emergency aid to long-term reconstruction, what we envision is a wholesale national renewal, a sweeping exercise in nation-building on a scale and scope not seen in generations. . . . Today, we have mobilized to give

Haiti and its people what they need most: hope for a new future. We have made a good start; we need now to deliver."

Delivery would indeed become the chief challenge if the capital really showed up in Haiti. Below the surface consensus, rifts began to appear regarding who would be in charge of the reconstruction dollars. The international financial institutions were vying for control, as were a few major donor nations and the UN. But the cast of characters raised the same question I'd had in Montréal: What about the Haitians? And which Haitians? It was an election year, and all involved feared that political turmoil would delay reconstruction.

These tensions, though hidden away, were fierce, and led to another proposal: a new approval body was needed to coordinate the coming surge in reconstruction funds. The Interim Haiti Recovery Commission (IHRC) would be co-chaired by Bill Clinton and Jean-Max Bellerive and made up of Haitian officials and representatives of donors that had pledged at least $100 million of reconstruction assistance or debt relief (the United States, Canada, France, Venezuela, the EU, Japan, the World Bank, the Inter-American Development Bank, and a few others). During its eighteen-month mandate, the commission would act as a clearinghouse for Haiti's recovery with the goal of increasing the efficiency and impact of allocations. It would also provide an infrastructure of transparency to reassure donors that funds were not languishing in corrupt or inept bureaucracies and to hold donors accountable to their pledges. Finally, the commission would find new ways of tracking, in real time, the implementation of projects.

The commission's evolution—from the doubts about Haiti's "absorptive capacity" (and veiled references to corruption) that surfaced in Montréal to the process of choosing who would be members among those gathered in New York—was fascinating to watch. The elephant in the room was that few donors trusted the Haitian government to disburse their money. But the government was by necessity a protagonist in Haiti's rebuilding effort, and almost three months after the quake, it was still sorely in need of funds just to keep its civil servants at their posts (mostly large tents or temporary buildings).[12]

To move relief funds quickly, donors had relied heavily on NGOs and contractors. For reconstruction to proceed in keeping with the action plan, the Haitian government needed to have an active role in vetting projects, inspecting progress, ensuring that laborers got their lot, and resolving land-title disputes. The public sector had not proven capable of performing these regulatory functions even before the quake, and now many donors deemed it even less able to do so. A history of outsourcing development projects to NGOs and contractors made trying to help the public sector now like trying to transfuse whole blood through a small-gauge needle, or in popular parlance, to drink from a fire hose. But leaving reconstruction solely in the hands of private contractors and other implementers (including large international NGOs) was a sure way to continue the same dysfunctional cycle.[13] The IHRC was meant to break through this impasse by providing a platform for collaboration and coordination, enhancing trust and inspiring what was termed donor confidence. However, as one could have guessed, the IHRC would be forced to live out its short life—eighteen months seemed short to me—in very adverse circumstances.

After many debates about governance, local control, transparency, and other issues, the commission did at last come into being by presidential decree and later parliamentary approval. The weeks ticked by during this long labor, which took us into May, and like any infant, the commission needed care and feeding. It needed funding. It had been clear in New York that some donors thought they should have more control over the flow of pledged resources. Bilateral agencies seemed unsure why they should abandon business as usual and go through a commission. Meanwhile, many Haitians were sure that the *blan*—foreign firms and contractors—would get all the money.

Clinton helped work through these disparate fears and concerns, approving projects that fit the national plan and bringing into the open who was doing what and with how much money, as we had tried to do in the Office of the Special Envoy. Staff and space and resources didn't show up until June, when Norway and Brazil sent $45 million and Mexican and Canadian philanthropists provided another $20 million in business loans. The Clinton Foundation chipped in $1 million to build urgently needed storm shelters in areas particularly vulnerable to hurricanes or heavy rains.[14]

A system of financial tracking and aid coordination that would build public-sector capacity seemed like a good idea. The Haitian government had tried to coordinate aid and NGOs in the past but with scant resources and personnel. (The two members of the NGO coordination unit had perished in the quake.) The UN cluster system was still struggling to keep track of all the groups working in post-quake Haiti. The Ministry we knew best, Health, lacked even the space and staff to vet offers of help—some great ideas, some goofy ones—that came in over the transom, if they'd still had a transom.

There had to be better ways to speed up implementation; money was clearly out there. In addition to the promises from officialdom, Haiti was also the object of a tsunami of generosity: it was estimated that 50 percent of American households donated to earthquake relief.[15] And families across Europe, including the U.K. and generous Ireland, responded with significant sums, too. Just as no previous natural disaster had wreaked such havoc in such a crowded space, neither had one prompted such an outpouring of solidarity. Where lay the disconnect between the great need on the one hand and the steady flow of aid and support on the other?[16] What would it take to transform these immediate expressions of solidarity or mercy or pity into the desired long-lasting outcomes—safe housing, clean water, good schools, health care, food security, and the dignity that comes from being liberated from the noxious cycle some describe as underdevelopment and others as structured dependence?[17]

One unanswered question was how much it would take to rebuild Port-au-Prince. The $9.9 billion pledged to Haiti in New York represented about $1,000 for every Haitian—not a lot if you're trying to rebuild a business or home, much less a safer capital city. And what if only 15 percent of the funds pledged arrived, as had occurred after the 2009 donors' conference? What little euphoria we felt right after the pledging conference gave way to anxiety and discord all too soon.

It was urgent that reconstruction start boldly and visibly. How would more than a million refugees make do in the spontaneous settlements throughout urban Haiti? We knew to expect strong winds and driving rain by mid-April, which threatened to strip the displaced of their tarps and tents and sheets, leaving the Haitians standing—if they still had strength to stand—on acres of mud and waste. People in the camps, some of them perched on steep hills, dreaded the rainy season and the flooding and mudslides that came with it. Every heavy rain that summer triggered anxiety and endless calls among groups seeking to provide care in the settlements. It proved far easier to demand better coordinated assistance, as John Holmes had done in February, than to really make it happen.

The coming rains also signaled the beginning of the planting season. The post-quake exodus from Port-au-Prince had placed great strain on rural host families, who had long struggled with food insecurity. They needed to turn their attention again to agriculture so that Haiti would not rely on imports for basic nutrition.

Back-to-school season was a sorry time. Many children in Port-au-Prince, especially those living in the camps, had nowhere to go; their schools had been damaged and many of their teachers killed in the quake. Schools needed to be rebuilt and temporary solutions were needed to keep children off the street and out of gangs. Before the quake, demographers and aid agencies spoke of the "youth tsunami" about to wash over Haiti, as if Haitian youth were more a threat than asset.[18] Human capital had long been Haiti's chief asset, and getting children and young people into safe schools that offered modern pedagogy was a top priority.

We spoke often of building back better, but what did it really mean? Literally, of course, it meant building disaster-resistant homes and other structures. It meant rendering the infrastructure of Port-au-Prince capable of supporting the millions of people who lived there. It meant building roads and bridges, improving water and sewage systems, and repairing old hospitals and building new ones. It meant making sure schools didn't suddenly collapse and mudslides didn't take down hillsides covered with houses. All these desired outcomes could mean creating jobs in the short term, and some of us felt that the most urgent task of all was the creation of jobs that would confer dignity to those in greatest need. With well-paid jobs, Haitians would themselves put safer roofs over their heads.

But only a minority of those displaced after January 12 would end up with more than plastic or canvas over their heads. By early summer, well over a million people were still living cheek-by-jowl in the camps, and moving people into safer housing was again declared a priority. Many Haitians were already patching up homes on their own. Haiti's government and the shelter experts had announced resettlement strategies by the dozen, but as usual, more design and planning occurred than implementation.

One project that attracted attention was a large resettlement complex proposed for Corail-Cesselesse, a windswept plain to the north of Port-au-Prince. This seemed an odd location because the region boasted little more than a few spindly trees. But we were eager to see people leave the muddy urban camps, and one of the most credible reporters living in Haiti had spoken of the project in fairly glowing terms: "The organized relocation camp at Corail-Cesselesse," he commented, "has thousands of spacious, hurricane-resistant tents on groomed, graded mountain soil. . . . Camp Corail offers a glimpse at what relief efforts can achieve; sturdy tents, adequate food, sanitation, and security."[19] Corail, we read, would be transformed from a model camp into a planned community with three hundred thousand spacious homes, restaurants, stores, and garment factories. Some began calling it a "Zen city," and "the key industrial city of the Caribbean."[20] Such hopes triggered a charrette of feverish plan-making and site design.

The promise of construction jobs lured thousands to the deforested plain of Corail to stake out a claim in this promising frontier settlement. But by July, the building process—the business of implementation—had stalled. Some disagreed about where to start construction; others about the right contractors for the job. Of the many planners, architects, potential builders, and engineers involved in the project, few seemed to be talking to one another. I asked one of them why the project was stalled, and he blamed the lack of clear title, an inept bureaucracy, fractious contractors, and a touch of sabotage. Then summer rains revealed the area as an immense floodplain; the proposed buildings would sink in the mud.[21] Corail was canceled. Many other resettlement initiatives lost steam as well, even as the rains continued to fall.

More modest efforts were easier to pull off, which is perhaps one reason why nimble NGOs seemed to thrive in Haiti. Although few displaced by the quake had the good fortune to end up under a real roof, among them were the more than fifty unaccompanied minors we'd come across in the General Hospital. Loune Viaud had been looking after them since the quake. With help from my Pétionville host Maryse, Loune sealed the deal on a property in northern Port-au-Prince, on the fringe of the quake zone. She hired health aides and rehab workers, mostly women rendered expert by their own experience as mothers, who were coached by professional physical therapists from Miami, Israel, and the Zanmi Lasante team. (Most of the children had severe disabilities.)

The place soon became a veritable oasis: a house full of kids and nurses surrounded by a few acres of well-tended land, lush with mangos and other fruit trees. It had a temporary library, a pool, and a humble fountain, which had been drained when they found the place but now flowed quietly. Chickens and guinea pigs were penned up around the periphery, and a tilapia hatchery and hydroponic gardens were being added in the backyard. Dozens of construction workers—there each time I visited, usually on weekends—were also putting up a large staff dormitory. The place was christened *Zanmi Beni*—"Blessed Friends"—and became an oasis both for the children and for a handful of displaced health professionals and volunteers.[22]

Three medical students, left homeless and school-less by the quake, were also living there in tents. For the first time in almost a century, the national medical and nursing schools would have no graduates. Although one class was receiving training in Cuba, few young health professionals would be entering service in the coming years. My colleagues at Harvard, Partners In Health, and Zanmi Lasante were trying to help fill this gap, including the Minister of Health's request that we triple the size of the Mirebalais hospital.

The Mirebalais expansion was already taking root, thanks to the hard work of volunteers in Chicago, Boston, and across central Haiti.

The medical students at Zanmi Beni reminded me of three Haitian medical students I'd met on that first night back in the darkened General Hospital. They hadn't eaten much since the quake, had lost their homes, and were there trying to help out at the hospital. But the only question they asked was: "How can we continue our medical studies?" Here was another role for American universities: to make sure that the current generation of trainees—in medicine and dentistry, nursing, pharmacy, and all the allied health professions— had a chance to complete their training. After Katrina, Harvard and other universities had taken students from Tulane, Dillard, Xavier, and the University of New Orleans, and now we need to help students from Haiti, too. Jim Kim, the President of Dartmouth, was up for it. At the Harvard Medical School Dubai Center, half a world away, health providers were being trained with the same methodologies we used in Boston. The goal was to realize the same standard of pedagogy and care at the two institutions. Most American research universities undertook similar "twinning" efforts in China, Singapore, and elsewhere in Eastern Europe and Asia and Latin America. But these sorts of collaborations were rare or weak in the poorer reaches of the world. The teaching hospital we were planning in Mirebalais would offer another home and a center of excellence, we hoped, for the next cohort of Haitian health professionals.

If we could build a major teaching hospital in the middle of central Haiti, seek the blessing of the Interim Haiti Recovery Commission, bring in new partners, and use private capital, we could help strengthen public health and medical care and medical education all at the same time. It was possible to imagine making a significant contribution to reconstruction, which was a lot more appealing than complaining about its glacial place and bemoaning failure.

I had personal reasons for wanting to work in Mirebalais, too. It was my first home in Haiti, where I'd first met Mamito and Fritz Lafontant. The summer of frustration, 2010, opened with a personal loss: Mamito died in June from a stroke. Mamito had taught me a lot over the previous twenty-seven years. She liked to give instructions, but her versions of "wipe your feet" or "clean up your room" were broader in scope, if equally to the point: "Make this house waterproof for this family; put tin on the roof and cement on the floor." She issued more typical maternal fiats as well, and everyone who visited Cange got a little dose of Mamito's mothering.

During the months after the quake, Mamito and her close-knit team received medical volunteers from all over and thousands of patients. She spent her days between the hospital and the church, which had remained an ersatz trauma ward for months. Well or unwell, she rose every day to give instructions to the planefuls of doctors and nurses and physical therapists who arrived in Cange. Mamito's job was to mother them a bit too: to make sure they ate enough and had clean scrubs and got a little rest now and then.

Her passing left a huge void in my life and the lives of many others. Didi flew back for the funeral, and then we returned to Rwanda for our daughter Catherine's confirmation. (Our work in Rwanda was going well; we were trying to hasten the completion of a flagship hospital in the northern Burera district.) I needed a break from Haiti and the grueling back and forth to Boston, and my coworkers did, too. The transnational doctors, a hardy lot, were weary—even the indefatigable Claire Pierre seemed tired. I was also falling behind in my Harvard duties and leaning on colleagues there to pick up the slack. But most of all, I wanted to see my kids.

Somewhere on the long list of reasons why the camps kept growing over the summer—the top reason being that the displaced had nowhere else to go—was that some supplies and provisions were reaching the camps, and the situation outside them was dire. By some reports, water insecurity had lessened throughout Haiti because aid groups were providing clean drinking water in the camps. One survey in Port-au-Prince suggested that diarrheal diseases had dropped 12 percent below the pre-earthquake level.[23] However, the massive importation of bottled water wasn't sustainable, and some local bottlers and merchants began urging aid groups to stop distributing free water. But given the lack of sanitation in many settings, the local water supply would be "sustainable" only if it did not become a conduit for waterborne disease.

By mid-July, most involved in quake relief—including officials from USAID, which in previous years had tried to skirt Haitian institutions—understood all too well the need for a new approach to delivering services. After reporting the improved water security in Haiti, Paul Weisenfeld, Haiti Task Team Coordinator for USAID, observed: "I think it's key to us that if we're going to have sustainability we are going to have to work through Haitian institutions, which requires strengthening them. Obviously [they've] been weakened tremendously by this earthquake, so at the same time that we implement reconstruction programs, we need to strengthen government institutions so that we can work through them."[24] The term "sustainability" has long been abused in development circles. It admits too many meanings. Sustaining lives in these camps would mean sustaining supply lines for as long as people lacked homes and jobs. Otherwise, we would see outbreaks of waterborne disease before the rains ended.

---

The greatest challenge of economic development in Haiti had always been massive job creation. By summer, more and more agencies were implementing "cash-for-work" programs. Such initiatives were surely one good way to move resources from the self-described donor nations to the survivors who were able-bodied and anxious to work. But the UN reported that these programs had generated only about thirty-five thousand jobs. What was needed was more on the order of five hundred thousand paying jobs, and soon. Haiti needed jobs that would confer dignity on the poor. As FDR said early in the Depression, "The Nation asks for action and action now. Our greatest primary task is to put people to work."[25] Martin Luther King and many others had echoed the view that paid labor confers dignity.[26] Most champions of rights for the poor, it seems, had come to this conclusion. A jobs campaign of this magnitude—with a focus on young people, especially young women—would not be a panacea for Haiti, but it would be a step forward on the long road to reconstruction.

While in Rwanda, I thought long and hard about that country's recovery from the genocide and about other recoveries of recent history. Bold rebuilding plans always include major public works projects. Haiti needed them, too. There were innumerable public-works jobs imaginable, from reforestation and rubble removal to building schools that were safe and well-supplied. Haitians needed a real health system, which would require massive investment in new clinics and hospitals, staff to run them, and health insurance—yes, "the public option." (Only three hundred thousand families in Haiti had private insurance.) These tasks were indivisible, as FDR noted at the outset of the Depression: "Public health . . . is a responsibility of the state as [is] the duty to promote general welfare. The state educates its children. Why not keep them well?"[27]

Job creation and improved health and educational services, with greater investment in the public sector, should have been a big part of the recovery plan. The Interim Haiti Recovery Commission needed to be swift and nimble; the rules of the road for development assistance needed to be rewritten, not to favor contractors and middlemen and trauma vultures, but to favor the victims of the quake. By summer, shovel-ready projects that could create tens of thousands of jobs (or perhaps more) were available. But most people were living in poverty without reliable jobs. Haiti's *ti machann* ("market women"), for example, seldom had access to capital or financial services and had been working against an undertow of unfair trade policies. But they were as entrepreneurial as anyone.

Projects of all sorts could be green-lighted by the recovery commission, but they would move sluggishly if the funds seeped in slowly or if strangling strictures were placed on their disbursal. The commission didn't even have its own project money. In the face of urgent need, were we well served by the fetishization of process that retarded the flow of capital into the hands of poor families?

Americans with long memories knew it was possible to move forward with a sense of urgency. During the Depression, job creation and improved services—from health care to education to rural electrification—were the focus of great efforts and significant enthusiasm. Roosevelt, then the governor of New York, called for "workfare" and welfare through the Temporary Emergency Relief Administration. This call was made on August 28, 1931, and the program was up and running by winter.[28]

Later, these lessons were brought to scale through many other programs, including the Civil Works Administration, which created millions of jobs and moved billions of dollars into both the public sector and the hands of the previously unemployed. Many civil works programs—dams, municipal water systems, public power plants, roads, reforestations, communications infrastructure, even blazing the Appalachian Trail—were completed in part because of the Civil Works Administration and other civilian jobs programs.

Certainly Haiti's need was no less great than that faced by the States during the Depression.[29] A better functioning tax base would have been handy. (The Haitian version of the IRS had never functioned well and, like the Ministries of Health and Education, had been destroyed in the quake.) But in principle, other capital was available: the world had responded generously, and now it was incumbent upon us to move these resources into the hands of the Haitian people. It was not a matter of choosing between public and private sectors, but of focusing resource distribution on the poor and displaced by providing basic services and by launching substantial job creation efforts. Only an infectious failure of imagination would slow such projects down or smother them in their cradles.

In Rwanda, I thought about the many meetings I'd attended since the quake. Some were less mind-numbing than others. Meetings involving President Clinton tended to be engaging because he always had good ideas and tried to boost morale. Other meetings seemed promising as well. On June 7, I was the lone American invited to a tripartite health summit between Haiti, Cuba, and Brazil. When I was informed by Claire Pierre that the meeting was to be held in the Hotel Montana, where Walt Ratterman and Mario Pagenel and so many others had died, I thought there had been a mistake. The Montana was down. But Claire would know; her mother had lived in an apartment there, which had been leveled. "Yes," she said. "That's where the meetings will be held. Some of the conference rooms under the hotel are intact."

On top of a hill overlooking the city and the bay and also the Central Plateau, the hotel grounds were an eerie perch. The building was little more than a pile of plaster and concrete and twisted steel. One of the owners limped over toward us. (She had been badly injured, I knew, and had lost one of her grandsons along with most of her guests.) She led us to a lower terrace under which lay, undamaged, a subterranean meeting room. The tripartite mission (Haiti-Cuba-Brazil) would meet there, she said. "And I have something for you," she told Claire. "Some things I found in the rubble."

When we emerged for a coffee break (and a break from translating between doctors speaking in French, Creole, Portuguese, and Spanish), the Montana owner gave Claire her sister's wedding album. "I found this in what used to be your mother's apartment." The album was water-stained and warped, but the pictures were mostly undamaged. It was one of the only times that I saw preternaturally cheerful Claire tear up. She hugged the album to her chest. "And for you, doctor," continued the owner, "I found this." She handed me a water-logged report of the health status of the Haitian people. Probably the work of some consultants who had stayed at the Montana, it was still wet and in worse shape than the photo album. I took it gratefully, and we returned downstairs to join the Babel of physicians from across Latin America, as they asked how a proper health system might emerge from the wreckage.

———

To those in the camps, and to many of my colleagues, the summer was one of lowered expectations. If help was on the way, it was travelling slowly and in the form of discrete projects visible to some but not to all. At least we knew the teaching hospital in Mirebalais—by far the most ambitious project we'd ever taken on—was moving forward. Many others labored mightily to improve conditions in one way or another. But projects without perceived national reach were not cheered by those untouched by them. As the rains fell, weeds appeared and began to cover some of the uncleared rubble. It was a summer of great discontent.

The months passed by in a blur—more meetings, yes, but also a frenetic push to get money and projects moving. It was during that summer that a group of us decided to pull this book together. We hoped it might lend clarity to the debates about reconstruction, and that it might serve as an account, however partial, of those first six months. But to write a book, or even a few chapters, required time alone. I hoped to find such time during a giant AIDS conference in Vienna in the third week of July. These meetings, which took place every two years, gathered twenty thousand people and were quite a spectacle. Although meetinged-out, I'd promised Clinton and some Haitian colleagues, including Dr. Pape and Father Eddy Eustache, that I would be there. Vienna was not a city I knew, but I'd imagined a tranquil week in a leafy city, when half my time could be spent writing. (Cassia Holstein promised to meet me there for this reason.)

We arrived in the middle of a heat wave, hotter than any I'd endured in Haiti or Africa, and there was a good deal less tranquility and writing than hoped for. President Clinton gave the meeting's plenary address, speaking of Haiti. The net movement, he said, was forward and positive. A few of us gave a presentation about medical care in Haiti after the quake. I was eager to hear Dr. Pape's opinions and projections. (GHESKIO's clinics and labs, which he had founded two decades previously, were smack in the middle of the quake zone.) He predicted that although Haiti's AIDS epidemic remained "under good control," the conditions in the camps, including the one abutting GHESKIO's downtown campus that we'd visited with Clinton in February, were ripe not only for epidemics of waterborne disease but for a rise in tuberculosis. Some of us, Pape included, remained worried about the introduction of cholera and other pathogens unknown to Haiti—as AIDS had been unknown a few decades before.

As in all such conferences, the most interesting conversations occurred *dans les coulisses*. Several of us met to discuss the Global Fund's grants to Haiti. The last real meeting on the topic had started at 4:00 P.M. on January 12, and the problems with the upper-level management of Haiti's AIDS programs remained largely unaddressed. It was also in Vienna that the Minister of Health in Lesotho, who had once worked with the Clinton Foundation, reiterated a promise to take in some Haitian students at their university. (The Rwandan government had done the same.) Didi agreed to spearhead that effort after her troubling visit to Parc Jean-Marie Vincent earlier that month.

One of my only celebratory breaks that summer was the July 31 wedding of Chelsea Clinton and Marc Mezvinsky. Chelsea and Marc had traveled to Haiti together shortly after the quake, and since then, Chelsea had been back to the camps, including Parc Jean-Marie Vincent. A student of public health, she had warned us of cholera and other waterborne pathogens. But on that day, we raised none of these topics. We tried to avoid saying the words "Haiti" and "earthquake" altogether. (It was a reminder that there might be other topics of conversation.) It was there, in a lovely town in upstate New York, that I finally started working on this book. The day after the wedding, to encourage myself to write—to stop and think and write—I made a brief pilgrimage to the graves of Franklin Delano and Eleanor Roosevelt.

———

Within a week, the proud father of the bride and I were back in Haiti, where it was almost as hot as the Austrian capital. Clinton arrived in Port-au-Prince on August 5 to help launch the newly baptized Interim Haiti Recovery Commission. As had been the case from the beginning, disagreements about the commission's role bubbled just under the surface. Some representatives of the development enterprise were resentful—why stand up a body like this, they asked, if there were existing bodies?—but most were worn out and ready to acknowledge that something new was needed. The diplomatic community was also in large part bound by the strictures of that world to at least feign enthusiasm for the commission. The Haitian politicians were, as ever, split—some denouncing the commission as a failure even before it met for the first time and others, including members of the Préval administration, obliged to be supportive. Many of the behind-the-scenes meetings were devoted to making the commission nimble, transparent, and strong without weakening the line ministries (the government agencies in charge of health, education, agriculture, et cetera). By this late date, most NGOs and aid groups allowed that efforts to bypass the line ministries had worsened Haiti's governance and fueled the overall lack of coordination. But how to repair this error while also speeding up reconstruction?

Claire Pierre was asked to head up the health sector of the commission. Could she be seconded by Harvard (and her hospital) to lead this small team? If anyone had the patience and competence for such a thankless posting, it was Claire. We were in full support, if she was willing to risk it. She was.

The next morning, Clinton traveled to Darbonne Sugar Mill in Léogâne, the town nearest to the epicenter of the quake. The only operational sugar mill in all of Haiti, Darbonne was always in the throes of closure because its output was as meager as its profit. Clinton was investigating whether investments in the mill might generate jobs and help stimulate biofuel production. We also came to see how Léogâne was faring: what had happened to schools and health centers, and what were the conditions like in its spontaneous settlements? I had worked in Léogâne's hospital as a medical student but had not been back in several years. (Léogâne was also the hometown of Edwidge Danticat, a friend and contributor to this volume.)

Léogâne is close to Port-au-Prince, but it takes hours to get there by road because of traffic south of the city; the road had also been damaged by the quake. Clinton and I were instead flying by Russian helicopter (manned by Ukrainian pilots eager to have their photos taken with him). The view from above was still difficult to bear. Seven months after the quake, less than 2 percent of the rubble had been removed from Port-au-Prince and the surrounding areas.[30] The heavy machinery needed to crush and clear rubble was in short supply. During most of the twenty-minute flight, there was not a glimpse of green. But the southern sprawl of Port-au-Prince gave way to farmland as we neared the temblor's epicenter.

Even in the farmland, many concrete buildings had collapsed, and from the chopper, pancaked buildings and slab roofs angled downward like wet cardboard. Decades of shoddy and helter-skelter construction visibly marked the social fault lines of the disaster. The building codes for Port-au-Prince were less than two pages long, and it was likely that Léogâne didn't even have those.[31] We'd heard that 90 percent of the town had been damaged or destroyed, but many people were probably living as they had before: in tin-roofed shacks that were almost too small to fail. So in another of Haiti's ironies, many of the poorer people's shacks were more or less intact, while concrete Léogâne lay in ruins. Debris clogged the streets, footpaths, and drains; people were pushing wheelbarrows and carrying buckets of water.

As UN officials, aid workers, and locals led President Clinton around, I hung back to get a quieter look at the temporary houses and shelters, called t-shelters. Close to a hundred thousand of them were supposed to be built in Léogâne—that had been the goal—but fewer than thirty had been erected so far. And although the name *t-shelter* itself suggested impermanence, they were something of a disappointment: solid two-by-fours were used as supports, but the walls were of white plastic; the roofs, cheap tin. Like the spontaneous tent cities, the t-shelters were poised in an uncomfortable space between the temporary and the long term. They were too flimsy to last for long and already threatened by the elements. When I'd worked in Léogâne two decades before, the rainy season invariably resulted in dramatic flooding throughout the city, including the hospital wards, when the local river jumped its banks. It didn't look like the t-shelters would be high and dry for long.

Soon, private musings about these shelters were echoed by publicly aired complaints from the beneficiaries. The model t-shelter Clinton visited was inhabited by a woman who had nothing good to say about her new home. She launched a stream of invective in Creole even as the disaster-relief folks were describing, in English, the sturdiness of the t-shelters—"these are built to withstand high winds and to serve as transitional shelters that can tide people over until more permanents shelters are built; they're much safer than tents." The model inhabitant scowled and complained. "Who would want to live in a house like this? The walls could be split open with a kitchen knife. It's tiny. I used to live in a three-story building!" The counterpoint was bizarre and discouraging for those who understood both versions of the tale. I was relieved not to be the translator. A Potemkin village this was not.

I was ambivalent about visiting the sugar refinery in Darbonne. Harvesting sugar cane is one of the most brutal forms of labor, and one historically linked to slavery from the sixteenth century on. Anyone who knew Haitian history, remote or contemporary, would be leery about the industry. The harvest was unpleasant in Florida, grueling in the Dominican Republic, and economically unviable in Haiti—again for reasons beyond the control of the cane cutters who were now greeting Clinton. And in all three countries, this harsh work was often done by Haitians.

But as we walked through the mill, my spirits lifted: a thirty-foot-tall portrait of Jean Dominique greeted us on one of the larger façades. For long years, he had fought the good fight and paid the ultimate price. He would've been disappointed by the slow pace of recovery after the quake and sent lots of young journalists out to document the reasons (and excuses) for delays. He also would have deplored contracts without benefits to Haitian firms. So it seemed right to see Jean Dominique smiling over an enterprise that promised to create better prices for the region's cane growers and cutters.

Haitians weren't the only workers in this mill, which reared up out of a green sea of cane. The Darbonne refinery had been, since its launch in 1983 on a loan from the World Bank, something of a white elephant. In its best years, it was only marginally profitable because cheap sugar imports—thanks to huge subsidies in the United States, especially—flooded Haitian markets. Another problem was the dwindling harvest: farmers on small plots of land were competing not only with U.S. trade subsidies but also with the technical advantages of agribusiness. Much of the harvest here was still done manually, which meant that cane cutters in Léogâne ended up doing the same sort of work whether in their home country or in any other. They would prefer, surely, to stay home, if they could make a living. After sputtering along for a few years, the Darbonne mill closed, to be re-opened in 2001 when Cuba kicked in $2.5 million in operating capital and a great deal of technical assistance. But the refinery still produced under capacity, providing only 2 percent of the sugar consumed nationally. Haiti, once the largest producer of sugar on the planet, couldn't compete with Dixie Crystals.

Then along came the call for biofuels, many of them made from sugarcane. Greg Milne, the young lawyer on our team, briefed me on the situation. Three years ago, an energy company invested in the mill to keep it from going under, and it soon generated three megawatts of electricity in addition to scaling up its sugar output (including syrup for alcohol fermentation). Maybe this white elephant would, with Cuban help and some investment, be given a second lease on life. Maybe it would help generate power for a region with little electricity.

At the time of our visit, the plant employed about 250 people. Greg Milne and others estimated that modest investments and upgrades could increase sugar and electricity output tenfold, especially if investments also went to local cane growers to increase their access to tools, credit, and better prices for their produce. Seeing Cuban and Haitian workers on the job, it didn't seem far-fetched to imagine that initiatives like this one—doing CPR on a moribund refinery—could guide our efforts to resuscitate the foreign aid apparatus. In any case, it seemed like a good use of Cuban expertise, and although the entire biofuels debate seemed impossibly complex, here was an agroindustrial effort that also generated electricity in a rural region that needed it desperately. This combination of potential positive outcomes, and Jean Dominique's symbolic approbation, made me feel better about visiting this outpost of an industry long associated with cruelty and coerced labor.[32]

Although my attention was focused on health care, I was learning a lot on visits like these. As hard as it was to be a cheerleader for sugar production or biofuels, it wasn't hard to applaud higher incomes for Haitian farmers, more electricity, and more processing capacity. In general, smaller-scale agriculture seemed to strike a better deal for the poor than did industrial and agroindustrial projects. With a fish farm or produce cooperative, farmers, *ti machann,* and others moving or selling their own produce might in principle enjoy more autonomy and higher incomes than factory workers. But the decline in agricultural production and continued ecological destruction made it hard for anyone tilling the soil or fishing to survive without improved processing capacity and ready access to credit. The microfinance boom had helped some families but had not prevented the rapid rise of food insecurity or the persistence of child servitude.

As noted, Haiti had been buffeted about in the global economy for centuries. Its first transaction, the Columbian exchange, wiped out the indigenous Taino population. (Léogâne, in fact, had been heavily populated by the Taino in 1492, when the global economy was born; its patron saint is the Taino Queen Anacaona.) As noted, the slave labor system put in place by the Spanish and French extracted immense profits from cash crops such as sugar and coffee. Such history tempers any romanticism about sugar refineries, coffee-washing stations, or even mango-processing plants. But on that August day, in the company of a couple of peasant cooperatives, some Haitian investors, a dozen Cuban technicians, and a former U.S. president, it felt good to leaven a visit to troubling temporary shelters with an effort to create jobs and electricity and processing capacity. Although anxious to return to medical tasks, I knew that poverty-reduction efforts, better wages, and improved access to the fruits of modernity would make our medical work easier and more effective.

Such were the insights of social medicine, a discipline I learned from Haitians and from mentors at Harvard. It was social medicine we tried to practice in Haiti and elsewhere in the world, from the poorer parts of Boston to the rural reaches of Rwanda, Malawi, and Lesotho. But the masters of this field were surely the Cubans, who, along with Aristide, had founded a new medical school in Haiti. The school was one among many worthy efforts shuttered by the 2004 coup. Most of the students had been able to continue their studies in Santiago, Cuba, however. At the close of a summer in which no students would graduate from Haiti's state medical school, sixty-seven newly minted doctors were due to receive their diplomas. One had been born and raised in Cange, and most others were from similarly humble backgrounds. I'd been one of the only American doctors involved in their first year of training and was honored to be asked to be the *parrain*—literally, the "godfather"—of their class. (The god-mother chosen was Marie-Laurence Lassègue, to whom I'd handed my satellite phone amidst the din of Toussaint Louverture Airport not long after the quake.)

I didn't know what to do for these young men and women other than to welcome some of them to our hospitals as interns. Claire and Loune suggested I give them each a stethoscope and one of my books. The ceremony took place at the Karibe Hotel, which, though damaged in the quake, was open for business. I didn't have to speak, and just sat there with Minister Lassègue and other dignitaries (the Cuban and Venezuelan ambassadors, and the leaders of Haiti's Ministry of Health), to celebrate the return to Haiti of this bumper crop of Cuban-trained doctors. Thirty of them approached me after the ceremony about forming a study group to stay in touch and keep learning. (They would be scattered across Haiti after years of study together in Cuba.) Most would have too little support—in the way of clinical supervision or didactic sessions—so some younger U.S.-trained doctors, including Natasha Archer and Michelle Morse, promised to help mentor them and connect them to a web-based platform we'd developed at Harvard. The students were full of trepidation and enthusiasm.

The graduation ceremony was one of the happier moments of the summer of discontent, and it made me all the more anxious to see the Mirebalais hospital up and running. It was possible, just then, to imagine a time when these young physicians could work in a hospital worthy of their talent and training.

⸻

The ceremony was also a reminder of my own students and the Department of Global Health and Social Medicine at Harvard, which I chaired. The work in Haiti was central to its mission, but the new academic year was about to begin. Classes would start soon, and I was unprepared. For the previous eight months, it had been all earthquake, all the time. It was daunting and emotionally difficult to think about teaching anything unrelated to the health challenges after the quake. What lessons could be drawn from the previous eight months? What links existed between short-term relief and the long slog of reconstruction? Observers and participants alike were struggling to make sense of what had transpired since the quake. There were plenty of stories and reports noting how little had been achieved. But most of the conclusions seemed premature: it was early to say much about the pace of reconstruction, other than that it was slow. And the pace would have been slow in less devastating circumstances, as we'd learned after the storms of 2008.

There were also other projects to keep going (and growing) in a dozen other countries. We were behind schedule to open the flagship public hospital in Rwanda's Burera district.[33] It would be smaller than the one we were starting in Mirebalais but was nonetheless the largest we'd built to date, and we'd poured blood, sweat, and tears into it. In fact, the hospital was a poster child for swords-to-plowshares projects because it lay on the site of a former military base near the Ugandan border. We launched the project with the Rwandan government and broke ground in the summer of 2008. We'd promised a glorious product by the close of 2010, and were a month or two behind. These promises, and others made outside Haiti, found their way back into my thoughts as August drew to a close.

I gave my first class of the year at Harvard College rather than the medical school (where I usually teach). The course was called "Case studies in global health" and, on September 2, I began with a presentation about the earthquake, the social roots of the disaster and the challenges to delivering care in its aftermath. To end on an authentic but optimistic note, I showed a brief video about Shelove and Carmen, both of whom stayed on in Cange and had been trained as physical therapy aides. At the time of writing, both had emerged as excellent *accompagnateurs* for other amputees—accompanying them on the long and painful road of recovery.

At my request, Shelove began looking after one patient: a young man named (believe it or not) Victory, who was suffering from tuberculosis and Hodgkin's lymphoma. When he arrived at the hospital, Victory weighed less than seventy pounds and was too weak to stand. After receiving treatment for both his afflictions, he was soon walking again. His progress was thanks mostly to his treatment but also to Shelove, who helped him get up on his feet again. Many in his shoes would be tempted to give up. But Victory received more or less the same medications he'd have received in Boston, plus something else: accompaniment by a survivor.

The video showed the women talking about the experience of losing limbs in the quake and of their new lives, making rounds with patients of their own just a few months after their amputations and rehab. Seeing Carmen trudge uncomplainingly to visit the homes of people disabled by all manner of ailments made me hope that the quake might have triggered a genuine disability-rights movement, long overdue in Haiti. I wanted to share with our students that there *had* been inspiring stories in post-quake Haiti—although they were rarely mentioned in the mainstream press, Haitian or American. The failures were always more noteworthy. "When I go to see patients, I show them how to walk," said Carmen. "I accompany them as they learn to use their wheelchairs. I talk to them. They ask me how I'm able to walk, if my prostheses hurt, if I'm able to run, if I can do whatever I want with them, and I say yes. I had thought I would never walk again, but now I can do whatever I want. My life has been changed."

Sanley, whose amputation had been delayed for weeks in vain hope of a limb-sparing procedure, was not featured in the video, but she has also done well. She remained in Boston with her mother; both were studying English. Sanley seemed like her teenage self again. When I'd last seen her in a cafeteria at Harvard Medical School, she was busy on a new computer using Facebook to find friends in Haiti. In the months after her rehabilitation, Sanley appeared on television with one of Boston's best-known chefs, a Partners In Health supporter named Jody Adams who'd participated in "Top Chef" to raise money for our work. In the cook-off, in which the chefs had been presented with a culinary challenge, Jody's included goat. She didn't win. A few months later, Sanley and her mother and Jody made a guest appearance on another show, seeking to improve Jody's goat-cooking skills. I didn't share Sanley's story with my students, but she was on my mind as I struggled through the lecture.

In keeping with the course's structure, the other faculty present responded to my remarks. The first respondent was Anne Becker, a psychiatrist with whom I'd trained in medicine and anthropology. After her first year of medical school, Anne had worked in the Port-au-Prince slum called Cité Soleil. She ultimately decided to do her doctoral research in Fiji, which turned out to have equally troubling, if less apparent, social pathologies as Cité Soleil. We'd been friends for more than twenty-five years. The second was Anne's and my mentor, Arthur Kleinman, also a psychiatrist-anthropologist, who had defined the field of medical anthropology through his long-term work in China. It was the third year we'd taught the course together, but the first time we'd shared a classroom since January. I regarded both of them as giants in the field of social medicine, and wondered what they'd say about the earthquake.

Anne Becker's comments were more informed by knowledge of Haiti. After the quake, she had returned to Haiti to visit one of the country's only psychiatric hospitals (her first trip back since the summer she spent in Cité Soleil). She expected, correctly, a near-total lack of medications in the damaged hospital, but this was not the problem the few caregivers there emphasized. "We need food and water," they said. "And mattresses and sheets and clothes for the patients." They also needed medications, of course, but were forceful in their ranking of needs.

Arthur Kleinman responded to my lecture by drawing on his prodigious knowledge of China. He told the class about the varied responses to two major quakes there. One, centered in Tangshan, may have killed as many as 750,000 people. But this staggering loss occurred in 1976, and the Maoist ideology then regnant led the state to bury many of the facts along with the victims. Its sorry history, Kleinman said, is only now being written. The Sichuan quake in 2008 claimed 68,000 lives and destroyed as many as fifteen million buildings.[34] It attracted significant media attention because, this time, the Chinese government allowed greater access to local and international press. The government also permitted volunteers independent of the party-state to participate in the relief effort. The response was massive: in addition to 130,000 soldiers and several thousand dispatched construction workers, some 150,000 volunteers from local and international aid organizations traveled to the quake zone to help.[35] "Never since 1949," noted Kleinman, "had the Chinese authorities allowed civilian volunteers to offer their services in a social space in which the state claimed capacity and authority."

Much had been made (in this book and in the meetings I'd attended) from comparisons to the Asian tsunami, but Kleinman's contrast of the two quakes in the same vast and changing nation was telling. The challenge was the same: which lessons were specific in their implications and which were generalizable? Since January 12, countries as different as Japan, Cuba, Mexico, and Brazil offered pragmatic assistance to Haiti by drawing on their own experiences with natural disasters. Some of this assistance had already proved helpful. But the circumstances in Japan and China and Brazil—and even neighboring Cuba—seemed so different from those in Haiti. Even when the acute insult—an earthquake or a hurricane—was the same, the chronic malady was very different. Haiti's problems seemed greater though this was not an easy point to make. I again found myself thinking of Rwanda, which seemed more like Haiti than did the other countries mentioned that day.

———

I was thinking of Rwanda for other reasons, too. En route to Kigali that evening, I had grabbed the previous day's *New York Times* in the flight lounge. Its lead editorial was titled "Katrina, Five Years Later." Positive notes were sounded, but with a warning: "The region faces huge challenges. The dearth of affordable housing casts a long shadow on the city's future. At the moment, nearly 60 percent of city renters spend more than 35 percent of their incomes on housing—normally about 40 percent of renters spend that much. These people skimp on nutrition and medical care, undermining the well-being of children, and are chronically at risk of homelessness." The editorial noted that, "with 55,000 abandoned addresses, New Orleans is probably the most blighted city in the country."[36]

I immediately thought of the students I'd taught that morning, wishing I'd shared this piece, because it said a lot (if indirectly) about the burdens of chronic weaknesses when dealing with acute problems. Anyone reading this article in Haiti would have thought of the camps. What might they look like in five years? What was the long-term prognosis for Haiti?

Certainly, there are platitudes and long-existing frameworks of interpretation regarding all that happens in Haiti and about the failure of the development enterprise there. Even over the past few years, several books have been written on these topics, and some tried to do the same decades ago.[37] One common platitude concerned the resilience of the Haitian people. The problem in dismissing the resilient-Haitian angle is that sometimes, as the stories of Shelove and Carmen and Sanley suggest, it was true. But then again, they had access to three things that many Haitians lacked: health care, training, and jobs. Those affected by the quake also needed these services, just as they needed water, food, and shelter.

As President Clinton predicted on the day of the quake, the shelter dilemma remained the ranking problem in Haiti. The number of people in camps—as many as 1.5 million—had not budged much over the summer. The reasons for the slow rate of resettlement were varied and complex, but chief among them were three. First, the majority of those in the camps did not own the houses that collapsed around them on January 12. They were renters, and in some cases squatters, who put huge fractions of their scarce resources—larger even than that invested by the people of New Orleans post-Katrina—into housing and food and education. Second, these services, as well as medical care, were difficult to access before the quake and at times were more readily available within the tent and tarpaulin settlements. Third, rubble removal had been slow. Omnipresent debris—"a cancer in the city," said Clinton during one August meeting—made it difficult for people to return even to intact houses. Thus did the camps stay full during the summer, even though the rains left them fetid and unsafe.

Tempers were increasingly short inside the camps. But what could be done to speed up reconstruction? The Haitian government wasn't idle on this front. By the March 31 New York donors' conference, an action plan (one cobbled out of several) for reconstruction was ready. In April, the Interim Haiti Recovery Commission created by presidential decree was passed by the fractious parliament. (Such work was conducted in makeshift buildings and shelters because both palace and parliament had been destroyed.) It took another month to stand up the beginnings of the commission within a tent (air-conditioned, but a tent nonetheless) and a month or so to organize the first meeting. Although it's unclear by what standards the speed of this response was being judged, an August 29 editorial in the *New York Times* sounded a rare optimistic note:

> The Interim Haiti Recovery Commission was set up after the Jan. 12 earthquake as a joint Haitian-international effort to effectively channel billions of dollars of donated reconstruction aid. Like everything else about the recovery effort, the commission, led by Prime Minister Jean-Max Bellerive and former President Bill Clinton, has been too slow off the mark. But we were encouraged by its second meeting in Port-au-Prince this month, where it announced dozens of new projects with clear benchmarks and the commitment of more than $1 billion to complete them.[38]

At the top of the list of projects was the removal of an additional one million cubic meters of rubble (as noted, only 2 percent had been cleared by mid-September[39]) and the construction of temporary hurricane shelters able to protect five hundred thousand people—both by November. These and other projects would require a smooth and rapid flow of capital and human resources, if they were to be completed on a tight schedule. On one point it's important to quibble with the *Times*: billions of dollars had been *pledged* to reconstruction rather than disbursed. No small amount of that capital was tied up by politics and by a concern with process that led to such caution and to a certain divorce from the sense of urgency appropriate to the raw need on the ground. Reconstruction funds were not, in fact, readily available in Haiti. This obsession with process, and the strictures of what the great sociologist Max Weber called "the iron cage" of bureaucracy, led to the rather underwhelming temporary shelters we'd visited a month earlier in Léogâne.

In the long term, meeting cherished social goals—from reconstruction to universal access to primary schools and health care—would require not just aid but also economic growth. In the short term, however, enough had been pledged so that many basic needs could be met if funds were disbursed and projects implemented. In health and education, implementation must be done through the public sector: how can there be public health or public education without a public sector?

How to break the vicious cycle of a functionally incompetent public sector leading to further inefficiencies and incapacity in providing public goods? This question is the subject of great and often ideological debates throughout the world, and we should mistrust those who profess overly confident answers. The answer surely is not to further starve the wounded public sector—however badly wounded it might be. Yet that's what was happening. By September, approximately 15 percent of the March reconstruction pledges had been met, and only 0.3 percent of the $1.8 billion in relief assistance went to the public sector. (The *Times* editorial mentioned that, in testimony before the U.S. Congress, I had complained that only 3 percent of this aid went through the public sector; I had overestimated by a factor of ten.) What was clear even before the quake was that this approach might sustain the NGOs and the multilateral aid machinery in Haiti but wouldn't suffice to build adequate capacity in the Haitian public sector itself. Nor would the established system of awarding contracts to beltway bandits (or even high-performing aid contractors) engage Haitian companies small or large.[40] If business continued as usual, neither the public nor private sector in Haiti was poised to accomplish much in the way of reconstruction, in spite of the best intentions of many of those caught up in Weber's iron cage of bureaucracy.

Finally, the *Times* editors also mentioned the Mirebalais teaching hospital, which had been one of the five health programs approved by the commission in its first meeting to consider such projects. Because we'd been involved in this city in central Haiti for almost three decades, and had for almost two years been pushing for a proper hospital there, I'd like to proceed by describing in more detail how this goal—to have a great hospital in central Haiti—was changed, indeed upgraded, by the quake. Some of the lessons we'd learned had been in Haiti, of course. But we'd also learned a great deal from Rwanda.

In 1995, Rwanda, still reeling from the genocide, was by many measures the poorest country on the face of the earth. It would be hard to imagine a tougher situation—even comparing it to Haiti after the quake. Although Rwanda lost neither a third of its housing stock nor all its federal buildings, it had surely lost more than a quarter of its civil service. Many of the other surviving civil servants were themselves deeply involved in or tarnished by the genocide. After the cessation of hostilities in Rwanda, scores of humanitarian groups and NGOs (small and large) jockeyed for position; most did not care to coordinate their efforts with other NGOs, much less with the interim government trying to restore order and basic services. To the west, in refugee camps in Zaïre, hidden among the real refugees, were many of the architects of the genocide. International arms dealers were still shipping them weapons, and cross-border raids and clashes were continuing apace. Rwanda's rich farmlands lay fallow and hunger was rampant. Many international observers were willing, in 1995, to write off Rwanda as a lost cause.

By 2010, the country would have been almost unrecognizable to the pessimists. Kigali, the capital city, was bustling and clean; new buildings were going up in droves. The country's GDP had more than trebled in the preceding decade. Education and health care had become, over those years, far more available to the average citizen, and an anticorruption campaign had yielded fruit: a good deal of investment poured in from abroad, from the large diaspora, and from within Rwanda itself. In 2010, hundreds of NGOs were still in the country, but coordination with local and national authorities was the rule in every sense of the word. The country's national development plan predicted that, by 2020, Rwanda would no longer require foreign assistance.

After working in Haiti and Rwanda for several years, I'd become accustomed to tracing a triangle between Haiti, Harvard, and Rwanda. In September, for long hours en route to Africa and back to Haiti, stuck in planes, I thought mostly about reconstruction. One vision of reconstruction that I've repeated *passim* at the risk of sounding like a broken record was rebuilding public infrastructure to strengthen sovereignty and basic social and economic rights. Although building back better seemed already a tired cliché, Rwanda had built sounder structures, reshaped its engagement with foreign aid, and expanded human capacity by investing in health, education, and gender equity. Could those billions pledged for Haiti's reconstruction be translated into  a plan like this one? Could some of the larger projects generate jobs that would transfer skills and draw some of the diaspora back to Haiti?

Questions like these led us back to our plans for the Mirebalais teaching hospital, our most ambitious effort to date. We sought commission approval not for funding—we had raised most of the money—but for legitimacy and coordination with other reconstruction efforts that fit into a national plan. The last stop on the triangle was thus central Haiti, where we were about to lay the hospital's cornerstone.

Mirebalais was, in a way, the birthplace of Partners In Health. Many of the founders (Ophelia, Father Fritz, and Mamito) and other supporters (including Didi and her family) had first met there in 1983. That year, almost three decades ago, we began to understand the poor quality of medical care available in rural Haiti. Although I hadn't yet started medical school, it didn't require an M.D. to understand that a five-minute exchange with a harried Haitian doctor with no lab or other diagnostics was not the recipe for delivering care. And it didn't require a degree in pharmacology to imagine that the various potions poured into corncob-stoppered bottles were not likely to have more than a placebo effect—or worse.

My experiences in Mirebalais that first brutal and instructive year inspired a life-long desire to see, in Haiti, a hospital worthy of its people. The devastating storms of 2008, and President Clinton's inclusion of Haiti at the 2008 Clinton Global Initiative, were links in a chain of events that led to an ambitious vision for the hospital. A young philanthropist, who was committed to the struggle against human trafficking, met with me and a coworker from Partners In Health and pledged, right then and there, a lead gift to rebuild the Mirebalais hospital. We suggested that some of her anonymous pledge supplement salaries for beleaguered health providers, train community health workers, and improve the existing facility (along with Cuban help). It would take at least a year to design the hospital and raise the rest of the necessary capital. "I trust you," she said, promising to visit in 2009. That visit was delayed until January 2010. She sent an advance team down to Haiti in preparation for her visit, and the team had the ill fortune to be in the Hotel Montana on the day of the earthquake. Both were injured badly but survived.

The quake made us rethink the project completely. With the nursing school destroyed and the medical school damaged and closed, with most of Port-au-Prince's hospitals down or in disrepair, where would the next generation of Haitian health professionals train? As noted, Alex Larsen, the Health Minister, asked us to make it a major teaching hospital. Partners In Health supporters, including new corporate donors, had sent thousands of donations for rebuilding. Why not try something really bold and beautiful?

The stars seemed aligned in other ways, too. Ann Clark, a classmate of mine from college, was now an architect and married to another architect; she had dragooned her small firm and family into redesigning the hospital plans.[41] One of my former students, David Walton, was committed to a thorough overhaul and expansion of the project. Both he and the architects hailed from Chicago and had rallied donors and companies there to the cause. Even more remarkable, a former construction company owner from Boston, Jim Ansara, had been practically living in Haiti since the quake, helping to assess the structural integrity of buildings and running from hospital to hospital. He was ready to pour time and resources and connections—his own and his company's—to make this one bigger and better. Together, this crew revised the plans more than a dozen times, ever growing their scope and making it, in the end, a 160,000-square-foot medical center. This was three times the size of anything we'd ever attempted to build before.

Mirebalais is the largest town in Haiti's lower Central Plateau. Even while shaking off jetlag, it was easy to sense the optimism of our Haitian coworkers and others who'd gathered there to lay the cornerstone. Heavy rains had fallen the previous night, and some of our coworkers (including David and Jim) had been temporarily stranded on the far side of the river that runs through the city. (The same bridge that had been destroyed by the 2008 hurricanes, now traversed by a simple concrete ford, often underwater.) But the waters receded and the morning of September 10 dawned hot and sunny; it was sweltering under the tent in which we gathered to launch the hospital. Part of the construction site had already been leveled, and more site preparation (moving more than an Empire State Building's worth of dirt) was needed before the foundations could be laid. Although this sounded dauntingly large, those gathered brought experience and a shared commitment to bear on a project that could help Haiti recover and maybe even flourish.

The Minister of Health was there, as were his senior leadership team, in part because the long-awaited hospital was also the first major health project approved by the Interim Haiti Recovery Commission. (Its logo showed up, among others, in the slideshow playing in the background.) Father Fritz gave the benediction. This was one of the first times he'd left Cange since the funeral mass for Mamito. The lead architect, my college friend from Chicago, presented the plans to an audience that included local officials, UN workers, the Cuban Vice-Minister of Health (accompanied by a handful of the thousand Cuban health professionals volunteering in Haiti), supporters of Partners In Health, and the Haitian medical staff. Construction teams from Haiti, the Dominican Republic, and Boston, including those stranded at the site the previous evening, were in attendance, as was Shelove, the proud physical therapist. Her limp was not perceptible; nor was my brother-in-law's. He had recovered quickly from his fractured ankle and had, since the quake, joined Zanmi Lasante's women's health team.

In spite of the heat, no one seemed to mind a long morning of pronouncements. After the opening invocation, the Mayor spoke, followed by Haiti's leading health officials. I had a chance to say my bit, too. For weeks after the quake, the best hospital in Haiti was floating in the Bay of Port-au-Prince. It was our hope that one day the best hospital in Haiti would be anchored on terra firma and followed by others in Port-au-Prince and elsewhere in the quake zone.[42]

But as ever in Haiti, feelings of pleasure and satisfaction were soon crowded out by anxiety and even dread: anxiety, for many of us, about how we were going to run such a hospital once it was built; and dread because a new epidemic, long feared, was about to hit Haiti. And it would first appear, in all places, in the city of Mirebalais.

# 7.

# RECONSTRUCTION IN THE TIME OF CHOLERA

*The third week in October* found me back in Kigali, where I received a message from Louise Ivers about a new problem emerging in Mirebalais and Saint-Marc. On the afternoon of October 19, our colleagues in Saint-Marc, a large coastal town where we've worked for only a few years, alerted us to the sudden arrival of scores of people suffering from acute watery diarrhea. Some patients were carried to the hospital on makeshift stretchers; others walked in unassisted but collapsed while waiting to be seen. After seeing similarly afflicted patients, a hospital further inland (the one where Shelove had been fitted for her prosthesis) issued a brief report predicting an outbreak of typhoid—a longstanding curse in Haiti, which just a few years ago was named the most water-insecure country in the world.[1] Upon hearing the details from Saint-Marc, I remember thinking, let's hope it's typhoid.

But this diagnosis seemed unlikely to me and to Louise, also an infectious disease doctor. Very few pathogens provoke the secretory diarrhea that was felling these patients in Saint-Marc and Mirebalais, and typhoid is not among them. For months we had been dreading the outbreak of a disease far more virulent than typhoid and known to mow through refugee camps and slums lacking clean water and sanitation—especially after wars and disasters natural and unnatural.[2]

After the U.S. Centers for Disease Control and Prevention had in March deemed cholera "very unlikely to occur" in Haiti,[3] why did we suspect that it was the cause of the influx of patients with acute diarrhea? First, cholera has an unmistakable clinical presentation. Infectious disease doctors would be hard-pressed to describe another diarrheal disease that can shrivel a hale adult in a matter of hours. (It makes even shorter work of children, the elderly, and the malnourished.) The last major epidemic in the Americas lingered in post-conflict Peru for three years, killing an estimated ten thousand before being brought to heel in 1994. (I'd seen the tail end of this epidemic during my first visit there.) Second, Haiti was an ideal host for cholera: even before the quake, it had little in the way of municipal water and sanitation systems, and had long been a mineshaft canary for epidemic disease. It was something of a miracle that Haiti had been spared cholera for so long.

Some had foretold the spread of such waterborne diseases years earlier. I'd issued this warning to the Senate Foreign Relations Committee in 2003, and again after the quake. When a series of Inter-American Development Bank loans to Haiti were blocked for political reasons in 2001, the projects they were intended to support—including one for water infrastructure improvements in Saint-Marc—lay fallow.[4] In 2008, we were still waiting. At the site of another delayed municipal water project in the north, the drinking water samples were polluted with human waste. (One of our young researchers there promptly fell ill with typhoid.) All this was years before the earthquake would render Haiti even more vulnerable to waterborne disease.[5]

In a sense, cholera had been waiting for us. We ought to have been more prepared. Once dreaded in cities throughout the world, including those in Europe and North America, cholera has become, with the advent of modern sanitation, a disease limited to developing countries—especially those riven by conflict. Today, it is the worst nightmare of doctors working in shantytowns and refugee camps.

The key to treatment is rehydration: replacing the fluids and electrolytes lost through explosive, watery diarrhea. Because cholera is
caused by a bacterium, antibiotics have a role to play, too. Sitting in
Rwanda, which has had its share of cholera, and thinking about the
outbreak in Peru, I hoped we could avert many deaths even if we
could not avert an epidemic.

Or perhaps this diagnosis was wrong, and the outbreak was not
caused by cholera. Perhaps we'd have a chance to pursue water and
sanitation projects more effectively. But late that October night,
Louise called me to say that, although the laboratory work had not
been completed, the news would be bad. After a century of reprieve,
cholera had returned to Haiti.

---

If the first nine months of the year were dominated by the earthquake, the last two seemed to consist of nonstop cholera. The earthquake laid down the conditions for an epidemic of waterborne
disease but by no means made it inevitable. Some conditions predated the quake; some became recognizable only in retrospect.
Cholera was the latest acute reminder of Haiti's integration into the
global economy and its paradoxical privation—of its place in a vast
transnational web and of its exceptional dearth of public services. In
the Republic of NGOs, private initiative could not conjure functioning municipal water systems and decent sanitation infrastructure out
of thin air. Without all the medical equipment, facilities, or medication we needed, without rapid integration of all necessary preventive measures and treatment, we would be in trouble.

By the last week of October we knew that four things were likely
to happen in short order. First, the epidemic would spread rapidly
across the country, since Haiti was fertile ground for any waterborne
disease caused by a bacterium that could survive, even briefly, outside a human host.

Second, effective means of treatment and prevention would be
quite limited in many areas and almost nil in others: those with
ready access to clean water would be spared, and those without

would not. Those with access to prompt diagnosis and proper care would survive, but many thousands without access to care would die. There was every reason to believe, from the first cases documented, that this would be a devastating epidemic that could not be limited to central Haiti, or limited to Haiti at all.

Third, we knew from previous epidemics that loss of life, especially among the young and previously healthy, would trigger cycles of accusation and counteraccusation. Blame was, after all, a calling card of all transnational epidemics, including the AIDS epidemic.[6] As with AIDS, the introduction to an island of a previously unknown infectious pathogen would implicate transnational spread. Cholera had to have come from somewhere.

The press to discover whence this new malady hailed would reflect the desire to know whose fault it was. Anthropologists often trace modern Haitian ways of explaining misfortune to the slave plantations from which Haiti was born. A wonderful essay about folk healing by Karen McCarthy Brown puts it this way: for the early Haitians, "natural powers such as those of storm, drought, and disease paled before social powers such as those of the slave holder."[7] Although explanations for the earthquake were natural (except among well-nourished American TV pastors), social responses would include local cycles of accusation, drawing on village-level feuds. Other accusations would be vaguely nationalist. Social turbulence around these themes would, predictably, complicate responses to the epidemic. Instead of "*What* brought this latest misfortune down upon us?" I expected to hear, "*Which foreigners* brought this latest misfortune down upon us?"

Fourth, expert opinion on cholera would be divided. Prevention experts would focus on their methods of protection (from water filtration to chlorination to vaccination) and treatment experts on their means of treatment (from oral rehydration to antibiotic therapy). There would be disagreements about priorities and investments. I'd seen these arguments during the Peruvian epidemic and read about them during the Zimbabwean one.[8] Conflicts of this kind seemed less to do with cholera than with long-standing divisions between medicine and public health. We'd encountered these same divisions when responding to AIDS and tuberculosis and malaria and cancer: instead of efforts to integrate prevention and care, there was brisk competition between those working in prevention and those seeking to provide care.

Some—like the Cuban brigade, GHESKIO, and, I think it's fair to say, Partners In Health—have long advocated the integration of prevention and care as leading to better prevention and more comprehensive care. But others pushed for their own areas of expertise and favorite solutions, leading to competition rather than cooperation; prevention versus care; water protection versus vaccination (or even chlorination versus filtration); regional versus national plans; oral rehydration versus antibiotic therapy; handwashing and small water-protection projects versus municipal water projects. This, in any case, is what we feared.

All four of these predictions came to pass. The cholera epidemic hit central Haiti—even more water insecure than the internally displaced persons camps—like a bomb, spreading from town to town and then into villages far from any clean or filtered water source. As for the rapidity of spread, the numbers spoke for themselves. No cholera epidemic stays local for long, and the Haitian one moved fast. I had heard of the outbreak in the third week of October from colleagues in Mirebalais and Saint-Marc, two cities connected by a river. It reached Port-au-Prince by November 9 at the latest, when cholera was diagnosed in a child who had not traveled outside the city.[9] Soon cases were reported across the nation. By the close of the year, almost two hundred thousand cases were registered in Haiti's ten departments, and nearly four thousand of those afflicted had died.[10] Given weak reporting capacity, these estimates were probably low. The Haitian epidemic is the most devastating the hemisphere has seen in decades.

The cycles of accusation and counteraccusation started, as predicted, on day one. Louise Ivers and David Walton had given me a heads-up, as I paced about in Rwanda. Although the world became aware of the epidemic when it reached Saint-Marc, there had almost surely been cases several days earlier far from the coast, in the region closest to the Nepalese peacekeepers whose base sits on the banks of the Meille River. Because that river flowed by the Nepalese encampment into the city of Mirebalais, a causal link was quickly posited, and not just by epidemiologists: much of the local citizenry believed that a new pathogen had been introduced by the foreigners in their region. Most of the foreigners in Mirebalais were UN peacekeepers, the great majority, in fact, from cholera-endemic countries.

Their numbers weren't small. In Mirebalais and elsewhere in central Artibonite Haiti were thousands of peacekeepers, some hundreds of them recently arrived, and within a few hours, accusations were flying. Some of the rumors were, as usual, absurd. But it was not unreasonable, epidemiologically, to assume a connection between the large and relatively new presence of people from South Asia and a new, externally derived epidemic—even before the infecting strain had been genetically typed and before it was known that waste management at the Nepalese base, managed by a private Haitian contractor, left much to be desired. In those first days of the epidemic, the chief task was to figure out where the epidemic had come from and to cut its spread by any and all means possible.

That's why, less than ten days after news of the first cases, I spoke to journalist Jonathan Katz, who was investigating how cholera had been reintroduced to the Americas. One of my suggestions was to identify the source of the Haitian epidemic and to study, genetically and epidemiologically, the introduced strain. On November 9, Katz wrote the following for the Associated Press:

> Public health experts, including UN Deputy Special Envoy to Haiti Paul Farmer, who co-founded Partners In Health, have called for an aggressive investigation into the origin of the outbreak. They say that should include looking at the unconfirmed hypothesis that cholera was introduced by UN peacekeepers from Nepal, a South Asian nation where the disease is endemic. Those peacekeepers are at a UN base on a tributary of the Artibonite River, which has been found to be contaminated with cholera.[11]

All this was technically correct, but it was certainly not my intention to fan the blame game. Still, it seemed important to understand the biosocial complexity of this rapidly changing epidemic. This meant understanding both the origins and genetic fingerprint of this particular strain, which would help predict its speed of spread, its appropriate treatment, and even its case-fatality rate. My Harvard colleague John Mekalanos, chair of the department of Microbiology and Molecular Genetics and a genuine cholera expert, made the same point even as we were studying the genetic fingerprint of the cholera strain: "It very much likely did come either with peacekeepers or other relief personnel. I don't see there is any way to avoid the conclusion that an unfortunate and presumably accidental introduction of the organism occurred."[12]

The popular press contained vivid accounts of the likely source of contamination. Katz did yeoman's work trying to figure out what was going on. This required him to visit the Nepalese base closest to Mirebalais, where I'd been received previously with great courtesy.[13] But Katz wasn't there to have a meal and a chat with the officers. He came to inspect latrines and septic tanks:

> When the AP visited on October 27, a tank was clearly overflowing. The back of the base smelled like a toilet had exploded. Reeking, dark liquid flowed out of a broken pipe, toward the river, from next to what the soldiers said were latrines. UN military police were taking samples in clear jars with sky-blue UN lids, clearly horrified. At the shovel-dug waste pits across the street sat yellow-brown pools of feces where ducks and pigs swam in the overflow. The path to the river ran straight downhill. The UN acknowledged the black fluid was overflow from the base, but said it contained kitchen and shower waste, not excrement.[14]

The circumstantial evidence was damning. Within days of the first cases, photos of raw human waste from the camps being dumped directly into one of the rivers connecting the camp to Mirebalais (and Mirebalais to Saint-Marc) covered the newspaper pages.

But the initial response of the UN was to deny any connection between the epidemic and the burgeoning presence of their troops from cholera-endemic regions. Katz put it this way:

> The mounting circumstantial evidence that UN peacekeepers from Nepal brought cholera to Haiti was largely dismissed by UN officials. Haitians who asked about it were called political or paranoid. Foreigners were accused of playing "the blame game." The World Health Organization said the question was simply "not a priority." But this week, after anti-UN riots and inquiries from health experts, the top UN representative in Haiti said he is taking the allegations very seriously. "It is very important to know if it came from (the Nepalese base) or not, and someday I hope we will find out."[15]

Umbrage was taken on all sides. The mayor of Mirebalais attacked the UN for introducing "yet another epidemic" to Haiti, echoing the views of many of his constituents. The Nepalese troops and the UN issued epidemiologically implausible, but socially and politically predictable, denials and hired a private Dominican laboratory to see if indeed any of their troops were sick.[16] Fortunately, they were not sick, but those who knew a bit about the microbiology of the causative organism, *Vibrio cholerae*, knew that it wasn't easy to grow in lab. They also knew that, as with most infectious pathogens, many of those shedding viable cholera bacteria would remain asymptomatic. As we would later learn, the South Asian strain of cholera active in Haiti has been shown to cause greater numbers of asymptomatic cases, to persist longer in the environment, and to exist in higher concentrations in feces.[17]

But political responses to the mounting epidemic ignored such clinical details. As the Haitians continued to demand explanations, the UN, and especially the Nepalese, continued to issue denials: "Nepal's UN office said in a statement Friday that its peacekeepers have never been linked to a communicable disease, and that tests done by the United Nations, Haiti's government, and independent groups prove that none of its peacekeepers now in Haiti has cholera.

Nepal firmly rejects such baseless, malicious, and unfounded reports put out by some media and individuals without any regard to the specific evidence to the contrary."[18]

Political protests against the peacekeepers occurred well before any of us spoke to the press. Categorical UN denials were only making the situation worse, we feared. Louise Ivers, the person I trusted most on this score, thought that an independent inquiry was needed. We began calling for strain identification to learn what antibiotics would be needed to kill the organism, predict the speed of spread, and estimate the chance of endemicity—settling in for the long term to plague an immunologically naïve population. Above all, pinpointing the source of the outbreak might have, early on, helped to stop its spread. But with many infected people traveling around the country, it seemed by mid-November that this window had closed.

Those seeking to deliver services—to diagnose and treat cholera, a disease about which they were learning, and to prevent it whenever possible—were of course affected by these social responses, which soon became violent. Within weeks of the first cases, the papers contained reports—some unconfirmed—of crowds throwing stones at UN peacekeepers' armored personnel carriers and, in one case, at UN helicopters seeking to land medical supplies in northern Haiti:

> Protesters have targeted the United Nations, as well as Nepal, all week. The world body claims demonstrators have attacked its peacekeepers, as well as prevented the movement of humanitarian aid and medical help by blocking roads, bridges and airports. "If this situation continues, more and more patients in desperate need of care are likely to die, and more and more Haitians awaiting access to preventive care may be overtaken by the epidemic," Edmond Mulet, the UN's special representative in Haiti, said in a statement. Small-scale skirmishes—involving rock-throwing and burning tires, then tear gas in response—erupted Friday in Port-au-Prince, relatively sporadic confrontations that paled in comparison with earlier violence. And eyewitnesses said that traffic was again moving in Cap-Haïtien, a

northern Haitian city that's the center of the outbreak, after four days of gridlock caused by massive protests.[19]

After returning from Rwanda, I wanted to discuss with Edmond Mulet why it might be prudent to investigate the source of the outbreak, and also to call for aggressive measures to prevent, detect, and treat cholera cases. Mulet wasn't at the UN log base when I arrived, so I left him a book I wrote more than a decade ago, which describes the predictable responses to epidemic disease that we were seeing with cholera. When I returned a few days later, Mulet had read most of the book, highlighting passages with a yellow marker. He was much taken by the similarities between the social responses to cholera and those registered in the eighties and nineties to AIDS and tuberculosis. Mulet estimated that half of all countries contributing troops to MINUSTAH (UN Stabilization Mission in Haiti) experienced regular outbreaks of cholera, and was disturbed by the focus on the Nepalese battalion. I understood his point and promised him that my comments were (to use the words of another UN friend, who had narrowly survived the quake), "eminently technical." We needed to identify the strain, get an idea of what it was likely to do in Haiti, and deploy every tool in the international arsenal against it. Mulet agreed. On November 20, he told the Associated Press, "We agree with him that there has to be a thorough investigation of how it came, how it happened, and how it spread ... There's no differences there with Dr. Paul Farmer at all."[20]

Gratified as I was by Mulet's clarification and support, we weren't seeking validation. We wanted to work together to strengthen efforts against a transnational epidemic. I was en route to Mirebalais to check on the hospital's progress, which had slowed after some of the Dominican engineers and contractors we'd hired left central Haiti during the cholera outbreak. But our Partners In Health and Zanmi Lasante teams had nowhere to go; we expanded our cholera work as we sought to keep the Mirebalais hospital on schedule.

The rural hinterlands and slums outside the quake zone suffered more than the camps, but all those unable to buy clean, filtered water would suffer. Although some found it perplexing that cholera largely spared the camps and instead laid waste to central Haiti, it was no surprise to those of us at Partners In Health and Zanmi Lasante. Our own small water projects over the years had humbled us about our ability to stave off epidemics of waterborne disease. We could protect certain villages, but the great majority of the rural population still lived without ready access to potable water and modern sanitation. Without a massive and coordinated scale up of such projects to help strengthen municipal water and sanitation systems, there was no way we could keep pace with cholera in rural Haiti.

Although prompt rehydration—simple fluid resuscitation with a well-known solution—could save almost anyone with cholera, most health providers were unprepared for the waves of people who walked, or were carried, into clinics and hospitals throughout central Haiti. The Cubans got right to work, as did some of the Médecins Sans Frontières groups. (There were so many borders between these doctors without borders that it was hard to figure out who was who.) Stefano Zannini, chief of a Médecins Sans Frontières mission in Haiti, called for more helpers and more collaboration: "More actors are needed to treat the sick and implement preventative actions, especially as cases increase dramatically across the country ... There is no time left for meetings and debate—the time for action is now."[21]

Working with the Ministry and other health-focused NGOs, my colleagues erected cholera treatment centers (or smaller treatment units) at each of our dozen hospitals and clinics across central and Artibonite Haiti. These sites were soon deluged with people standing, or trying to stand, in line for intake into these centers. Such rapid treatment responses saved lives, probably thousands of them. But thousands more would be lost, we feared, in what was likely to be a long struggle against cholera in Haiti.

For me, the fourth predicted struggle—that between experts—was the most enervating. Although I'm trained in infectious disease management (and the social responses to epidemics), and although I was one of the few doctors in Haiti who'd ever seen a case of cholera,

I'm no cholera expert. But several of my colleagues, including John Mekalanos and one of my classmates from Harvard Medical School (Ed Ryan), were world-renowned cholera experts. Their genetic analysis of the Petite Rivière strain revealed an El Tor biotype of *Vibrio cholerae* serogroup 01, which had, in other parts of the world, proven virulent and hard to slow down.[22] If the history of similar El Tor strains in Bangladesh and Nepal offered any indication, the disease would likely become endemic in Haiti. These academics who mapped the strain were also strong proponents of rapid implementation of both prevention (from clean water to roll-out of vaccine) and care (from rehydration to antibiotic therapy).

It was the public health experts, Haitian and especially transnational, who were in discord. In keeping with widespread pessimism about the potential for health delivery in post-quake Haiti, many argued that it would be too difficult to launch comprehensive prevention and care efforts in Haiti. Vaccination was especially discouraged.[23] These "minimalists" were often the leading figures in international health. Others—and we were in this group—argued that there was no time to waste. In about forty days, cholera had caused more than two thousand deaths in Haiti, almost half the number reported during Zimbabwe's year-long epidemic.[24] There would, of course, be implementation challenges to rolling out vaccine in Haiti. But Zanmi Lasante had achieved a 76 percent completion rate for a three-dose course of HPV vaccine in rural Haiti. That is almost twice the rate of completion for similar courses in U.S. settings. Moreover, the earthquake occurred between the second and third dose for many of the girls enrolled.[25]

The battle lines were well worn: on the one hand, the minimalists favored heavy investment in health education and massive distribution of chlorine tablets for drinking-water disinfection. On the other hand, the "maximalists" argued that, although there might be no way to stop cholera in its tracks in Haiti, *all* the tools for preventing its spread (from improved sanitation, including chlorine tablets, to effective and safe vaccines) and for treating those already stricken (from rehydration and replacement of electrolytes to antibiotics) needed to be promptly integrated with the more restrained public health responses. Interventions such as exhorting people to drink clean water and wash their hands, or distributing chlorine tablets, were necessary but would never stop the epidemic. Having watched with horror as cholera ripped through the Mirebalais prison, killing five young detainees in as many days, we also wanted to review the evidence for antibiotic prophylaxis in certain instances.[26]

Three weeks after the first cases came to light, Jeffrey Sachs called, as he had more than a decade previously regarding AIDS: "Why aren't we responding to this epidemic more aggressively, with integrated prevention and care? Aren't there vaccines and also antibiotics? Isn't this a bacterial disease? Why aren't we bringing in the private sector, including companies that can help us get filtered drinking water and soap and antibiotics scaled-up more widely?"

Why indeed, I thought, as I often did during discussions with Sachs. He was well aware of the politicization of water aid that had occurred between 2001 and 2004, when the quality of the Haitian water supply was held hostage to the United States' displeasure with President Jean-Bertrand Aristide. He'd been one of the few aid experts willing to testify before Congress regarding this sorry affair.[27]

Sachs had already contacted Unilever, a company with significant production capacity in the Caribbean, which made soap, hand sanitizer, and water filtration units. We agreed to set up a conference call with Unilever by the third week of November, and then another with cholera experts at the start of December. The first promised to be uncontroversial: the company pledged to donate many of its products and also some expertise on clean water and sanitation.

The second conference call, including the academics and the public health experts, was harder. It seemed that the latter were reluctant to commit the necessary resources; it also turned out that they had underestimated the dimensions of the Haitian cholera epidemic. On November 25, a *Wall Street Journal* article, "Cholera Spreading in Haiti Faster than Thought," noted that official projections about the peak size of the epidemic had more than doubled. Nigel Fisher, a smart humanitarian and a top UN official in Haiti, summed up the revised estimates: "When we were in the initial stages of planning, we had said there would be 200,000 cases over six months. Today the figures are 425,000 over six months, of which 200,000 will be before year's end, with a peak before Christmas."[28] I was grateful for Fisher's candor.

The second call, set for December 3, would bring together academic cholera experts, vaccine researchers and manufacturers, clinical trial gurus, and several implementing bodies working in Haiti. We agreed that Harvard Medical School, rather than the UN Office of the Special Envoy, should host the call, in part because of the clear policy disagreements and in part because of the fractious relations between the MINUSTAH troops and Haitians in cholera-affected regions.

The close of November, between the two calls, found me back in Haiti. In Mirebalais, the Cubans and Zanmi Lasante teams were managing to save almost all patients who showed up to the cholera treatment center there. The great worry was for all those falling ill far from towns with cholera treatment capacity such as Mirebalais. My colleagues from Zanmi Lasante spoke of scores of deaths in rural hamlets. "These deaths aren't even counted," they told me.

So the second conference call really mattered. The agenda was modeled on the effort we tried to engineer a decade previously, when the same sort of arguments—pitting AIDS prevention against AIDS care—were dominant. Back then, Jeff Sachs, still at Harvard, had helped bring us together. Now based at Columbia, he insisted that I take charge and try to assemble a group of cholera experts. We thought perhaps a few dozen specialists would join, but more than eighty people called in from Haiti, across the United States, Geneva, and as far away as Korea (where John Clemens, one of the world's leading cholera vaccine experts, was working). Our Partners In Health and Zanmi Lasante teams were present, as was Bill Pape. We discussed the ranking problems facing cholera prevention and care, and also the priorities for the coming months and years. Disagreement surfaced about the problems and the priorities, but the debate seemed constructive.

To continue the conversation after the call, we began work on a "consensus statement," as we'd done for AIDS a decade previously. We learned a lot about the minutiae of cholera prevention and care and about the importance of sparking greater public concern about the epidemic. The cholera experts were the most helpful: they shook the public health minimalists out of their torpor. No one working in the western hemisphere had seen anything like the Haiti epidemic in decades. "This is not your grandmother's cholera," David Sack had said.[29] He didn't specify whether he meant this in terms of virulence or infectiousness, but we feared it was both.

We weren't sure we'd be able to complete a consensus document in short order, although we had committed to trying. The maximalists among us decided that, rather than languishing in the bitter debates over the origins of cholera in Haiti and the role of prevention "versus" treatment, we would write our own pieces for medical journals and for the popular press. Within a month, Louise Ivers, David Walton, and our Haitian colleagues had written pieces in the *Lancet* and the *New England Journal of Medicine*.[30] A few days after these pieces appeared, on December 10, 2010, Partners In Health hosted a press call. By then, we'd developed treatment capacity at all our sites in the rural Lower Artibonite and Central Plateau, and set up a fifty-bed cholera treatment center in Parc Jean-Marie Vincent. We were also carrying out intensive education and prevention campaigns. We'd already spent a million dollars and planned to spend more than twice that amount again by the end of the fiscal year. The United States had, by some reports, committed more than $57 million to fight cholera. The idea that it was impossible to launch a comprehensive, integrated response, including ramping up vaccine production (or even building a new factory to manufacture vaccine) in the face of such investments was absurd. The Haitian cholera outbreak also afforded us the long-overdue chance to build a global stockpile of vaccine that could be deployed during this epidemic and the next.

The conference calls seemed to have positive effects. Jonathan Katz reported a growing consensus about the need for vaccines in Haiti, for example. He noted that I had endorsed broader use of the vaccine [in Haiti], and called for creating emergency stockpiles of millions of doses to keep cholera from spreading to other countries. He endorsed measures like searching Haiti's central mountains for people too sick to reach clinics, using antibiotics even in moderate cases, and rebuilding the water and sanitation networks shattered by January's earthquake. Other cholera experts [also on the conference call], including a different team from Harvard Medical School, where Dr. Farmer teaches, have also called for stockpiling millions of doses to stop outbreaks, as is now done with measles vaccine and the flu drug Tamiflu."[31]

For a time it didn't seem that we were alone. The *New York Times* ran a piece suggesting that some of the people from the Pan American Health Organization, who had initially opposed large-scale vaccination as impractical, had changed their minds. For example, PAHO's John Andrus was quoted as saying, "We recognize that it's time to rethink our position. We don't want to miss an opportunity."[32]

But as 2010 drew to a close, it seemed that the opportunity had slipped away. The consensus statement was underway, but the minimalists and the maximalists were often deadlocked. We went to friends in the popular press, and managed to get a piece into the December 20 edition of *Newsweek*:

Cholera demands ... fully integrated prevention and care, using all the tools available and raising our goals. Twelve years ago we argued that AIDS treatment using antiretroviral therapy was possible even in rural Haiti—and the results have justified that approach. The Haitian cholera epidemic exposes the fallacy of setting goals based on a country's GDP. Pathogens like HIV, cholera, and dengue move within a complex web of global social connections, binding the richest and the poorest countries together in vulnerability. But while those microbes jet around the world, their remedies remain stuck in customs. There's no excuse for allowing Haiti's cholera disaster to escalate. We already have preventive measures—from improved sanitation to vaccines—and effective treatments: rehydration, replacement of electrolytes, and antibiotics. We must move swiftly, aggressively, and together. If we insist that prevention and care are complementary, and we draw on any and all means available globally, we can beat this emergency—and whatever problem comes next.[33]

The week before Christmas, I visited a few of the cholera treatment centers in central Haiti. Our colleagues were doing stellar work. They followed strict infection-control procedures, spraying our shoes with chlorine solutions that made our eyes burn and filled the air with an unforgiving scent. But these procedures suggested that no transmission would occur in these sites. We also knew that almost all those seeking care there would survive: in Mirebalais, the case-fatality rate—the percentage of people presenting with cholera who died—had essentially fallen to zero. These centers were run by Haitians from Zanmi Lasante and by members of the Cuban medical brigade (one of whom was Bolivian). The numbers of new patients were dropping, but the tents were still full.

We also visited the nearby Mirebalais construction site. David Walton and Jim Ansara were there and showed us around their ambitious project. The site was nothing if not inspiring: acres of buildings were going up. But we were only a few hundred yards from a site where young people and old were lying on stiff cholera cots. They weren't dying, thank God, but they were still suffering from an eighteenth-century illness.

We also visited the cholera treatment unit our teams were running in Lascahobas. Almost no one was dying from cholera there, either. But the beautiful courtyard garden was brown and shriveled by the chlorine solution that had been used for infection control.

On the flight back to Boston, I shared my anxieties about Haiti's long-term challenges with an American family with whom we'd been traveling. (They'd been strong supporters of Partners In Health's efforts in the past.) Although the entire family had been to Rwanda, their eighteen-year-old son had never been to Haiti before this trip. It was a lot to take in: the cholera centers, the crowded hospitals, the capital still strewn with rubble, an accident in which a cyclist had been fatally struck minutes before we drove by.

I was worried about the five Haitian students heading to the Rwandan National University. Their tuition would be free, courtesy of the Rwandan government, but we hadn't purchased their plane tickets yet; nor had we obtained visas so they could travel through the United States. And the Rwandan academic year started in January—less than a month away. As I discussed these issues with the family, the young man—a senior in high school—said quietly that he wanted to sell some stocks he'd been given years ago to help buy the tickets. It turned out that he owned enough stock to purchase all five of them.

So one anxiety was allayed when I headed back to peaceful Rwanda with my brother-in-law, an obstetrician, who'd helped write the *Newsweek* article. It was a joy to be reunited with our children— my three and his two made five. It was a merry Christmas dinner. But it was clear, as the evening wore on, that Haiti was on our minds. A handful of us were still up at two in the morning, arguing heatedly about what should be done about cholera and about reconstruction. We didn't get very far, except as regards annoying our non-Haitian hosts and friends.

The consensus statement on cholera was still stuck on the differences between the minimalists and the maximalists.[34] How to integrate vaccination into the response was the chief sticking point. The minimalists argued that there was insufficient data to show that vaccine would confer protection in a "setting like Haiti" (whatever that meant: either that its population was immunologically naïve or that infrastructural obstacles doomed the effort in advance). Nor was there sufficient stock in the world, they said. But without consensus, who would begin ramping up production?

Cholera case-fatality rates were still highly disparate. In Mirebalais, there hadn't been a cholera death in several weeks; in other stations, one out of ten cholera patients diagnosed with the disease died. By early 2011, almost two hundred thousand cases and four thousand deaths had been reported.[35] One modeling exercise under review suggested that cholera would not peak in certain regions till almost a year after the first cases were reported in October. For example, the model predicted that the epidemics in the Grand'Anse,

Nippes, and Sud departments would peak in December 2011, with an incidence of 200 cases per 100,000 population.[36] That would mean, in just three departments, almost 3,000 people would become ill with cholera in a single month. A *Lancet* study conducted by Jason Andrews, a young researcher at Harvard Medical School who had helped us in Petite Rivière de l'Artibonite, predicted at least 779,000 cases and 11,000 deaths by the end of 2011.[37] As we rang in the New Year in Rwanda, it was hard to feel triumphant about our efforts in Haiti, because the cholera epidemic was, in our view, completely out of control. Other experts (most of them trained in public health) disagreed: we were being alarmist and counterproductive, they said.

If the public health and clinical experts couldn't agree, it's not difficult to imagine the discord among NGOs and other implementers. Just before the dawn of the new year, a disgruntled doctor from Médecins Sans Frontières (the home base of disgruntled doctors, some might say) lamented in the *Guardian* the poor coordination among groups trying to respond to cholera. I quote the piece at length because it was a pretty apt, if dismal, description of the problems we faced:

Ten days after the outbreak hit Port-au-Prince, our teams realised the inhabitants of Cité Soleil still had no access to chlorinated drinking water, even though aid agencies under the UN water-and-sanitation cluster had accepted funds to ensure such access. We began chlorinating the water ourselves. There is still just one operational waste management site in Port-au-Prince, a city of three million people. On the one hand, Haitians were deluged with text messages imploring them to wash before eating, while on the other they had to bathe their children in largely untreated sewer water. Before the quake, only 12% of Haiti's 9.8m people received treated tap water, according to the US Centres for Disease Control (CDC) ... Throughout the 1990s, the UN developed a significant institutional apparatus to provide humanitarian aid through the creation of the Department for Humanitarian Affairs in 1992, later renamed OCHA, all the while creating an illusion of a centralised, efficient aid system. In 2005, after the Asian tsunami, the system received another facelift with the creation of a rapid emergency funding mechanism (CERF), and the "cluster" system was developed to improve aid efforts. The aid landscape today is filled with cluster systems for areas such as health, shelter, and water and sanitation, which unrealistically try to bring aid organisations— large and small, and with varying capacities—under a single banner. Since the earthquake, the UN health cluster alone has had 420 participating organisations in Haiti. Instead of providing the technical support that many NGOs could benefit from, these clusters, at best, seem capable of only passing basic information and delivering few concrete results during a fast-moving emergency. Underscoring the current system's dysfunction, I witnessed the Haitian president, René Préval, personally chairing a health cluster meeting in a last-ditch effort to jump-start the cholera response.[38]

On one hand, we could point to certain successes. We'd been able to reduce case-fatality rates to zero wherever we had the tools of our trade and the ability to pay the nurses and doctors and infection-control staff we'd trained in preceding months. On the other hand, some public health experts had underestimated the dimensions of the cholera epidemic and had actively discouraged more aggressive interventions. Estimates of two hundred thousand cases had once been decried as hyperbole; some still denied the need for vaccine. As noted, almost a million new cases have been predicted by the end of 2011. It was impossible to know if this was an overestimate, but we maximalists faced the New Year with nothing less than shame. If our goal had been to scale up on integrated and comprehensive cholera response using all available interventions, including vaccine, we had failed miserably.

I found myself talking about cholera every day and mostly lamenting our failure to bring all the tools of our trade to bear on the epidemic. My eldest daughter, Catherine, reminded me that my sorrow bordered on obsession: "Dad, can we not talk about cholera at the dinner table?"

No, not yet.

As the anniversary of the quake approached, it was difficult not to stop and take stock of the situation: How much had been accomplished, and how much remained to be done? What would Port-au-Prince look like on January 12, 2011? The medical metaphor of acute-on-chronic seemed still useful when considering these questions. I've argued that the early rescue and relief efforts described in these pages were not a failure. Although too few were saved from the rubble and too many were still living in squalid camps almost a year after the quake, there was, until cholera hit, no second spike in what epidemiologists call "crude mortality rate."

Humanitarians often took credit for averting secondary waves of mortality, and justly so in some circumstances. Haiti's well-managed internally displaced persons camps were a good example: such camps saw fewer cases of cholera because their residents had access to clean water and modern sanitation (especially compared to many rural regions outside the quake zone and outside the realm of modernity). But cholera was far from under control.

Vulnerability to cholera and other stuttering secondary catastrophes remained extreme in urban Haiti. On September 24, a month before the first cases of cholera, a violent thunderstorm lasting less than thirty minutes killed six people and ripped down the flimsy shelters of almost twenty thousand families.[39] It tore through the General Hospital, laying waste to the fragile tents sheltering tuberculosis patients. If a thirty-minute storm caused such damage, what would happen if a larger one struck?

Some reconstruction was underway, and more was promised. The day after the thunderstorm ripped apart the tuberculosis ward in the General Hospital, Bernard Kouchner, the French Foreign Minister, announced a twenty million euro rehabilitation and reconstruction project at the hospital.[40] Our colleagues at the General Hospital, including Alix Lassègue and Miss Thompson, were grateful for France's help but were holding the applause until the work began in earnest. (It was our worry that the Mirebalais hospital would be completed first, becoming the *de facto* national referral hospital.)

Major infrastructure rebuilding proposals were heartening but slow to get moving. The grace and comity that had animated the Haitian and international response efforts immediately after the quake had largely evaporated even before cholera struck. Every day the press reported stories of struggles over scarce resources, within the camps and without. People in the camps were frustrated: persistent vulnerability frayed nerves. They complained about the lack of services, especially the lack of schools available for displaced children. Dramas occurred as a few landowners tried to push the displaced out from under their tarps, tents, and beat-up sheets of tin or plywood. At the close of September, the *New York Times* ran a long report about efforts to enforce property rights instead of sheltering homeless people. On the leafy grounds of one church mission, foreign and homegrown clergy seemed set on pushing refugees out of the camp that was set up there immediately after the quake. "'This used to be a beautiful place, but these people are tearing up the property,' said . . . a Church of God missionary living at the site. 'They're urinating on it. They're bathing out in public. They're stealing electricity. And they don't work. They sit around all day, waiting for handouts.'"[41] Surely the missionary intended no irony by applying a phrase like "tearing up the property" to people displaced by an earthquake that quite literally tore up the Haitian capital, their homes, and their lives.

The cholera outbreak created yet another set of obstacles on the rubble-strewn road to reconstruction, and made the persistent lack of readily available funds for large infrastructure projects such as municipal water systems ever more crippling.[42] Although the United States, Cuba, and many other government and nongovernmental groups had invested in cholera treatment and prevention, none of us mistook these frantic efforts for reconstruction. An Associated Press story documented the slow pace of reconstruction:

Not a cent of the $1.15 billion the United States promised for rebuilding has arrived. The money was pledged by Secretary of State Hillary Rodham Clinton in March for use this year in rebuilding. The United States has already spent more than $1.1 billion on post-quake relief,

but without long-term funds, the reconstruction of the wrecked capital cannot begin.[43]

Other accounts disputed the exact numbers and the causes of delay. (Some simply invoked the word "bureaucracy" as an explanation.) But one thing seemed certain: the holdup stemmed from
fundamental weaknesses in the machinery of foreign assistance, often having more to do with donor-country problems than Haitian
ones. The \$1.15 billion the United States pledged in March for recon-
struction had stalled because of partisan politics in Congress.[44] In its
sluggish delivery on aid promises, the United States was far from
alone. Our UN office reported that, as of December 2011, 52.9 percent or \$2.38 billion of the reconstruction pledges for 2010 and 2011
had arrived.[45] And of the money that had been disbursed according
to official reports, some was a phantasm born of bookkeeping wizardry (retooled aid dollars or tardy delivery of already promised
loans to the government of Haiti).

When funds were, at last, released from the bureaucratic snares of
foreign assistance, there was no guarantee that they would reach the
most deserving projects. There was stiff competition for contracts,
from the quake's immediate aftermath to the long road of reconstruction, and as noted, the Haitian companies seemed to be losing these
fights.[46] Unless the rules of the road for foreign aid were changed,
the anemia of reconstruction projects in terms of creating local jobs
and strengthening Haitian capacity (including that of small construction firms) seemed likely to persist.[47]

Although many NGOs still preferred to work on their own or in
collaboration with other members of "civil society," some of the big
players were beginning to rethink the merits of public sector engagement. Try as they might, the dozen or so NGOs working at the
General Hospital could not keep the place afloat. The hospital,
months after the quake, still faced the double burden of the biggest
caseload in the country and perhaps the biggest facility funding
shortage. But international NGOs had raised millions of dollars for
earthquake relief. Trying to connect the dots, we went to the Amer-

ican Red Cross and asked them to invest money in salaries for nurses, janitors, surgeons, and others at the General Hospital. It took convincing by a number of people (including President Clinton), but they said yes. The Red Cross provided—through what was for them a modest grant—invaluable medical equipment and staff salary support.

NGOs had many other opportunities to accompany the public sector as it struggled to rebuild the shattered health system. The story was the same in public education and, as cholera reminded us, public water and sanitation. But beyond the cluster system, how could the machinery of foreign assistance better coordinate funding flows and the division of labor to strengthen public institutions and generate long-term reconstruction?

The Interim Haiti Recovery Commission sought not to be yet another cog in the vast machinery of foreign aid, but rather to introduce some transparency and coordination to the process. It leant a seal of approval to projects—whether from NGOs, contractors, or line ministries—that fit within the national plan, and then tried to patch together funding for approved initiatives. The commission would also track pledges and disbursements to prevent donors from defaulting on their promises and grantees from failing to make efficient use of funds.

These failings of mainstream aid in Haiti were, of course, well-known.[48] The rebuilding efforts (or lack thereof) in Gonaïves after it was ravaged in 2004 by Tropical Storm Jeanne were a case in point. As bad as parts of New Orleans looked four years after Katrina, the city of Gonaïves was, on the eve of the 2008 storms, almost completely unrestored by the money pledged after Jeanne. It was never clear how much of it ever reached Gonaïves, or Haiti for that matter, because there was little in the way of tracking mechanisms at that time.

The end of 2010 was too early to tell whether the new Recovery Commission would work. If it fails, it would probably be because the body lacked teeth and had to rely on the goodwill of all parties. In its first three months of existence, the commission approved reconstruction projects worth $3 billion, but unmet pledges meant that most of these projects remained incompletely funded or not funded at all. It wasn't clear why, other than the usual bureaucratic siloing, major funders had not put more resources into the commission. Some argued that the commission existed only to green-light projects lacking sufficient resources. But this was circular reasoning, especially when made by those who themselves control many of the resources: what good was a stamp of approval if projects lacked funding for implementation?

Case-by-case investigations of where the money was stuck revealed, as noted, foreign-grown political obstructions and bookkeeping tricks but also the very real lack of what aid specialists call "absorptive capacity." Haitian institutions, public and private, have been long starved of resources; a massive influx of funds, unless carefully distributed and monitored, could have overwhelmed them. But some of the build-up was merely the wait-and-see approach characteristic of the foreign aid enterprise. If the commission were able to shepherd some large-scale projects forward in the early days of reconstruction, it could grease the skids for future projects and begin to serve its purpose—improving aid efficiency and effectiveness and transparency and speed.

If the commission fails, and if development assistance in Haiti remains mediocre, it's easy to guess who will be blamed: those who stuck their necks out for a more nimble and transparent process. But the default mode is to blame the Haitians: their culture, institutions, and lack of ownership over reconstruction and development schemes. And as of late October, the way aid was flowing—or rather, the way obstacles were appearing to curtail its flow—seemed to augur a future in which Haitians not only lack sufficient resources for a massive, New Deal-style job-creation campaign, but also are themselves held accountable for any failure. (Such accountability becomes a further reason to deny them support.) That was what happened after the four storms of 2008, after the flooding of Gonaïves in 2004, and after so many disasters natural and unnatural over the course of Haitian history. At the close of the year, the Haitian government was receiving few foreign assistance dollars and collecting little in the way of taxes.

―――――

Knowing that billions of dollars have been spent in Haiti over recent years can lead to cynicism about aid effectiveness. Tim Schwartz and several others have offered scathing assessments of the failure of development assistance in Haiti. The challenge before such critics— and I'm one of them—is not just to diagnose the problem but to fix it. Some aid agencies and foundations, paralyzed by failure, have been, at times, reluctant to work in Haiti. But they returned soon enough after the many crises of the past years—storm, flood, famine, quake, displacement, epidemic disease. The trouble was that no famine or refugee crisis or cholera epidemic was solely a *natural* disaster. They were always social disasters, and almost never local in their etiologies.

This insight is not new: Mike Davis made this point about what he called the "late Victorian holocausts"—a series of famines that occurred not in isolated backwaters but rather in settings firmly integrated into the British Empire.[49] These famines were the result of policy decisions made far from the famine-affected areas, just as the late-twentieth-century collapse of Haiti's rice production was triggered by biased trade rules set in North America and Europe. Small-scale Haitian farmers could not compete with huge First World agricultural subsidies after Haitian import tariffs were removed as part of strangely labeled free-trade agreements.[50] These policies were of course designed without the agreement of Haitian farmers, who then watched their livelihoods slip away within the space of a few years.

Unfair trade policies were nothing new, as any Haitian historian could tell you. What was new, or newly significant, was the rise of a massive machinery of humanitarian assistance, much of it rooted in the private sector. In the last few decades, the number of NGOs exploded, in large part because of the great and unattended needs of the increasingly unequal world. In a damning new book, *The Crisis Caravan:*

*What's Wrong with Humanitarian Aid?*, Linda Polman dates this explosion not to the nineteenth century, when the Red Cross was founded, but to the Biafran War of 1967–1970, which led to the first televised famine and as stirring an international response as had been seen since protests over Belgian rule in the Congo a century ago.

Polman offers an unsparing ethnography of humanitarian assistance: "Wars and disasters generally attract a garish array of individual organizations, each with its own agenda, its own business imperatives, and its own institutional survival tactics."[51] The Haitian earthquake certainly attracted an array, garish enough, of organizations, each with its own imperatives and plans. By the fall, some of these organizations had already moved on to the next disaster. But plenty more were in Haiti to stay, joining an already dizzyingly complex mix of international NGOs, local NGOs, church groups, and mainstream purveyors of development assistance. Writing just after the quake, Mark Danner called Haiti "the great petri dish of foreign aid."[52] Few would agree that it has been a successful experiment.

The pitfalls of humanitarian aid are becoming better known. Indeed, careful consideration of more recent humanitarian disasters, especially those linked directly to strife, offers scant hope for the business-as-usual approach to disasters natural and unnatural. Philip Gourevitch reviews Polman's grim book and several others in a recent *New Yorker* essay, "Alms Dealers." He summarizes the arguments of the now "groaning bookshelf" of aid critiques by echoing Polman's argument: "Sowing horror to reap aid, and reaping aid to sow horror, [Polman] argues, is 'the logic of the humanitarian era.'"[53] The logic of assistance that focuses on funneling resources to the NGOs large and small, and its unintended consequences, were played out in dramatic terms in Africa (Nigeria in the late sixties and the Great Lakes region and Horn of Africa from the eighties until today) and in Southeast Asia (Cambodia).[54]

Those first weeks after the quake, when rescue and relief workers poured in, seemed animated by a different spirit than that evoked by Polman and other aid critics. There was much goodwill and generosity; and there still was almost a year later. But we ignore these critiques at our peril. It's useful to consider each of Gourevitch's examples and reflect on the current Haitian dilemma. Doing good is never simple. He invites us to "consider how Christian aid groups that set up 'redemption' programs to buy the freedom of slaves in Sudan drove up the market incentives for slavers to take more captives." This dramatic example has echoes in modern Haiti: the political economy of servitude underpins not only the Haitian *restavèk* tragedy, linked as it is to both poverty and the lack of public education for all, but also the hardship of the *braceros* who cross the Dominican border to harvest sugar cane under conditions denounced as slavery as recently as 2003.[55] Growing inequality, both within countries and between them, is the linchpin of modern servitude and weakens the ability of those with the best of intentions to avoid perverse consequences. Efforts to prosecute those who rely on children for domestic labor are less likely than structural interventions— making sure that children go to a school where they might receive sound instruction and at least one decent meal—to lessen the *restavèk* problem, a symptom not of Haitian cultural uniqueness, but of poverty and inequality.

The militarization of aid is an equally complex topic. "Consider how," Gourevitch continues, "in Ethiopia and Somalia during the nineteen-eighties and nineties, politically instigated, localized famines attracted the food aid that allowed governments to feed their own armies while they either destroyed or displaced targeted population groups."[56] Since 1995, Haiti has had no army. Its dissolution was not mourned by many: as the citizenry and historians know, the modern Haitian army was created during the U.S. occupation by an act of Congress. It never faced a non-Haitian enemy. Dissolving it as a body did not remove the army as a political risk, however, as was clear in the years leading up to 2004, when the elected government was dislodged by a violent process still willfully misunderstood in spite of abundant proof that weapons and other material were supplied to former soldiers massed on the Dominican border.[57] Among the effects of the 2004 coup was, predictably enough, the further weakening of the public sector.

But few of those working in Haiti after the quake mistake these struggles over the control of the state apparatus with the logistic help provided by the U.S. military and others, a topic discussed in this book by Louise Ivers and others. When we start conflating the help offered by the USNS *Comfort* with struggles to topple sovereign governments, we have lost the gift of discernment.

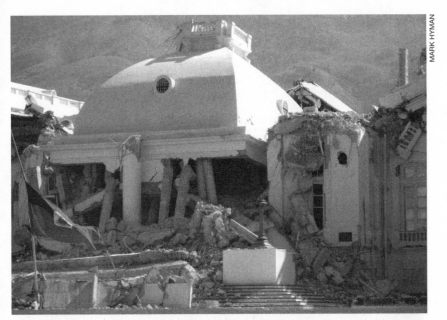

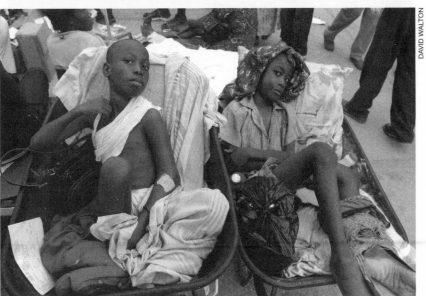

The century-old National Palace, destroyed in the earthquake
(as was almost all other federal infrastructure)

Injured boys in wheelbarrows at the General Hospital

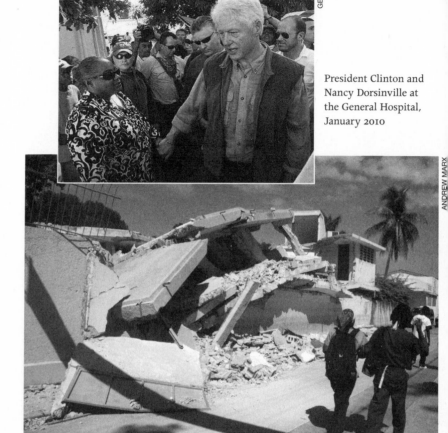

President Clinton and
Nancy Dorsinville at
the General Hospital,
January 2010

The nursing school
in Port-au-Prince

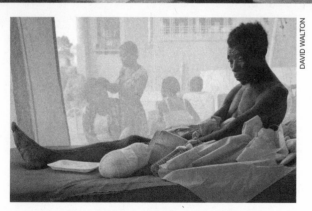

Injured man in tent clinic outside the General Hospital

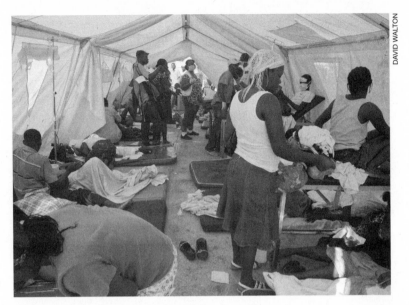

Tent clinic outside the General Hospital, five days after quake

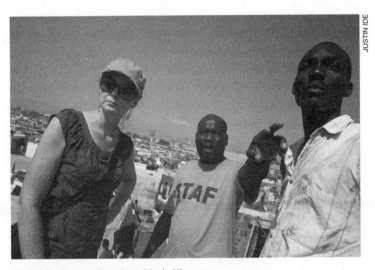

Dr. Louise Ivers at Parc Jean-Marie Vincent

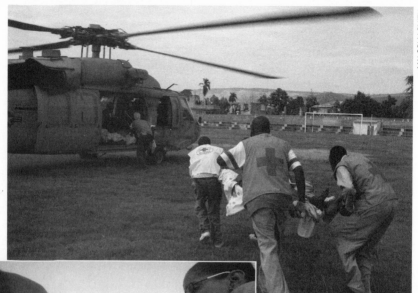

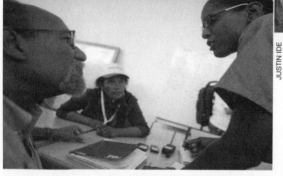

Patient being evacuated from Saint-Marc to the USNS *Comfort*

BELOW: The USNS *Comfort*, the U.S. Navy floating hospital, steamed into Haitian waters on day 8 after the earthquake

Dr. Alix Lassègue, Director, and Marlaine Thompson, Chief of Nursing, with Harvard medical resident, Dr. Natasha Archer, at the General Hospital

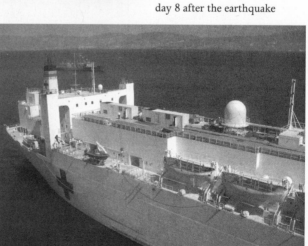

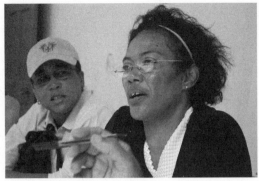

Marlaine Thompson, Chief of Nursing at the General Hospital, with Loune Viaud, Director of Strategic Planning and Operations for Zanmi Lasante

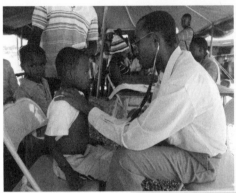

Dr. Dubique Kobel providing primary care services in Parc Jean-Marie Vincent, where 50,000 people were living in February 2010

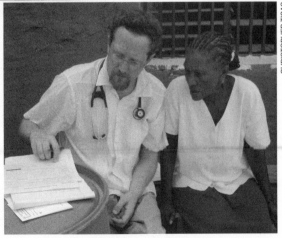

Dr. Evan Lyon with patient at the General Hospital

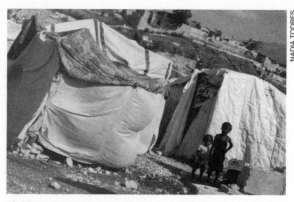

NADIA TODRES

Children in Parc Jean-Marie Vincent, March 2010; 1.3 million were living in similar conditions throughout the quake zone

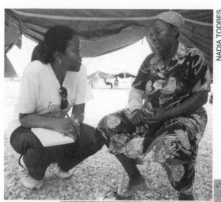

NADIA TODRES

Didi Bertrand Farmer speaking with a woman in camp Carradeux (3,500 people, 680 families, 1 water source, 7 latrines), July 2010

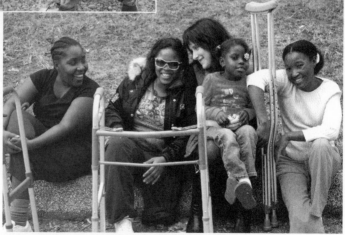

BETH ROSENBERG

Naomi Rosenberg from Partners In Health's Right to Health Care Program with quake-affected patients, Philadelphia, March 2010

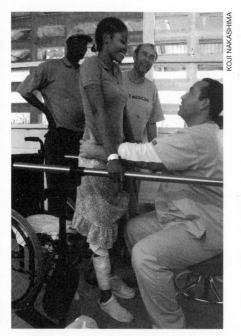

Shelove Julmiste in rehabilitation, Hôpital Albert Schweitzer

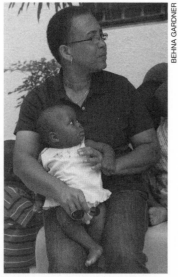

Loune Viaud and baby Rose at Zanmi Beni. ("I have a dream for every one of them.")

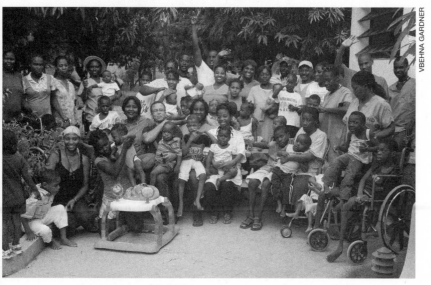

The caregivers and children at Zanmi Beni, November 2010

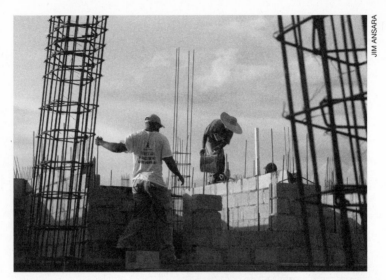

JIM ANSARA

Dr. David Walton at
the Mirebalais hospital
construction site,
January 2011

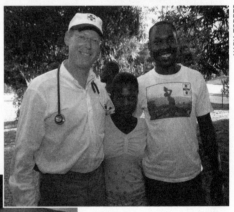

NADIA TODRES

Dr. Paul and Dr. Christophe
with Roseleine after
treatment, Lascahobas,
January 2011

DAVID WALTON

A cholera patient receiving intravenous fluids,
Lascahobas

# 8.

===

# LOOKING FORWARD
# WHILE LOOKING BACK
## *Lessons from Rwanda*

*T*o *advance a process* of discernment is one of the only reasons to publish a book like this one, written as events continue to unfold. It's difficult amid such suffering to find hopeful and relevant examples of building back better. But Rwanda offers more than a glimmer of hope, and we have more years of perspective with which to render judgments about central Africa. The legacies of colonialism and failed humanitarianism are still evident there as they are in Haiti.[1] When Philip Gourevitch (following Linda Polman, Fiona Terry, and others[2]) asks us to consider "how, in the mid-nineties, fugitive Rwandan *génocidaires* were succored in the same way by international humanitarians in border camps in eastern Congo, so that they have been able to continue their campaigns of extermination and rape to this day,"[3] he is making a claim of causality regarding the disastrous consequences of a series of decisions made far from the scenes of suffering witnessed in the Congo.[4] Crossing the Rwanda-Congo border to Goma offers a lesson in contrasts: on one side of the frontier are Rwandan resettlement towns and planned villages, called *imidugudu*. On the other side, many of Goma's buildings are partly buried in the hardened lava that poured forth from the giant Nyiragongo volcano in 1977 and again, more apocalyptically, in 2002. The Congolese side remains vulnerable to the raids of armed bands comprised of some of the same people who fled these camps when Rwandan forces finally invaded in 1996. This is the wild, wild east of Congo: almost as crowded as Rwanda, straddling the same volcanic hills, but immeasurably more lawless.

What makes the difference? One answer is circular: the Rwandan side of the border has more security. Other assessments note a heavy Rwandan hand in recent extractive endeavors in the Congo. Another reason, and one with more lessons for Haiti, is a rationally planned development strategy directed by the Rwandan government. Rwanda remains a political flashpoint in international circles, generating almost as many discrepant views as Haiti. But its renaissance is increasingly recognized as an example of building back better. In 1996, two years after the genocide, Rwanda was still strewn with mass graves. With a million dead and two million recently repatriated refugees, it still ranked among the poorest countries in the world.[5] Although Kigali's infrastructure escaped major damage during the civil war and genocide, it was then a small city without the capacity to welcome even a fraction of the returnees. Many development experts were happy to write off Rwanda as a lost cause: the next in a long line of failed states doomed to ongoing conflict and underdevelopment.

Fifteen years later, Rwanda has been transformed. If, as Jared Diamond has suggested, the collapse of Haiti and Rwanda were rooted in desperate competition for scarce resources, it's worth noting that Rwanda by 2000 was no less crowded and cramped than before the genocide.[6] But the strife within its borders had lessened even before the wheels of economic growth started turning. I'd like to consider some of the policies that may have led to this upward trajectory— some of them surely relevant to Haiti's own rebuilding challenges.

In many ways, post-genocide Rwanda looked much like Haiti: a mountainous and densely populated country with high birth rates, intransigent poverty and consequent health problems, a history of post-colonial social strife (albeit shorter than Haiti's), weak or discredited public institutions, low levels of literacy, and scant formal employment. The parallels should not be taken too far, however, because in other ways the countries diverge. No significant ethnic division haunts Haiti (although some remnants of European racial hierarchies are alive there to this day); Haiti is not packed with *génocidaires* and the families of their victims. Nonetheless, the similarities warrant a closer look.

Over the five or so years after the genocide, the transitional government of Rwanda—led by Paul Kagame, the former leader of the Rwandan Patriotic Front whose military campaign is widely credited with ending the violence in 1994, at least within Rwandan borders—honed a development plan, later named Vision 2020.[7] The plan called for investments in agriculture, infrastructure, and private enterprise; it laid out targets for the health and education systems, and for decentralization and coordination of development assistance. Vision 2020 also called for an end to dependence on foreign assistance by that year. The plan did not reject such aid—two decades is a long time for a proposed divorce—but rather stressed sovereignty as a precondition to long-term reconstruction and growth. But rebuilding the country's institutions could not start in earnest until the massive numbers of repatriated refugees were resettled, even as the guilty among them were brought to justice. And each of these steps to recovery required a modicum of security in the broadest sense of the word.

Roadmaps such as Vision 2020 are a dime a dozen (the Corail-Cesselesse charrette, for example); implementing them effectively is another matter. The transitional government knew it needed new resources to reinvigorate public institutions. It quickly set about collecting taxes—one of the more thankless tasks facing post-disaster administrations—and sought, fitfully at first, to fight corruption.[8] The contours of this effort had sharp edges. Many bureaucrats and local officials found themselves in trouble when asked for transparent accounting and reporting. Zealous protagonists of transparency waged a high-stakes public relations battle well before the infrastructure of transparency—electricity, computers, accountants, et cetera—was widely available, even in Kigali. The authorities also sought to settle disputed land claims in a manner that might encourage private investment and the return of more of the diaspora. Investment was a widely recognized prerequisite to growth among economic policy advisors; repatriation, however complicated a process, was indispensable because many of the Rwandans who had fled during the civil war and the preceding decades of ethnic tension were highly educated, internationally connected professionals.

The ungainly coalition of rebuilders had no shortage of external detractors, including some within the governments of Belgium and France—the colonial and neocolonial powers in Rwanda, respectively. Most supporters of the pregenocide Rwandan government pitted themselves against the interim government.[9] Surviving architects of the genocide were scattered around Africa and beyond; most were fleeing justice, but some managed to infiltrate various international organizations, as Gourevitch and others reported. However, there were many untainted critics among the "expert" ranks of human rights lawyers and humanitarian groups purveying basic services to refugees.

Resettlement of refugees was a key issue. Today, many Africans displaced by conflict have languished in refugee camps for well over a decade.[10] To avoid condemning its diaspora and returnees to a similar fate, the interim government of Rwanda hatched an audacious repatriation and resettlement strategy, building thousands of small settlements called *imidugudu*. These hastily confected villages distributed the influx of repatriated Rwandans throughout the country to avoid fueling urban slums such as the ones marring cityscapes across Africa (and Haiti). By all accounts an ambitious plan, it was showered with scorn by some refugee and shelter experts (they were already in existence by then) and lauded by others.[11] In the months immediately after the genocide, the interim government negotiated the return of fifty thousand Hutu refugees from Burundi. Denouncing this scheme as forced repatriation, humanitarians and human rights lawyers predicted violence and misery. But the plan went over without major problems.[12]

The interim government needed a bolder strategy to repatriate the millions of Rwandans still in the Congo, many of whom were openly hostile to the fledgling government in Kigali. The entrenched humanitarian enterprise—aided in a sense by Mobutu's dictatorship, which had also sent troops in support of the *génocidaire* régime[13]— was also complicit, as studies later showed, by feeding and housing and caring for *génocidaires* in their midst. Well fed and confident of their return, these *génocidaires* were clearly the biggest threat to the interim government and to security across Rwanda. For almost two years, the leadership in Kigali, facing a complex public-relations battle they often lost, demanded that the camps be dismantled and the refugees repatriated. With each cross-border raid from the Congo, Kigali continued to warn the UN and humanitarians that they would invade to shut down the camps if the attacks continued.

In mid-1996, Kagame launched a wildly improbable mission. His armies dismantled the refugee camps on the border, then pressed through the Congo—ninety-four times the size of Rwanda and as large as Western Europe—to Kinshasa, toppling Mobutu and his thirty-year stranglehold over the country. Much to the world's surprise, the plan seemed to meet its objectives, although it was widely denounced as forced repatriation or worse.

Public-relations battles aside, what did this massive repatriation, forced or unforced, mean for overcrowded Rwanda? Stephen Kinzer describes what must have been a shock to the system: "Like a single organism, this huge mass of people left the squalor of refugee life and trudged toward an uncertain future at home . . . During those weeks in the autumn of 1996, more than a million people returned to Rwanda along the same roads they had used to flee two and a half years earlier."[14] The *imidugudu* absorbed many of the returnees, countering the low expectations of the international community and shelter experts.[15] There were snags—overcrowding, joblessness, discord—but the interim government persisted, pushing development partners to build schools and health centers around the settlements. Little by little, over the years, that's what came to pass.

Within Rwanda, reconciliation would take more than providing cheap housing, building schools, and strengthening the health sector. Stiff competition for scarce resources remained. The sheer number of competing land claims was a recipe for ongoing strife.[16] A means of adjudicating such claims was needed, as was a means of meting out justice to those who had participated in the genocide and again lived in close proximity to the survivors and relatives of the victims.[17]

To address competing claims on land and other property, including businesses, the interim government held a number of town-hall meetings in which a plan for resolving property disputes was discussed. This went on for months and finally led to the creation of regional offices with the authority to settle disputes and to disburse funds for reimbursements in the event that previous administrations had seized private property.[18] Many plots were returned to their former owners; some were given to the displaced; some were added to the holdings of other homesteads.[19] It was a messy formula but seemed to work better than predicted.

What to do with the guilty and accused was an even greater challenge. A few architects of the genocide were put on trial at the International Criminal Tribunal for Rwanda, in neighboring Tanzania, and still others in official courts in Kigali. But these processes were lengthy, costly, and required an impartial legal system with an adequate and trained staff. Such legal infrastructure did not exist in Rwanda. The prisons were crammed with tens of thousands of accused *génocidaires,* and few resources were available to pursue the sort of truth and reconciliation process followed in South Africa.[20] Even in 2005, when Partners In Health arrived in southeastern Rwanda to rebuild medical infrastructure, Rwandan prisons remained full of the accused and untried.

Rwanda needed an alternate legal mechanism to reach justice after the crimes of the 1990s, and it found one in tradition: the *gacaca* courts, long used for settling village disputes. *Gacaca* literally means "short grass" because in precolonial times such hearings took place in open areas where entire villages could convene. The interim government adapted the *gacaca* system after the genocide: "We took this concept [of *gacaca* courts] and developed it because it would reach people, and they would see themselves in it," explained Kagame. "It's the way our culture traditionally resolved problems. We have picked it and developed it to deal with present-day problems."[21] Tribunals would occur in public and near the scenes of the alleged crimes; both victims and witnesses had a chance to speak; sentences were limited to thirty years (half the time was spent on parole). Ultimately, about 80 percent of defendants were freed by the *gacaca* tribunals, not because they were guiltless but because there was strong pressure for self-incrimination. Confessions were met with shorter sentences, many of them deemed to have been served already.[22]

The *gacaca* courts did not fail, as some predicted, and by 2007 they had cleared out the prisons through alternative sentences, including community service. The processes seemed to allow some semblance of social recovery to occur. Although the painful process of genuine reconciliation might take generations, physicians working in the prisons (as we did) saw the reduced number of inmates diminished the likelihood of epidemics within such institutions.

For foreigners like me, it wasn't clear who was Hutu and who Tutsi, and we were not invited to inquire. "Ethnic divisionism" was banned in Rwanda, making it increasingly different from its former twin, Burundi, where we've also worked and where people are more open about their so-called ethnicity. In his book *The Antelope's Strategy: Living in Rwanda After the Genocide*, intrepid researcher Jean Hatzfeld cites one Rwandan's testament to this uneasy comity:

I joined two agricultural cooperatives with the sugarcane planters along the Nyabarongo River: that's eighty-three Hutu and Tutsi farmers in all and, with the farmers growing foodstuffs, one hundred and thirty growers. We organize raffles to help with purchases, we stand one another to drinks, we talk together quite properly. But speaking in friendship, that's another matter. The state played its role to keep revenge from overtaking reconciliation. One cannot erase vengefulness completely from the minds of survivors. I know I have been forgiven not by them but by the state. The survivors, even if they do their share, they don't feel safe next to the killers, they're scared of being pushed around again. Trust has been driven out of Rwanda. It will wait behind many generations."[23]

As a physician working in the public sector, or as a foreigner living in Rwanda, it was hard not to give thanks for the *gacaca* process
and the imposed prevention of revenge. Just as it was hard to claim
that the *gacaca* courts had failed, so too was it hard, within a decade
of the genocide, to argue that the rebuilding of the civil service had
failed. Rwanda was, by then, almost the mirror opposite of a "failed
state," to use the term favored by experts and echoed in the popular
press. The country was able to draw on its diaspora (sizeable, if
smaller than Haiti's) to rebuild. Other technicians of various nation-
alities were drawn into government ministries to help build Rwandan capacity. The state also made great strides in promoting gender
equity among its civil service, recently passing Sweden as the country with the highest proportion of female representation in the
world.[24]

The machinery of humanitarian aid and reconstruction was welcomed into Rwanda post-genocide but with more substantial strictures than in Haiti (or in the Congo). The policy was clear: NGOs and
aid institutions were welcome if they squared their plans with the reconstruction priorities of the government. Some NGOs left, protesting
that the Rwandan government was heavy-handed, controlling, and
antidemocratic. (Such critiques were not often heard in the years before the genocide, as Peter Uvin's work attests,[25] when aid groups
were given a carte blanche to work in Rwanda.) The post-genocide
government did not mourn their departure because it regarded some
of the NGOs, and much of the humanitarian machine, as part of the
problem. The feeling was mutual, often enough.

Debates about these issues continue to this day, but their urgency
is lessened by both security and continued economic growth. Mass
violence has not recurred in Rwanda, and the GDP has trebled over
the past decade. This year, the summer before elections would formally grant Kagame a second and final term, a number of articles appeared in the international press arguing that his was an
authoritarian government with slender commitment to democratic
rule. But critical re-readings of the evidence will require a careful
evaluation of the views of the many polities and organizations committed to self-exculpation regarding the genocide and its echoes in

the eastern Congo. For example, the recent United Nations draft report was damning to Rwanda. The official Rwandan response, published simultaneously, wrote the same history along very different lines.[26] One thing is sure: mutually contradictory claims of causality and assessments of blame will continue to be advanced with great confidence for years to come.

One thing that isn't open to much debate: Rwanda in 2010 is a far cry not only from Rwanda in 1995 but also from Rwanda in the years just before the genocide. In *Aiding Violence*, Uvin explained how he and others in development circles failed to note the rise of genocidal ideology because of their exclusive focus on certain indicators: GDP per capita, inflation, corruption indices, and demographic trends. In effect, Uvin argues that he and his colleagues were blind to the palpable frictions erupting around them because their attention was fixed narrowly on the "development model."[27] The risk of making a similar mistake remains today. But armed with cautionary tales from Uvin, Polman, Terry, and Dambisa Moyo (indeed, the entire "groaning bookshelf" of critiques), it would be a shame to shirk the hard tasks of analysis and discernment, whether the topic at hand is central Africa after war and genocide or Haiti after coups and storms and the quake of 2010.

One thing Haiti could use right now is analysis informed by discernment and a pinch of optimism about rebuilding. Facing a challenge of this magnitude, taking the side of critique (and, sometimes, despair) is certainly easier. Many in Haiti (and some outside) appear content to forecast failure unendingly. But as Michèle Montas and others contributing to this book show, cynicism about reconstruction is less common among the Haitian poor—the majority of the country's population—than might be expected. Many Haitians interviewed after the earthquake or during the interminable wait for rebuilding to begin still believe that *Ayiti p'ap peri*—"Haiti will never be finished." Many believe that Haiti can change, in spite of the fact that they themselves have, so far, been given little role in helping to rebuild their own civic institutions and infrastructure.

Haitian history is rife with examples of exclusion and its constant counterpart: resistance. The country was born through violent resistance to an oppressive social and economic system, the "peculiar institution" of slavery.[28] In the years following independence, many Haitians voted with their feet, removing themselves from ruined plantations to small plots of land and rejecting, when possible, any and all systems of coerced labor. As steep mountainsides were cultivated, population growth and ecological decline (due to deforestation and erosion) set the stage for the late-twentieth-century collapse that itself set the stage for both urban migration and increasing vulnerability to storms and other disasters.

The collapse has been ecological, economic, and political. The war of independence, the forced popular movement that created a nation in 1804, had no triumphant follow-up. Instead, the country divided into north and south, and the bulk of the state's effort focused on self-perpetuation. Coup followed coup, as politicians either conscripted the remnants of the revolutionary army or created their own militias to seize power. This was, as the anthropologist Michel-Rolph Trouillot has observed, a case of "state against nation."[29] By the late nineteenth century, Haiti had become a predatory state, like Rwanda pre-genocide: weak and unable to meet the basic needs of its people but strong enough to prey on them. The Duvalier régime (1957–1986) was less an aberration than the ultimate expression of a predatory state based on patronage and violence.

This was all supposed to change in 1990, when Latin America's oldest republic held its first free elections. The Haitian people, previously excluded from the political process, participated in great numbers, electing a representative of the renascent and unforced popular movement. That government lasted only seven months before it too was unseated by a military coup in September 1991. But the participatory impulse was too strong, and the military régime too violent, to return Haiti to the status quo ante. Since the 1986 fall of the Duvalier dictatorship, no unelected régime has lasted long, and each elected government (there have been, really, only four) has emerged from the popular movement. Only two people have ever been elected to Haiti's highest offices in democratic elections: Aristide and his former prime minister, René Préval. Their original platform, laid out hastily in the troubled interregnum that followed the end of the dictatorship, was to promote basic social and economic rights and to allow wider civic participation in governance.

This movement, too, has fallen prey to the fissioning tendencies of Haitian politics. By the time this book is published, another election cycle will have taken place. Haiti's many misfortunes and persistent poverty, which together have dashed some of the hopes shared after the fall of the Duvalier dictatorship, and exclusion of the political party identified with Aristide will mean less participation in the electoral process. But a strong government requires strong civic support and not only from the vocal members of "civil society"—code, as noted, for the non-poor. The non-poor are a minority in Haiti, a tiny economic élite and small middle class. A book about Haiti after the earthquake is perhaps not the place in which to reflect on theories about human rights, but struggles about voting rights and subsistence rights are intimately related to debates about development and humanitarian assistance. These debates have been playing themselves out in Haiti for decades.

Now, as cholera spreads rapidly through rural Haiti and menaces the camps and slums in urban areas, Haitians like the ones I've had the privilege to serve as a doctor continue to press for a stronger and more competent government; they continue to question mainstream views of both development and human rights. Like many Rwandans, most of the Haitians interviewed for the Voices of the Voiceless project want to live in a country no longer dependent on foreign aid. They want to live in a country with food sovereignty and basic services. They want decent jobs and to participate fully in the reconstruction of their country. The events of the past year have thrown the alternatives manifested by these debates, and the problems underlying them, into stark relief.

Listening to the poor helps us frame these alternatives clearly. Will we promote genuine development in the manner wished by the Haitian majority? Or will we stay pinned to the same, tired approaches that haven't brought us much closer to the stated goals of either development assistance or the Haitian people? Fair trade, food

sovereignty, access to health care and education and clean water—
these social goals can surely be linked to economic and political
strategies that lead to growth, better governance, and reconstruction. Will trade policies punish Haitian farmers, as before, or will we
insist on arrangements that help expand the economy and the number of decent jobs in the country? Will food assistance develop markets for locally grown produce, or continue to rely on imported
surplus from U.S. or European agribusinesses that decry subsidies
for others while ardently defending their own? Will we fight to make
sure that quality primary health care and primary education, at the
very least, become readily accessible to all Haitians, or will we remain ensnarled in uncreative financing models that impose users'
fees and thereby ensure that the poorest have no access? Will we invest in municipal water projects throughout rural and urban Haiti,
or will we continue to privatize a system that is already fractured by
private interests? Will the response to the shelter crisis remain every
man for himself, without plan or code, and with little chance for the
poor to benefit from the coming building boom? Or will the next
years include pro-poor strategies that help create more and safer
housing with modern sanitation for those now sheltered under tents
and tarps and bits of tin?

———

A year after the quake, Haiti looks almost the same as it did for the
six-month anniversary. But what will the next years bring? Let's say
the date is now January 12, 2015. What has happened to the rubble,
the camps, the promised efforts to rebuild? What has become of the
threat of worse environmental disasters? What has happened to the
cholera epidemic? Has reconstruction remained stalled by petty political squabbles, a lack of vision, and far too little focus on implementation of goals, whether modest or ambitious?

No crystal ball is needed. Another quake could skew any prognos-
tication; with greater probability, the tail end of a hurricane season
like that of 2008 could recur between the time this book goes to
press and when it sees the light of day. But because Haiti's problems
are old and reconstruction too slow, it was never difficult to forecast

likely futures, especially in the short term. The answers to these questions will depend to a large extent on programs and policies enacted and then implemented in 2011 and shortly thereafter—programs and policies decided within Haiti and without. Let's imagine the discrepant possibilities.

**Reconstruction.** In scenario one (at the optimistic end of the spectrum), the reconstruction phase is in full swing by 2015. After a faltering start, an increased fraction of the resources pledged to reconstruction flowed to projects employing large numbers of Haitians and creating new Haitian businesses; indeed, the number of decent local jobs created was one of the metrics by which all proposals were judged. By 2015, more than two million Haitians have participated in public-works projects, bringing unemployment below 50 percent for the first time in decades. Thousands of skilled Haitian laborers returned from the Dominican Republic, the Bahamas, and other countries in the region after they learned that they could expect better wages and working conditions—and more compelling projects—at home. Millions of tons of rubble were cleared from Port-au-Prince, and much of it was recycled and sold.

Construction, including public works, hasn't been the only growth industry. An integrated natural-defense plan linked reforestation, watershed protection, and small-scale agriculture together into one massive endeavor. A Green Haiti Pact brought together donors, regional and local governments, women's groups, peasant organizations, and young people. Projects included ready access to credit and tools for small farmers and fairer prices for their produce.[30] The initiative offered subsidies for alternative energies like liquid propane so that Haiti could wean itself from charcoal. (Alternative cooking energies included briquettes made from agricultural and other waste.) The use of charcoal and wood in bakeries, laundromats, and other industries was banned as cleaner energy became a growth industry in Haiti. Wind turbines have been erected in several sites across the country and are maintained by well-trained locals who are paid for their labor and who share in the turbines' output; small hydroelectric plants gave a green boost to rural electrification projects without flooding large tracts of fertile land; these plants now also power dozens of food-processing plants that add value to farmers' produce and ready it for local markets or export. Solar panels manufactured in Haiti have appeared on roofs throughout the country as increasing numbers of small businesses and homeowners found them affordable, dependable, and safe; several Haitian factories now manufacture these solar panels both for local use and for export to the United States and elsewhere. Within a few years, Haiti, once the world's largest assembler of baseballs and brassieres, is on the way to becoming one of the top ten exporters of solar panels in the hemisphere. Haiti is also well on its way to fuel self-sufficiency. The fraction of people connected to the electric grid has gone from under 10 percent in 2010 to over 30 percent in 2015, and as many more are generating their own power with solar panels and wind turbines.

In a bleaker version of events, 2015 has brought more heartache to Haiti. Although several projects have been completed, national reconstruction remains stalled as recriminations and backbiting dominate the political scene and the local media; frustrations on all sides lead many international partners to scale back efforts and focus on other trouble spots. Foreign aid was not reformed substantially, and uninspired bilateral arrangements (some favorable and others less so) remain the order of the day. Credit remains out of reach for most living in poverty and hampers the growth of small businesses. Charcoal, still the only cooking fuel within the grasp of poor Haitians, remains a cash crop as the deforestation of the country draws toward its endgame. The 2014 rainy season was marked with mudslides, flash floods, and great damage to property and livestock; thousands of lives were lost. The coastal fishing industry, smothered by erosion, saw dropping yields and still lacks modern storage and processing capacity. The hurricane season has just ended without another direct hit; Haitians pray that the storms spare the country again next year. But most know it's simply a matter of time before heavy rains or worse wash more lives and livelihoods onto the now lifeless reefs abutting Haiti's estuaries.

**Housing.** In either scenario, safe and affordable shelter will be another of the weighty matters that continue to preoccupy those living in Haiti. It was understood shortly after the quake that people could be pulled out of the camps by opportunity or pushed out by force. In the optimistic scenario, in which pull forces predominate, massive investments in housing stock have been made in well-chosen sites throughout the country. Such housing units were planned and built, complete with basic services—clean water, modern sanitation, and of course health care and education—and with proximity to a growing number of jobs in the formal economy (which boosts tax receipts) and, for farmers, to processing plants, warehouses, and customers for their produce. By 2015, the number of people in camps has been reduced by two-thirds, and large planned communities are taking final form in half of Haiti's departments. A dozen smaller developments, the fruit of participatory community planning, are underway in the other half. The rate of home ownership has risen steeply, and many poor families can now hope to avoid informal settlements and slums without sanitation, electricity, water, and roads.

In version two, push forces have dominated: sharp clashes between landowners and the displaced continue. Haiti's police are called to forcibly remove more than one hundred thousand "squatters" (less than ten percent of the million and more in camps) and violence leads to scores of deaths. Multinational troops are called in on the side of the landowners, and in 2015 Haiti is again declared an unsafe destination by many other countries (some of them with far higher rates of violence in their own cities but less vulnerable to travel bans). Those forcibly removed find themselves in equally grim settings, and resentment toward the police and other representatives of the state reaches an apogee. For many of the displaced, the concept of the rule of law lacks all legitimacy because law has been used so many times against them and almost never for them. The class divide in Haiti has deepened further, both in terms of economic disparities and in terms of the loss of shared purpose. Social capital has been squandered.

In a pessimistic view, the year 2015 also brings a steady drumbeat from the development community, foreign and homegrown: in an effort to avoid creating dependency upon such extravagancies as food and water, the argument was made that basic service provision to those living in camps needs to be cut back. This policy was recognized by most camp dwellers as an effort to push them out by making the camps uninhabitable. Cholera and other waterborne diseases, only recently brought under control, returned with a vengeance, not only in the camps but across the country. These diseases brought great suffering and death and also lower profits for farmers in cholera-endemic areas, whose products are spurned on local and international markets because of misguided fears about transmission.[31]

**Health and education.** As early as 2009, it was clear that two-thirds of medical care and more than 80 percent of primary and secondary education were delivered in the private sector—a fact linked, in the eyes of many, to poor health indices and low rates of literacy. What will the next five years bring?

Well before 2015, the public hospital in Mirebalais will have been completed and launched. This will come to pass in either scenario, I dare say. But in the brighter scenario, it came to fill a better role not simply as a teaching and referral hospital but also as a source of care for the large number of families coming to central Haiti to work in schools and health care institutions as well as in agricultural regions opened up by better roads, improved irrigation, and ready access to credit. Nonstate providers (from NGOs to religious groups) continue to furnish many of these services but are now doing so in a more coordinated manner, one that builds local capacity by training workers and by moving resources to where they are needed most. The medical center in Mirebalais, drawing on educators from North America and Cuba and the Haitian diaspora, has been training not only doctors and nurses but also a broad range of allied health professionals able to strengthen health systems throughout the country.

The cholera epidemic was brought to heel in 2012 after a coalition of Haitian and international players fought for ramped-up vaccine production in India, leading to the world's first cholera-vaccine stockpile. The vaccination campaign was linked to renewed efforts to make safe water and modern sanitation widely available across the country. Haitians were at the center of this effort, as they had been years before in the delivery of integrated AIDS prevention and care that halved the size of epidemic in Haiti. Cholera treatment centers closed as the number of new cases dwindled to a few a day; patients were expertly treated in the public-private health centers and hospitals in each department.

In this optimistic scenario, building back better has been applied to both infrastructure and human capital. The long-term development plan, Haiti's version of Vision 2020, led to a policy known as *investir dans l'humain*—"investing in people." The renaissance in public education opened up primary and secondary education to all and helped prepare young Haitians for full participation in the governance of an increasingly decentralized economy and the global knowledge economy. The *restavèk* problem has diminished as all children are finally accorded a chance to go to a good school, regardless of their parents' ability to pay school fees. Each year, the quality of pedagogy has improved as more teachers are trained and retrained—and as their salaries rise.

In a pessimistic version of events, 2015 marks the fifth year of a cholera epidemic that won't be leaving Haiti anytime soon. Several hundred thousand Haitians have fallen ill with the disease; international experts were never able to agree on the need to deploy cholera vaccine and more aggressive treatment. Thousands of small water projects lessened the number of cases, but the hybrid El Tor strand is now endemic in Haiti and across the Caribbean. (Cuba and Jamaica were largely spared due to aggressive prevention measures.) The occasional case in Florida or New York has led to scapegoating of Haitians and calls for more aggressive responses to the disease in Haiti. But too few robust programs were implemented, and the lack of ready access to potable water and modern sanitation meant that, in 2015, scattered outbreaks of cholera again occurred in each of Haiti's departments. Dithering about the role of cholera vaccine and proper management of these cases in such resource-poor settings continues in meetings, and in meetings about meetings.

**Governance.** Haiti, increasingly vulnerable to hurricanes, also faces other kinds of storms: 2010 was an election year. Political discord continues to roil Haiti, as it must when so many are excluded from full participation. By 2015, the country has a new president and a new legislature. Their legitimacy in the eyes of the Haitian people, surely more important in principle than their legitimacy in the eyes of a vaguely defined international community, will depend on the manner of their advent to public office.

In version one, increasingly unlikely, there is continuity with the popular movement that grew in the late 1980s, and 2011 will have marked the third time in Haiti's long history that power is transferred peacefully from one civilian and elected government to another. In this optimistic (if improbable) vision, continuity with 1990—the Great Rupture with autocratic or military rule—is clear. At every level of government, from the capital to the ten departments to all of Haiti's towns and villages, there is a growing consensus regarding a sound plan for sustainable development. Continuity with the other great moment of Haitian history—the fight against slavery and for independence—is palpable, as people are engaged in their own development and in a shared vision of fundamental freedoms, including freedom from want and servitude. The watchword of this participatory democracy comes from the former slave Toussaint Louverture, whose famous line upon being captured by Napoleon's forces is known by every Haitian child lucky enough to be in school: "In overthrowing me, you have done no more than cut down the trunk of the tree of black liberty in Saint-Domingue. It will spring back from the roots, for they are numerous and deep."

In version two, willed or unintentional exclusion of the popular movement, having led to low voter turnout, leads to a government with scant legitimacy in the eyes of the majority. Without genuinely participatory government, sustainable development will be difficult in Haiti. "Participatory" does not mean the fetishization of some superficial process contracted out to a consulting group charged with interviewing "the community" about how it feels about one or another plan for breaking the cycle of poverty, storm, disease, and cronyism. Nor does it mean a ceremony involving ballot boxes and candidates flown in to greet the populace after having charmed alien donors. "Participatory" means, rather, a transfer of at least some resources from rich to poor. This is a transnational process, and it means a historical reckoning with what has happened to Haiti's once abundant resources, including those taken from the Haitian people over three centuries of coerced labor, unequal development, local misrule, gunboat diplomacy, military occupation, dictatorships family and military, and persistent attempts to undermine the popular movement.

When Franklin Delano Roosevelt wrote of the four freedoms, "freedom from want" was central to his platform. That speech was delivered in 1941, but the same concern for human security—housing and food security, education, and jobs—led to his election amid the economic disaster of 1932 and to his reelections in 1936 and 1940. Roosevelt's audience did not anticipate that the Four Freedoms (freedom of expression, freedom of worship, freedom from want, freedom from fear) might once again become the Two Freedoms under subsequent American administrations. Haitians have long known that rights are worth fighting for and more than words on paper. In the past three decades, as in the late eighteenth century, they have been seeking both formal and substantive rights: as the saying goes, *san pè nan vant, pa gen pè nan tèt* —"when we live with hunger, we will not live in peace." Until the basic needs of the Haitian majority are met—food and shelter, education and health care, jobs that promote dignity—there will be scant peace in Haiti.[32] This was true before the quake, and it remains so after.

# EPILOGUE

## *January 12, 2011*

*I*t's hard to know where to end an account like this one, but the one-year anniversary of the earthquake seems as good a time as any. We've all been forced to think hard about the past year, and to consider the next steps. Discussions are underway about the future of the Office of the Special Envoy (this decision will be up to President Clinton and the UN), about the rebuilding of the health system (this discussion should be the purview of the Ministry of Health but remains subject to the will of the donors, who control so much of the funding), and about reconstruction (this should be in accordance with a national plan, endorsed by those most affected, although this goal remains elusive).

The one-year anniversary also meant, for me and for thousands of coworkers, difficult decisions for Partners In Health and Zanmi Lasante. So much changed with the quake: one day, we were heavily concentrated in rural regions and working to provide health and social services across central and lower-Artibonite Haiti. Within a week or so, we were struggling to provide basic services in four camps in the heart of the city, including sprawling Parc Jean-Marie Vincent.

We were all ending a year of incalculable loss and facing one of great uncertainty, sure to be deepened by the upcoming runoff elections for president and then another season of rains and hurricanes. The death of Tom White, a founder of Partners In Health and the first to invest in our endeavor—"to make a preferential option for the poor in health care"—closed out our own year of loss. I was once again en route between Rwanda and Haiti when Ophelia Dahl gave me the news of Tom's death. I headed back to Boston immediately. Tom's widow, Lois, asked me to give the eulogy during his funeral on January 11, one day before the anniversary of the quake. Somehow these sad anniversaries were all jumbled together for me: in speaking about Tom in a packed Jesuit church at Boston College, I was speaking about Haiti, too.

The service drew a big delegation from Haiti, including Father Fritz. There were mourners from a dozen countries: a map of his generosity. Mapping or measuring largesse is hard, quite apart from personal loss. How do you measure compassion and goodness? As fond as Tom was of precision, his stock in trade as a builder, he was deeply mistrustful of confident answers to this question. Long before he knew success in business, Tom was asking hard questions about how to live in a world in which it was simply not possible to be free of anxiety. For someone who loved numbers and worked closely with engineers to build sturdy bridges and tunnels and buildings, he was always the first to admit there was no unfailing algebra of decency, no geometry of the heart or calculus of compassion. If I may paraphrase Tom's son Peter, Tom's determination to realize *eudaimonia*—human flourishing—had inspired all those gathered, as I noted in my eulogy:

> Tom knew his math but also taught many of us (to borrow from Ephesians) that we sometimes see best with the eyes of the heart. He did not, in his charitable work, take short cuts or avoid the hard process of discernment. Tom knew that everyone in this world can and does suffer, but he also knew that some suffer more than others and that many suffer injustice.
>
> Tom's generosity did not require proximity. His imagination, and the eyes of his heart, allowed him to understand suffering unlike any he had seen, even in the theatre of war. That's why his generosity was legendary not just in his hometown but around the world. I hope I might be forgiven for mentioning his work in international health,

since that's what we did together for almost thirty years. It was something of a lost cause until Tom lent us his time and backing. Since Tom's death, Partners In Health, which Tom founded *and* funded, has received messages of sympathy and support from Peru, Rwanda, Lesotho, Russia, and especially, from Haiti. Allow me to indulge in what Tom would term running the numbers: by our count, the organization he founded has built or refurbished some sixty hospitals and clinics, scores of schools and community centers, and employs, in over a dozen countries, more than thirteen thousand people. As Jim Kim noted in speaking to the Boston *Globe*, Tom's early investments in taking on the care of people living in poverty and with chronic disease led directly to major changes in the way global health is delivered, saving millions of lives already and promising to save millions more.

Within hours of leaving Saint Ignatius, my brother Jeff and I were headed back to Miami and then I was on to Port-au-Prince. We needed to mark the one-year anniversary of the quake.

I grabbed a copy of the Boston *Globe* in Logan airport, and on the front page was a thoughtful and well-researched article about Partners In Health by Stephen Smith. Caught up in eulogizing Tom White, and in seeing, at his funeral, many of my friends and coworkers for the first time since the earthquake, I was reminded by Smith's piece that, although we were working in a dozen countries, it was Haiti that had consumed us the preceding year. Haiti would be central to our work in the coming years, too. Smith's article captured the struggles we'd been facing (and sometimes avoiding), and also made clear just how generous our supporters had been:

With thousands of bodies and minds shattered—and the emergence of a lethal cholera epidemic—the Partners In Health workforce in this country, constituted almost exclusively of Haitians, soared from roughly 4,400 before the catastrophe to 5,500 now. Fueled by donors who showered it with $89 million, Partners In Health hired mental health specialists, recruited amputees to visit the limbless, and sheltered forsaken children. And, in its most prominent bricks-and-mortar expansion ever, it is building a $15 million, 320-bed hospital in the hills north of Port-au-Prince.

So much growth so fast has sparked soul searching, even trepidation, at an aid agency that as recently as eight years ago worked in just one bucolic village, Cange, and scavenged for donations. Much as Haiti stands at a crossroads, so, too, does Partners In Health.

Will it remain for the long haul in the capital city, where it sees 7,000 to 10,000 patients a week in camp clinics? And how will it sustain the post-earthquake expansion as interest in Haiti wanes and generosity flows elsewhere?

The answers to those questions will resonate across a country whose medical system was fractured even before the earthquake: Partners In Health plays a singular role, collaborating with the cash-strapped Ministry of Health to treat more patients than any group in the country.[1]

Smith echoed many of the questions we had been wrestling with since the quake—questions of scale and scope, of our strategy in the spontaneous settlements and in cholera treatment centers across the country, and of the future of our work in Haiti when the world's generosity turns its eye to the next disaster natural or unnatural.

That next day, the twelfth of January, we were back in Haiti, some in central Haiti (in the "bucolic village" of Cange—a former refugee camp) and some in Port-au-Prince. The capital city still looked as if it had just been leveled by an earthquake. But many of us remembered how different the cityscape looked the year before.

The city was full of people marking the anniversary with solemn ceremony, quiet prayer, and even protest over everything from the slow pace of reconstruction to the results of the recent presidential primaries, which at one point counted more than thirty candidates. The political class was locked in old struggles for power over an increasingly debilitated state. The popular movement, to a considerable extent excluded from formal participation in the elections, was scattered and leaderless in Haiti. (Its leader remained exiled in South Africa.)[2] Unsurprisingly, voter participation hit an all-time low in November, and was followed, also unsurprisingly, by dispute (some of it violent) over the election results. As cholera spread and as re-construction faltered, many delegations and gatherings of important personages commented on which two candidates received the most votes in the first round of what were clearly flawed elections—flawed in concept (again, because the elections were not fully inclu-sive of all political groupings) and in execution (people in the camps had a predictably hard time voting even when they wanted to). As Claire Pierre said to me, "It's been a long, sad road from 1986, when everyone who is now bickering was in agreement about ending the Duvalier dictatorship and building a democracy."

Little did Claire know that the Haitian political scene would soon become even more shambolic: on January 16, Jean-Claude Duvalier himself showed up in Haiti, stepping off a French commercial flight. It was unclear why he had returned. But it was unnerving to many, especially to his former victims. There was talk of his facing charges. But for all the bluster—and there wasn't much of it, given how worn down people were and how many Haitians hadn't even been born when Duvalier fell—the Haitian justice system didn't even have the organizational capacity to bring charges against the aging dictator. If, as Marx averred, history repeats itself first as tragedy, second as farce, it was hard to know where Duvalier's return fit in the spec-trum.

Farcical electoral disputes had, as usual, consumed the attention and time of the Haitian political class and of the "international com-munity" in Haiti. That meant that less attention was being paid to problems like cholera, which continued its grim march forward in the absence of consensus regarding comprehensive prevention and care. Electoral squabbles also took away energy that should have gone to resettlement and rebuilding. By the one-year anniversary, the numbers in camps had declined, but between eight hundred thousand and a million Haitians remained without safe shelter. Al-though Parc Jean-Marie Vincent was now full of makeshift restau-rants and beauty parlors and cell-phone distributors, it was as teeming and precarious as ever.

The Port-au-Prince–based team, including Drs. Louise Ivers, Anany Prosper, and the Kobels, was still working in the camps. But conditions were difficult. We did not have, as Stephen Smith had discovered in his research for the *Globe*, any sort of exit plan. Yet we were sick of hearing the words "exit plan" from disaster-relief NGOs and "shelter specialists" and "internally displaced persons experts." How could we leave when most of the conditions that had first led us to work in the camps persisted a year after the quake? Then again, we had also failed to install proper sanitation in the camps.

We disdained glib talk of exit plans and "sustainability" but still lacked a sound strategy for delivering better services as the crisis caravan moved on to the next humanitarian disaster. The actor Sean Penn, working since the quake in the only camp larger than Parc Jean-Marie Vincent, had better ideas and more commitment to implementing them than did many of the self-described experts. One of our modest ideas—to find educational opportunities for young Haitians in African universities—was already bearing fruit: the first five Haitian students were already enrolled, by January 12, 2011, in the National University of Rwanda. But south-south collaboration of this sort would not solve the problems in the quake zone.

We needed new ideas, as our colleagues said to Stephen Smith. The *Globe* article described the dilemma of seeking to deliver better services in temporary settlements:

> "You have to adjust to the situation; you have to have new ideas," said Dr. Anany Gretchko Prosper, the Haiti-born physician who runs the medical operations of Partners In Health in Port-au-Prince. "The priority is to keep the patient alive."
>
> The clinic treats babies, children, pregnant women, adults, the mentally troubled. A pharmacy dispenses drugs; a lab performs tests.
>
> But the staff works in a clutch of steamy tents, with no prospect of anything more permanent. When Partners In Health approached the government about erecting a more substantial structure, Haitian officials demurred, wary of anything that suggests the tent camps are enduring fixtures.
>
> And the clinic lacks the full complement of social and economic services that are the hallmark of Partners In Health in the countryside, where the diseases of poverty are treated, as well as their festering

causes. Internally, the charity is grappling with its long-term presence in Port-au-Prince.

"Some people inside of PIH, like me, we think that if we stay in Port-au-Prince, we have to implement the full package," Prosper said, citing surgical and orthopedic services as examples. "We cannot continue to give health care under a tent. At midday, it's [more than 100 degrees] inside, you understand?"

---

I was full of admiration for Anany and the Kobels and for all our colleagues working in these steamy tents day after day, month after month. I though of them often on the anniversary.

The first ceremony I attended that morning took place in an empty lot downtown, where the Haitian version of the IRS had stood before the quake. Any evidence of the big white building that once filled the site was gone: the lot was razed and raked flat. A couple of tents had been erected for the ceremony. It wasn't yet 100 degrees underneath them, but it would be soon. President Clinton, Laura Graham, and others on Clinton's staff were there, as were President Préval and members of his government. A bugler, perhaps one of the surviving members of the military band mentioned by Oscar Arias in his long-ago, upbeat op-ed about the dissolution of the Haitian army, played taps; two women in traditional white Haitian dresses sang a mournful song written for the occasion; several speeches struck a solemn note. Distracted and thinking of all I had seen over the preceding 365 days and wondering what other friends and colleagues were doing to mark the anniversary, I knew I wouldn't remember the speeches. (Tom White's funeral service had been only 24 hours earlier, and it seemed long ago and far away.)

Claire Pierre and I left the formal ceremony early to visit the General Hospital, only a few blocks away. It would be President Clinton's next stop and we'd promised to meet him there. We passed the site of the Ministry of Health; it too had been cleared of debris, belying oft-heard claims that no rubble had been removed. The ruins of the palace, on the other hand, looked untouched, and most estimates concluded that less than 20 percent of the quake debris throughout Port-au-Prince had been cleared.[3]

The General Hospital was bustling that morning. Dr. Lassègue and Miss Thompson were there, as were a handful of die-hard American volunteers, including a former student from Harvard Medical School who is now an infectious disease doctor, marking a year of service to the hospital and its patients.[4] Most of the disaster relief organizations were long gone. The hospital showed no signs of reconstruction, only a new tent—the cholera treatment unit. President Clinton came by to cheer the staff and volunteers, and to pledge support for the planned reconstruction promised by the governments of France and the United States. "It looks a lot better now than the last time I was here," he said. It was true. Clinton's public comments at the hospital were largely about AIDS and tuberculosis drugs, but he also praised the American Red Cross and Dr. Lassègue for working together to help keep the General Hospital employees at their posts during the tough year since the quake.

I didn't say so then, but knew, as President Clinton did, that only steady and patient accompaniment of the Haitian officials in charge of the hospital would get it rebuilt and improve the quality of the care and training there. Patient accompaniment had never been a strong suit of foreign aid—much less the crisis caravan—but that didn't mean, as Clinton reminded us, that we couldn't change the aid system itself. If billions of dollars had been raised for Haiti by private charities and relief groups, there had to be better ways of getting money into the hands of those working in tough postings like these.

The rest of the day went by in a haze. The indefatigable President Clinton went on to two more commemorative events—at one of them, Prime Minister Bellerive spoke of 316,000 dead—and then to visit a women's economic recovery initiative. But for those of a less formidable constitution, it was time for solitary reflection. Not feeling prayerful, I retreated to Maryse's house to contemplate the year quietly and alone.

The next day, I boomeranged back to Boston after Loune, my brother-in-law, and I made a brief visit to the beautiful school

Maryse and her husband had helped build not far from one of the planned cities that had still not been started. We'd hoped to make it to Mirebalais, but were short on time: our colleagues and supporters in Boston were also gathering to mark the one-year anniversary. We expected a big crowd, including some Haitians who, like Sanley, had received care in Boston. Claire wanted to go too, but she was working full-time as the health lead with the Recovery Commission, and so stayed behind.[5]

The theme of the Boston commemoration was "Remember, Reflect, Respond." The remember part was difficult. The invasive images and sounds and smells and textures of those first few days after the quake had faded, which was good and bad and surely necessary. All of us tried to forget. But some memories were well worth summoning because they could remind us how much humans can offer one another in times of distress. These memories included heroic attempts at rescue and relief, and (when successful) the beauty, skill, and passion of these efforts. But they also included things no one would wish to encounter again: images we see in nightmares and intrusive thoughts; sounds like the slow creaking of a roof starting to fall, then the thunder of its rapid collapse upon the living, the cries of pain from underneath the rubble, the persistent groans of the injured and dying; and lingering impressions of touch, which in those days ran the gamut from the punch of bone-breaking cement, to the urgent tug of hands seeking to save those trapped, to the gentle or sometimes sharply honed touch of skilled medical care. Some, spared against long odds, can still taste January 12 as the unfamiliar flavor of relief or gratitude. Most still taste the bitter dregs of sorrow.

Whether gathered in Port-au-Prince, Cange, Kigali, or Boston, we survivors contemplated the pain of others. Some lost limbs, many lost family, and perhaps everyone lost a bit of innocence about the possible dimensions of a collision between bad luck and longstanding unfairness. Others found themselves transported over and over again to a house of pain, pinned under the fallen beams of oppressive memory.

Pragmatic solidarity from many corners of the world came to lift the weight of disaster from its victims. Haiti's plight inspired many efforts, some chronicled, however incompletely, in this book. All the doctors and nurses and first responders were grateful to those whose generosity allowed us to serve as best we could. We could have done better, certainly, and can do better in the future. We *must* do better at reconstruction than we have to date. We need to draw on every noble sentiment and every bit of technical skill to make Port-au-Prince a livable city and to make "build back better" more than an empty slogan.

Some recovery efforts are well underway. The new teaching hospital in Mirebalais is a third of the way completed, with hundreds of workers on site already. To some, the hospital is just a building in progress, one project among many. But for me it's emblematic of both our aspiration to rebuild better and our respect for the Haitian people and their story. We hope it will be a temple that will reflect both our respect and love for the fallen, those named and unnamed, and our desire to make the fruits of science and the art of healing more readily available to Haitians. The scars left by the earthquake are lasting; may the effects of the solidarity it provoked be permanent as well.

*Port-au-Prince and Boston*
*January 12–15, 2011*

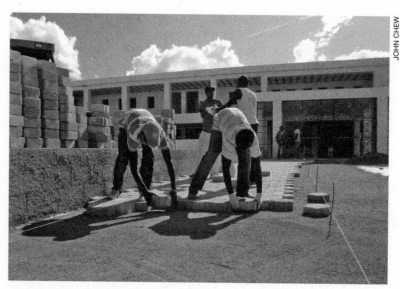

*Construction workers laying the front walkway to the Mirebalais hospital, January 2012*

# AFTERWORD
## March 31, 2012

*B*y the time these words are printed, two and a half years will have passed since the earthquake. The second anniversary of the quake was marked by solemn ceremonies in Port-au-Prince and elsewhere. Having attended some of these, and been part of the somber parade of survivors and still-grieving families, I was anxious to mark the date with something other than, or at least in addition to, crepe and mourning. To this end, I left one such ceremony, a chance to mourn friends and colleagues lost two years previously, and headed back to Cange.

Cange was, on January 12, 2012, much the same as ever: crowded with patients and doctors and nurses and teachers. All of us allowed ourselves more than a bit of optimism, since our colleague Garry Conille, a fellow public health physician and leader of the UN Office of the Special Envoy for Haiti, had been named Prime Minister in October 2011. He was the third candidate advanced by Michel Martelly, a well-known singer who had won the presidency with 700,000 votes less than a year after the quake. It was a tenuous union, we would later learn, but an asset to our efforts to improve the public-sector health system. We needed a proper Ministry of Health to do our work, and Conille named a Minister, Dr. Florence Guillaume, shortly after he was approved by the Haitian parliament. These were welcome developments, in part because we knew that Guillaume is committed to building robust health infrastructure for the entire nation. Along with the Prime Minister, she was skeptical about NGOs operating on their own but completely sanguine about the need for them.

All of us who had labored after the quake, in the General Hospital and in camps, had hungered for expert assistance. We had hungered for saviors. Although they never really appeared, we still hoped for major recovery efforts, for vast public works, for deep private investments in infrastructure. Personally, I kept thinking of the city of Kigali, with its skyscrapers and cranes and clean streets and bustling small businesses. I wasn't confident that Port-au-Prince should be a city of high-rises; not at all. But all of us were anxious for some tangible evidence of recovery and renewal.

Conditions in Haiti are harsh, but improving, and that's cause for some satisfaction and perhaps revision of the skepticism that runs through the preceding pages. It's only fair to acknowledge that I may be saying this to give hope to those who read this afterword, especially those working to help rebuild Haiti. We all know the phrase: hope is not a plan. But hope is, in this line of work, a necessary ingredient. My time in Port-au-Prince, Mirebalais, Cange, and Saint-Marc, and meetings with Haitian officials in the trailers that still serve as the offices of the country's leading health and development experts, and even the recent commemorations of the two-year anniversary of the quake, gave me hope—hope worth sharing with all those who support a vision of building back better in Haiti.

The latest figures tracked by our UN office show that 52.9 percent of the funds pledged to Haiti for 2010–2011 have been disbursed.[1] Disbursement is a far cry from implementation, but that's not bad compared to the record after the 2008 hurricane season (15 percent of pledges disbursed) or to other pledging sessions before that. Many more of these recovery funds—about 10 percent—have gone through channels managed by the Haitian government, compared to initial post-quake humanitarian aid (0.3 percent). These seem like steps in the right direction, even if we've a long way to go.

As I write in March 2012, Haiti is again in a fragile political situation. Our colleague Garry Conille, who served as President Martelly's Prime Minister for the past four months, has just stepped down. The Interim Haiti Recovery Commission, envisioned as coordinating international assistance, was not renewed by parliament when its mandate ended in October 2012. Ongoing political skirmishes test the confidence of many supporters and investors.

Yet there are also reasons to be hopeful. Yesterday, I traveled around the country with President Clinton and a group of renewable-energy investors and entrepreneurs. President Clinton, who remains a stalwart and pragmatic advocate, secured the promises of a half-dozen top executives to invest in Haiti's infrastructure and then announced that he will be back in a month or so with a group of investors interested in tourism.

Although the streets of Port-au-Prince are still strewn with rubble (about half of it had been cleared by the two-year anniversary), ambitious infrastructure projects have cropped up across the city. Most are private-sector endeavors, such as hotels and small businesses. With investments from the United States, the Inter-American Development Bank, and a South Korean textile company, ground has been broken on an industrial park outside the northern city of Cap Haïtien. The project will create, we're told, tens of thousands of permanent jobs in the garment industry and other manufacturing sectors, in addition to the construction jobs it will generate.[2] It is the hope of progressive and engaged allies of the Haitian people that these jobs will be well paid and that these plants, unlike most of their predecessors, will be "green" and pro-poor. Certainly, with unemployment still in excess of 50 percent, there will be long lines when the factories start hiring.

New jobs in manufacturing are one thing, but what about the vast machinery of foreign aid and humanitarian work? Two years after the earthquake, and nearly thirty years after I first came to Haiti, I believe that the only way to create durable and transformative change—to break the cycle of disease and poverty holding hostage the lives of millions of Haitians—is through the approach that my colleagues and I have termed *accompaniment*. During his short tenure as Prime Minister, Garry Conille had committed to this approach. He would say in meeting after meeting that the goal of any international assistance should be the "transfer of functions" to a Haitian counterpart. He asked for direct investment in Haitian organizations and government agencies. When he met recently with the largest international NGOs in Washington, D.C., he listened to their concerns about weakness and lack of expertise in the government and then asked them to help be a part of the solution. He wanted them to pay for senior staff and advisors in the ministries, in order to develop platforms for improved management and transparency and expertise within the government so that they could do the jobs for which the population is holding them accountable.

A brigade of people now share this understanding that what Haiti needs most is accompaniment. Many of the most effective *accompagnateurs* are mentioned in this book—President Clinton chief among them, but also those like Loune Viaud, Denis O'Brien, and Louise Ivers. Some others I have just come to know—including President Martelly and the first lady, the leaders of the UN in Haiti, UN Resident Coordinator Nigel Fisher, and UN Special Representative to the Secretary-General, Mariano Fernandez. These colleagues and scores of others have stated their commitment to Haitian institutions and leaders, and are pushing themselves and everyone they work with to think in large-scale and transformative ways. If these lessons have been learned, it is nonetheless true that there's a long way to go before they're implemented. On many scores, progress seems slow: the collapsed portions of the General Hospital haven't been cleared, much less restored, and efforts to rebuild the nursing school and other training infrastructure have yet to be launched. When I feel discouraged about the pace of building back better, I return often to one project described throughout this book: the Mirebalais teaching hospital.

First envisioned as a community hospital, the Mirebalais facility has been transformed—in most senses, by the quake—into a national teaching and referral hospital. It will be prepared to receive patients by mid-2012. To see, in the largest city on the Central Plateau, a gleaming hospital and medical campus taking shape across what was once a bit of broken terrain running from steep conical hills down to an unproductive rice paddy—more of a swamp, really—would be a stirring image for any visitor. But it is especially moving for anyone who remembers Partners In Health's modest and often discouraging beginnings a few hundred yards down the road almost thirty years ago. Mirebalais was just a sleepy town when we started trying to deliver quality medical services to people in great need of them.

It is not easy to admit, even today: we tried and mostly failed. Sometimes we succeeded: a child with acute malaria who received chloroquine, a man with scabies who received the right topical medication, a woman whose fractured bone was set with competence and compassion. But when we look back honestly at our first years of hard work and eighteen-hour days, we cannot claim to have done a good job delivering quality health services. We were delivering something as hard and fast as we could. But surely the quality of the deliverables matters more than the good intentions of the caregivers or the pace of their work.

Haunted by mediocrity, we keep returning to the task of improving the quality of care. But good medical care cannot be readily delivered in poor-quality hospitals and clinics. After the quake, all of us were forced to rethink our plans to build another hospital that would be good by Haitian standards, even if not by the highest international standards. Back to the drawing board: this is what is meant by "build back better." Health care and education are far from the only services needed, of course, but they remain important entry points for development. The Mirebalais hospital has created thousands of jobs, many of them permanent. It will also introduce new technologies into Haiti's public sector: when completed, it may be the largest solar-powered hospital in the developing world.

Those who have worked to bring Mirebalais into being have high aspirations for rebuilding in general. What needs to happen to make building back better more than a slogan? Sticking with the example of a hospital is illustrative of challenges in all sectors. We can take on ambitious projects and see them through to fruition as long as we have three kinds of resources. Financial ones, of course. How else could we build (let alone run) a modern hospital in a place where clean water, electricity, and modern infrastructure are all but absent? Modern medical resources, obviously enough. How could we deliver modern medicine without clinics and hospitals and the tools of the trade—preventives and diagnostics and therapeutics—readily available to those who need them, regardless of ability to pay? But we also need human resources: committed doctors and nurses and managers, and those who comprise the greatest number of employees on our payroll—the people who run labs, take x-rays, and deliver services within the homes and villages of our patients, and those who transport patients and specimens, who service and repair equipment, who tend to the needs of patients and fellow employees alike.

The human resources challenge is perhaps greatest. Rural Haiti has long lacked trained medical professionals; even before the 2010 earthquake, most studies on this topic suggested that the majority of Haiti's physicians and nurses had left the country altogether and that those who remained were concentrated in the capital city. (The dean of Haiti's oldest and largest medical school said publicly that 80 percent of medically trained Haitians now reside outside the country.) The loss of Haiti's nursing school to the 2010 quake, along with heavy damage to other institutions of medical education, worsened the situation.

But launching new programs in a district or two is never enough: once services are offered to the poor anywhere, the notion of "catchment area" or "district" falls apart until such programs are brought to national scale. This is the great dilemma of every Minister of Health, including Dr. Guillaume and Dr. Agnes Binagwaho, Minister of Health in Rwanda. They can and do encourage pilot programs and local initiatives, but they must also imagine, or reimagine, health care delivery at the national level.

Every effort to lift the standards of medical care available to the poor brings new challenges. Hospitals, along with health centers and community-based care, are the bedrock of every health system, but they are large, expensive, complex institutions to run. The complexity of hospital-based care is one of the reasons global public health starts with the low-hanging fruit. Low cost, high return: that's why public health practitioners are always pushing bednets, vaccines, family planning, prenatal care, hand washing, and latrines.

But the more difficult health and development problems, the higher-hanging fruit—from drug-resistant tuberculosis, mental illness, and cancer to lack of education, clean water, roads, and food security—cannot simply be wished away by the gurus of cost-effectiveness (the ones with the tiny resource pies). The low-hanging fruit hangs, after all, under a larger canopy of fruit. Do the models now dominant in global health and development permit us to harvest the higher-hanging fruit? Can we address more of the need?

The short answer: of course we can, with innovation and resolve and a bolder vision than has been registered in decades.

For one thing, practitioners of development too often lapse into competition when partnership and cooperation are needed. This fairly recent history highlights that we are all—the poor and those who serve them—socialized for scarcity. To return to Mirebalais: some part of the brain assumes that if a new hospital gets the lion's share of attention—if it actually becomes a flagship project—then another effort will suffer. But in our best moments, all of us know that this sort of thinking is wrongheaded. A teaching hospital in Mirebalais will not drag down the quality of care in other settings but, rather, will lift it up. We are so socialized for scarcity that we assume that if we focus on educating doctors, we will neglect educating nurses (to say nothing of other health professionals, from laboratory technicians to community health workers to teachers); that if we focus on cholera vaccination, we will neglect water and sanitation; that if we focus on research and teaching, service will suffer—when, again, we know in our best moments that simply adding training and research components to a service project, even one as straightforward as treating acute childhood malnutrition, will improve outcomes.

Investing in small business or new health infrastructure or schools in resource-poor settings again breaks down the notion of "catchment areas." Where joblessness is the status quo, building a new hospital can bring disappointment to some because so many people in the district, and the surrounding ones, want to work there—and usually not because they want a better job but because they want a job, period. Poor Haitians are of course also socialized for scarcity: they assume that if someone else gets a job, even someone in their own family, then they themselves will not.

This sort of limited-good, zero-sum thinking is to be expected among the poor, who know firsthand that the good usually is limited in impoverished settings. But it is unacceptable among goodwill groups (foreign and homegrown) and development experts seeking to attack poverty. Few of us have endured real scarcity or lived on the edge of survival. Yet many "experts" display a worshipful regard for cost-effectiveness analysis, often without rigorous assessment of either cost (how big or rigid is the pie, really?) or effectiveness (how might we measure the long-term impact of harvesting high-hanging fruit?). Those of us who consider ourselves public health experts need to scrutinize the movement of capital as closely as we do the movement of microbes. If we've learned anything from the past decade, it's that the resource pies dedicated to fighting global scourges like AIDS or poverty are not fixed, but can and must be expanded.

Finally, a word about cholera. As noted in Chapter 7, it was obvious in the weeks after *V. cholerae* hit Haiti that international and Haitian medical and relief teams needed to mobilize all effective deliverables and pull together all potential partners to prevent a major epidemic in the Americas. We failed to do that, and Haiti is now home to the world's largest cholera epidemic in recent history. Socialization for scarcity has had its usual pernicious effects in responding to cholera: water projects have been pitted against vaccination, one form of treatment against another. Has the window closed? As we've argued from the beginning of the epidemic, an aggressive and integrated approach might lead in a decade or so to the eradication of this disease, which was previously unknown in Haiti and the Dominican Republic.[3] An integrative approach could help in other cholera hot spots around the globe, too.

The Haitian Ministry of Health has vocally supported the modest vaccine roll-out that Zanmi Lasante is initiating in April 2012 in concert with the ministry and with GHESKIO. Integrating vaccination into an ambitious water and sanitation effort would surely reduce fatality rates and slow the epidemic. That in itself would be a victory. But it is also necessary to bring down the price of the vaccine and relevant medications and to help develop a global stockpile of vaccine. We hope to show how this cholera vaccine roll-out might strengthen the national vaccination program and generate new knowledge about combating cholera and other vaccine-preventable diseases in Haiti and elsewhere in Latin America, Africa, and Asia.

This won't be easy. The rainy season begins in April; we will need to do meticulous monitoring and evaluation. But we are confident that service delivery, coupled with training and research, and enriched through partnerships—with the Ministry of Health, with GHESKIO, with U.S. research universities of global repute—offers a way forward with more than a small chance of meeting some of our goals.

I am reminded daily that a lethal and growing epidemic is raging in Haiti—sickening and killing thousands of people (mostly the poor, of course). It is no surprise that there is a good deal of discussion about blame and recrimination.[4] None of it interests me as much as taking immediate, bold action to stop the spread of cholera, which we know how to do. We will all be to blame if we fail to take this moment to show that we can think and act differently, to show that we can respond collaboratively, using the best technologies available, to an urgent crisis. Over the past year, global bodies have spent over $150 million on cholera treatment and prevention efforts—important work, but unlikely to stop the epidemic and eradicate it from Haiti. What's needed are two critical additional measures: one difficult and expensive—the creation of a safe water and sanitation system for Haiti (something that the international community has promised for decades and never delivered)—and the much simpler intervention of providing an adequate amount of the oral cholera vaccine, which has been proven safe and effective.

Obviously, building the infrastructure for a clean water supply would cost a great deal more than that, but we should not forget that $2 billion was pledged after the quake and has not yet been disbursed. There are aid agencies, NGOs, and philanthropists spending money on other projects, and pots of money that have yet to be allocated. In fact, some of these funds are committed to disparate water projects, but what is needed, as argued in this book, is a massive effort to bring modern sanitation and water systems to every city, town, and village in Haiti.

———

No project of any kind should be circumscribed by the fallacious notion that goodness is a limited commodity. We need to expand the notion of good and the standard of excellence. We need to embrace the idea that one flagship project might raise the aspirations of all of our efforts.

On a philosophical level, none of this is news. In his superb biography of William James, Bob Richardson (husband of American writer Annie Dillard, and a wonderful writer in his own right) quotes James saying:

> Spinoza long ago wrote in his Ethics that anything that a man can avoid under the notion that it is bad he may also avoid under the notion that something else is good. He who acts habitually *sub specie mali*, under the negative notion, the notion of the bad, was called a slave by Spinoza. To him who acts habitually under the notion of good he gives the name of freeman. See to it now, I beg you, that you make freemen of your pupils by habituating them to act, whenever possible, under the notion of a good.[5]

Acting under the notion of good does not provide us with a ready-made strategic plan. But it does help us cultivate the hope and optimism—the "meliorism"—that underpin efforts to raise the standard of living available to all Haitians; to launch, continue, or finish ambitious rebuilding projects; and to stand with Haiti as it struggles to recover after the earthquake in the coming decade—and the ones beyond it.

That there will be more shocks, of one sort or another, is clear enough. As of March 2012, we have found much to deplore but also much to celebrate—even if there is not, technically, a government in place. President Clinton was there to push renewable energy—solar and wind, especially—as a means of bringing electricity to even the most remote villages. He also reminded us that Haiti's electrical costs were among the highest in the world. And we went to some of those remote villages and towns. This trip was particularly gratifying for me. We returned to Boucan Carré, with its array of solar-powered hospital, clinics, and schools. I was thinking, of course, of Walt Ratterman, whose commitment to "solar," as he called it, lived on in those who, since his death, had outfitted a dozen more schools and clinics in Haiti alone. I was thinking of my protégé, Mario Pagenel, who would've been thrilled to see Mirebalais hospital—and even more pleased, I'd bet, to know that we had launched a new training program in family practice, as he had exhorted us to do.

Soon we left Boucan Carré for Mirebalais, which meant we would cross the modest bridge, which said so much about the potential for partnership. The Mirebalais hospital sprawled across a small dell like a temple, gleaming white and girdled by black Haitian ironwork. Clinton spoke about the hospital as an example of what could be done in short order, and against long odds. We returned to Port-au-Prince for a dinner with leaders in the renewable energy sector. The mood, at least then and there, was upbeat. Suddenly, conversations were interrupted by a low rumble, and the ground shook for a second. Many of the first-time visitors to Haiti did not realize that this was yet another aftershock, but the Haitian waiters and those who'd been living and working in Haiti rushed out of the building. Within minutes, someone reported that the temblor had measured 4.7 on the Richter scale.

Haiti is not of course the only country visited by earthquakes. This particular aftershock caused no damage, but it occurred almost a year to the day after a quake wreaked great havoc in Japan. Evan Osnos, writing in *The New Yorker*, had this to say about that disaster and its storied aftermath: "The moment that Japan remembers as 3/11 was not one disaster but three—an earthquake, a tsunami and a nuclear meltdown. And then there was the repercussion that nobody expected in the rush of stoicism and sacrifice that so impressed the world. As evidence piled up of government failures—coverups, bureaucratic paralysis, an industry that disguised honest assessments of risks—Japan's confidence in the political establishment that has created its modern miracle collapsed: the 'fourth disaster of March 11,' as one commentator puts it. . . . The Fukushima meltdowns shattered trust in nuclear power in Japan and elsewhere, and it's not clear how much of that will recover."[6]

Haiti has not, of course, experienced any miracles in almost two centuries. But it was and will always be the locus of a genuine miracle of modernity: the fight against slavery and for equality. The cost of this fight was great and enduring, as any Haitian will remind you. Although Haiti has no nuclear industry to damage, it too has known a collapse, decades old, in confidence in its political establishment; and it has yet to find confidence in the broader political and economic world in which it is enmeshed. The 2010 quake has been followed by other disasters, including a runaway cholera epidemic and a failure to invest sufficiently in rebuilding the institutions that any country needs to protect its citizens from want and danger. This work, the project of the Haitian people, continues to call out for unstinting support undergirded by respect and solidarity. There is little doubt that such a project is well within the reach of all people of goodwill.

*Port-au-Prince*
*March 31, 2012*

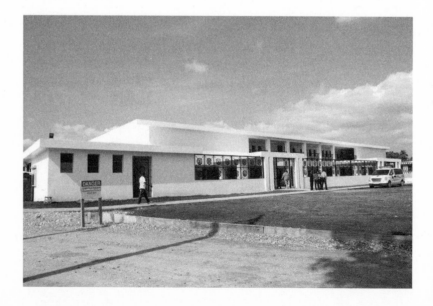

# Other
# Voices

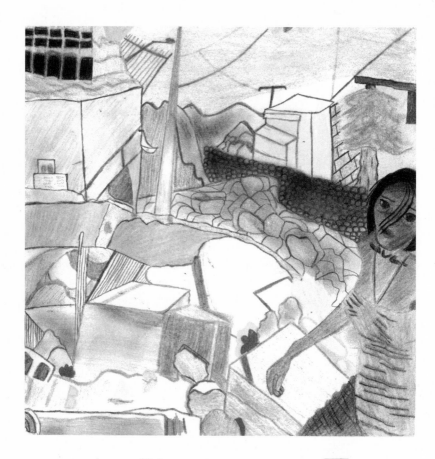

## Haïtian Distress

I drew this picture for my father's book about the Haïtian earthquake. On the girl's face, you can see the expression of worry. She has lost her whole family, and she is looking for their bodies in the rocks.

—CATHERINE BERTRAND FARMER

# LÒT BÒ DLO, THE OTHER SIDE OF THE WATER

## EDWIDGE DANTICAT

I was in a supermarket in Miami's Little Haiti neighborhood with my two young daughters when my cell phone rang.

"Edwidge, are you home?" asked my former sister-in-law, Carole, whose birthplace—Kingston, Jamaica—has a history with earthquakes.

"No," I told her. "I'm in the supermarket with the girls."

"You haven't heard then?" she asked.

"Heard what?"

"There's been an earthquake in Haiti."

"An earthquake in Haiti?" I said this so loud that a few people stopped to look at me. Being in Little Haiti meant that many of the people working and shopping at the supermarket were Haitian. One or two nodded as if to confirm what I was hearing. They already knew, I realized. Others immediately began dialing their own cell phones as if to get further clarification for themselves.

Although I had been hearing and reading about a possible massive earthquake in Port-au-Prince for years, it always seemed beyond the realm of possibility. It simply seemed inconceivable that an earthquake could rattle the country—my country, even though I had not lived there consistently for thirty years, since I was twelve years old.

"I'm watching CNN now," Carole said. "They're saying the earthquake is 7.0."

The significance of that number did not immediately register. A 7.0 earthquake might cause little damage in one place, while it could devastate another. It all depended on the population density and the capability of structures to withstand the shaking.

"They're saying it's catastrophic," Carole explained.

Catastrophic, I could understand.

"Just get home," she said. "I'll call you later."

Soon after she hung up, my cell phone started ringing nonstop.

My husband, ever so cautious, asked when I picked up, "Where are you?"

"In the car," I said, not sure how I had gotten myself and the girls and the groceries in there.

He wasn't sure I knew and he didn't want to worry me. I brought it up myself while keeping my ears tuned to National Public Radio.

"I'm calling everyone in Haiti," he finally said, "but I'm not getting through."

During the drive home, I looked out the window but could barely see the brightly colored homes and storefronts of Little Haiti. Dusk comes quickly on January nights, and this night was no different. Still, it felt as if dark clouds had swallowed the day a lot faster than usual.

My heart was racing as I started running down, in my mind, a list of the people that I would need to call, e-mail, text, or fax to check on in Haiti. At that moment, the list of aunts and cousins and friends in different parts of the country seemed endless. Most of them lived in Léogâne (the epicenter of the earthquake), Carrefour, and the eye of the storm—because of its population density and its ever precarious buildings—Port-au-Prince.

I tried to think of the most efficient way to learn about the greatest number of people. It would be best, I told myself, to call several people who would have news of everyone else, the family leaders, if you will. My cousin Maxo was one of those people.

Maxo had lived in the United States for nearly twenty-five years before returning to Haiti in the 1990s. At sixty-two, he had been married several times and had eleven children ranging in age from forty-two to fifteen months. He was a generous, lively, and over-indulgent soul who had taken over the family homestead after his dad had died in 2004. Maxo and five of his youngest children and his wife were living in Bel Air, the poor hillside neighborhood where I grew up. Maxo's was the first number I dialed at a red light on the way home. I heard a strange sound on the other end of the line, not quite silence, but not quite a busy signal either, something like air flowing through a metal tube or thick cloth.

When I got home, my husband was in front of the television watching CNN as he dialed and redialed his mother's cell phone number in Les Cayes, a southern town more than a hundred miles from Port-au-Prince. The television screen showed a map of Haiti with a bull's eye on Carrefour, where my husband's two uncles live. There were no images yet of the devastation, just phone and studio interviews with earthquake experts, journalists, and the occasional survivor (often via Skype) by the ever-changing news anchors. The Haiti-based eyewitnesses were describing a catastrophic scene, in which the presidential palace and several other government build-ings had collapsed. Churches, schools, and hospitals had also crum-bled, they said, killing and burying a countless number of people. Aftershocks were continuing, prompting a tsunami warning. The earthquake, we learned, had probably been caused by a strike-slip fault, where one side of a vertical fault slides past the other. It was barely six miles deep, leaving little cushion between the fault and the houses precariously perched upon the earth. (Later, we would find out that the earthquake was caused by a previously undetected fault, leaving the potentially cataclysmic danger of the other faults intact.)

"It was as if the earth itself had become liquid," one survivor said, "like the ocean."

On Twitter, the Port-au-Prince-based hotelier and musician Rich-ard Morse announced that the Hotel Montana was gone. My hus-band and I had stayed at the Montana several times, often with our oldest daughter in tow. Entire neighborhoods had slid downhill, others reported, each row of houses pressing down on the next in a deadly domino effect. Daniel Morel, a veteran Haitian photojournal-ist, sent out some of the first pictures online: pancaked buildings and dust-covered silhouettes stumbling out of the rubble, many bloodied and nearly dead.

My husband and I kept dialing the phone numbers of friends and relatives in Haiti and getting no response. While keeping an eye on the television and an ear to a local Haitian radio program, we managed to get some dinner together for the girls, who at first did not seem to understand what all the fuss was about.

Before falling asleep, however, my oldest daughter, Mira, asked if her grandmother was okay. We tried to reassure her as best as we could, but we did not know ourselves whether my mother-in-law— who often traveled from Les Cayes to Carrefour—was alive, or whether anyone we knew was alive.

The routine became (1) dial phone numbers of friends and relatives in Haiti; (2) go online—including social networking sites—for a bit more information; (3) dial friends and relatives all over the United States and Canada, who were also dialing and checking networking sites, and ask, "Have you heard from anyone?" They had not.

No new information was coming through the radio or television. The news was breaking all evening, but the same information was being repeated. U.S. State Department spokesman P. J. Crowley told CNN that we should expect "serious loss of life."

Occasionally, my cousin Maxo's phone would ring when I dialed it.

I tried texting.

No reply either.

I then got a call from the producers of AC360, CNN anchor Anderson Cooper's signature show. They had found me through my publisher and wanted to know whether I would come on the show.

"What will I say?" I asked my husband.

"What you feel," he said.

What I was feeling was nearly indescribable even for a writer. I was extremely worried about my loved ones, but I was also feeling a deep sense of dread, a paralyzing fear that everything was gone, that Haiti no longer existed, that the entire country had been destroyed.

We had been watching Haiti's ambassador to the United States, Raymond Joseph, on CNN and other media outlets. He had explained not only the gravity of the current situation but also a bit of Haiti's history and how Haitian fighters, after they had gained their independence from France in 1804, had traveled throughout the world, including to Greece, Latin America, and the United States, and had helped others gain their independence.

"This is the worst day in Haiti's history," he said. Haiti has helped the world before. Now it was the world's turn to help Haiti.

"Ask for help, too," my husband said. "The country's going to need lots of help."

Ask for help, I kept telling myself, as I sat in the satellite studio in Miami Beach waiting to go on Anderson Cooper's show. I had no word from anyone in Haiti. The phone calls were still not going through. We had only heard rumors of some famous Haitians having died in the earthquake. Many of those rumors would later prove untrue.

Also on AC360 was Wyclef Jean, the internationally known musician, who had also moved from Haiti to the Unites States as a child. I felt like sobbing when Anderson Cooper turned to me on the monitor and said, "Edwidge, I know you have been trying to get in touch with your family as well. Have you had any luck?" I explained that I had not.

In some circles, many of us who were asked and went on television that night, the next morning, and in the days that followed were accused of trying to make heroes of ourselves. However, I will never regret this particular media outing because one of my maternal cousins would later tell me that he had somehow managed to see that program on his cell phone while lying on a blanket on the street in front of his flattened house in Léogâne. Before that, he said, he'd thought that the earthquake had happened all over the world and had feared that even if we'd managed to survive it in Miami, we might still be in mortal danger from the announced-then-called-off tsunami. He had been as worried about me as I'd been about him. We laugh about this now, but it makes perfect sense because one of the first videos broadcast after the earthquake was of a young girl watching a cloud of dust rise up to the hills from a broken Port-au-Prince and screaming, "The world is coming to an end!"

"This is probably one of the darkest nights in our history," I managed to tell Anderson and his viewers that night. "We're going to need an extraordinary amount of help in the days and months and years to come. I think the whole country basically is going to need rebuilding. And people who are the poorest of the poor, least able to withstand something like this, are suffering. And we absolutely need help. We desperately, desperately need help."

After the program ended and other programs began, the dark night dragged on. My brother-in-law came over with some friends and we put together a kind of command center, trying to make our efforts at reaching loved ones more efficient. We were still watching the television news programs, but some of us were now delegated to the phones and others to the computer and the radio stations.

Around midnight, we managed to reach my mother-in-law on her cell phone in Les Cayes. There had been  no damage where she was in Les Cayes, but she was still feeling tremors.

"The ground is shaking," she kept saying. "The ground is shaking."

Her radio transmission had gone off that afternoon and she knew very little about what was happening in Port-au-Prince and the surrounding areas. We told her the little we knew and she was shocked. Before she could ask about her brothers in Carrefour, we were cut off. We would not be able to reach her again for five days.

With daylight the next morning came the first vivid images of the devastation. Piles of rubble were everywhere, many with both frozen corpses and moving limbs peeking out of them. Watching a video of one trapped little boy reaching for his mother from a pancaked house, I saw the little hand and cried. Little did I know then that my cousin Maxo and his ten-year-old son Nozial had already died and that three of Maxo's other children—including the fifteen-month-old—would be trapped in the rubble for two days before being rescued.

Perhaps because the images of the helplessly trapped were so hard to take, a lot of the television news coverage quickly shifted to successful foreign-led professional rescues. Many months later, I was surprised to learn that fewer than two hundred people had been rescued by professional rescuers. The rest, like Maxo's wife and children, had been saved by their Haitian friends and neighbors.

As for the foreign-led rescues, even if the rescued person died an hour or a day later, that person's predicament needed a dramatic arch, not unlike the short stories and novels that someone like me might write. The viewer needed an ending, and it had to be uplifting so that he or she could continue to watch the heart-crumpling rest. Of the many stories that might have been too devastating to watch are some that my family members told me: of hundreds of people who individually or in small groups kept vigil near a pile of rubble and spoke to their buried loved ones as they slipped away, dying an agonizing death so close, yet beyond reach. Of the trapped loved ones who exhorted their family members to go and leave them behind, to go on with their lives. Among the many things that are haunting about this disaster is to think about how many people could have been, might have been saved, if only love and good will could have rescued them all, if only there had been the right equipment ... if only ... if only ...

Since January 12, 2010, I have often been asked what it was like to experience the earthquake from a distance. Was it traumatic?

Frankly, I have seen too many people who've been irreparably scarred by both physical and psychological wounds to say that I have suffered many. It would be disrespectful to equate my pain and bereavement with that of those who nearly lost their lives and sanity to the devastation.

The Sunday following the earthquake, I took my girls to a service at a large Protestant church in Little Haiti. I had not attended church for some time and was craving that sense of community and solace that it could offer at moments like this. An earthquake survivor, a Baptist minister, had found his way to us and was telling what had now become the familiar story of hundreds of thousands of corpses, most of them picked up with earthmovers to be carried to mass graves.

As the minister was speaking, the woman sitting in front of me, in her early forties and the mother of two small children, like me, became increasingly upset until she was doubled over and convulsing with grief. That woman had lost twenty-five family members. Because she was not a legal resident of the United States, she couldn't go back to Haiti and try to find and bury her parents, without risking not being able to return to Miami.

There are degrees of trauma and loss I suppose and if you get invited on television programs and are asked to write articles about yours, it seems bigger. However, so many people have suffered much more, are still suffering much more, and I surrender all the blank spaces in and around these words to them. I surrender these spaces also to the dead, to the lives unfulfilled, to the stories untold. We will never know all the stories. Mine is only one—and it is from far away, from *lòt bò dlo*, "the other side of the water," three Haitian Creole words which evoke both migration and death. Separation, no matter how it happens, is earth shattering. But even for families accustomed to necessary ruptures, this was the most catastrophic. Like the woman in church, they would never be able to say good-bye and would never even learn the fate of their loved ones who were buried, unidentified, in mass graves.

In the weeks and months following the earthquake, many journalists, visiting dignitaries, and even casual observers praised the extraordinary resilience of the Haitian people. Indeed, that resilience is inspiring. For the first hours and days after the earthquake, Haitians were pretty much on their own. Their government, paralyzed by its own losses, was incapable of assisting them, so they dug their loved ones out of the rubble with hammers and axes and even their bare hands. As food and water became scarce, they divided small rations among themselves.

Haiti, which is often referred to as the poorest country in the Western Hemisphere, had yet another crucial lesson to teach the world: a lesson in resilience. If some of the more sensationalist broadcasts were any indication, the world was expecting something else. Journalists eagerly jumped in the middle of chaotic food and water distributions, allowing themselves to be bumped and shoved for the cameras. Such was the fear of looting that Haitian policemen shot hungry young men to death over bags of rice. However, the massive, large-scale looting that was anticipated never took place. Instead, Haitians buckled down for what will surely be a long and difficult road. They set up temporary shelters with sticks and bed-sheets, making public places their homes. When it rained, they stood up and let the muddy water flow between their legs.

After three post-earthquake visits to Haiti, I began to ask myself if this much-admired resilience would not in the end hurt the affected Haitians. It would not be an active hurt, like the pounding rain and menacing winds from the hurricane season, the brutal rapes of women and girls in many of the camps, or the deaths from cholera. Instead, it would be a passive hurt, as in a lack of urgency or neglect. "If being resilient means that we're able to suffer much more than other people, it's really not a compliment," a young woman at the large Champs de Mars camp in downtown Port-au-Prince told me.

As friends and leaders both in Haiti and in the international com-munity shape their reconstruction plans for the country, they will be remiss if they misinterpret as complacency the grace, patience, and courage that Haitians have shown for more than a year and a half since the January 12, 2010, earthquake. Haitian history teaches us otherwise. Haitians were resilient against the brutal Napoleonic code of French colonial slavery until they started a revolution that created their republic in 1804. Haitians endured thirty years of the Duvalier dictatorship until they ousted Jean Claude Duvalier in 1986. It is now only a matter of time before their post-earthquake endurance justifiably wears out.

In the meantime, that resilience has shown itself in many home-grown efforts, in the beauty parlors and barbershops in the camps, where people who wake up and go to sleep in the midst of inevitable squalor refuse to let it define them. In the letters dropped in the sug-gestion boxes in which tent city residents plead for food and water and jobs and schools for their children. In the faces and voices of the men and women who read to, sing with, and draw with the or-phaned children in the displacement camps, where they are also liv-ing. Often unrecognized, some extraordinary leaders are rising out of the makeshift displacement camps. I know a woman who from one day to the next had a hundred people in her yard. She would have never considered herself a leader before the earthquake. She is sixty-nine years old and has lung cancer. Another man was feeding and organizing an entire neighborhood after the earthquake. He is a painter. Haitian-Americans have also stepped up to the plate. Some have rushed to Haiti with larger aid organizations, and others have just picked up and gone on their own. From the young doctors and nurses who arrived that first week, to the teachers and therapists for whom going back and forth to Haiti has now become routine. And yes, also the artists, singers, painters, poets, and novelists too.

For us creative types, especially those who have spent most of our lives outside Haiti, yet still consider ourselves bound to it as the umbilical cords that joined us to our mothers, another Haiti occasionally sparks our imagination. Whenever I am asked to lay out my own personal "vision" for Haiti's future, I think of that place. It is a place where every child (both boys and girls) goes to school, where every person eats everyday and has a roof over his or her head. It is a place where women and girls are fully protected, where there is no rape, no kidnapping. In that place, there is no *peyi andeyò*, no unsurmountable rural-urban divide.

It would be great, however, to see a society emerge out of the rubble that comes closest to the ideal vision that the majority of Haitians, who are mostly poor and marginalized, have for Haiti's future. All of Haiti's children, including my two daughters and all of those who have crossed both earthly and cosmic barriers to *lòt bò dlo*, will be counting on it.

# SIM PA RELE*
# (IF I DON'T SHOUT)

## MICHÈLE MONTAS-DOMINIQUE

### The voices of the voiceless

When my friend Paul Farmer asked me first to participate in, then to write about, the collective effort we undertook last February and March to give voice to the silent majority of Haiti, my answer was immediately yes.

Yes, because I owe this small contribution to so many friends forever silenced. I owe it also to the hundreds whose bodies I saw lying on the sidewalks of the Canapé Vert and Martissant roads, in Port-au-Prince the day after that fateful January 12. Each one was covered with a clean white sheet, in a sign of ultimate respect from an unknown survivor to an unknown victim. I owe this small contribution to the mother I saw at 5 o'clock that terrible morning of the 13th, carrying on her back a wounded son twice her size, rescued from the rubble. I don't know her name. I don't know if she ever found a hospital. We never spoke. But I know in my soul how much her voice should count.

In the midst of the mind-boggling devastation that was my city—the dead bodies and more than a million displaced people living in makeshift camps—I felt compelled once more to help echo the voices

---

*From the title of the 1995 report of Haiti's National Truth and Justice Commission that investigated the massive human rights violations of 1991–1994.

271

of those who are never heard, those who are never consulted, and those who never participate in the life of their own country except when they are asked to cast a ballot for one candidate or another, as was the case last November.

I worked for many years doing just that, before the quake shattered all our lives, as a radio journalist at Radio Haiti. Since the midseventies, we had lent our microphones to coffee growers and factory workers, peasant associations and newly formed labor unions, trying to break the wall of silence imposed by a dictatorship. We were there again in 1987, after six years of forced exile, recording and broadcasting the voices from the slums of Port-au-Prince and Gonaïves and from the villages of the Artibonite valley.

Back then, the words from peasants, artisans, and market women expressed the aspirations for change. Our mission was about participation, justice for all, and transparency in government. It was about *chanje leta,* changing the state, from a predatory one into one that provided services to its population. We would make sure, in our newsroom at Radio Haiti, that every day would have one major story from *andeyò,* the "outside country," as every place besides the centralized Republic of Port-au-Prince is called.

In the last few years, however, the voices from below have become muted or irrelevant to the decision makers. The airwaves are filled mostly with politicians speaking about the government and about other politicians, with little reporting from *andeyò.* I wonder how much effect the voices we so often aired had in shaping our postdictatorship Haiti. Has our oral society absorbed the calls for change so that we can produce real change? Was voicing our demands a good enough substitute for action?

Now that the dust has settled, the hidden realities of Haiti are emerging. "Beyond the mountain, there is another mountain," says the Haitian Proverb. The quake that killed tens of thousands of the people we loved has brought together in the tent cities not only the victims of those thirty-five apocalyptic minutes but also those who have moved from the slums of La Saline, Cite Letènel, or Jalouzi to find, in the camps, the basic services they were denied for decades. The deep-rooted social injustices of the past have now caught up with us, no longer hidden, exposed now on every public square and every vacant lot in this broken city.

Another reason why I said yes to Paul is because I felt that I was in a privileged position to better echo these voices. I had been working at the United Nations, before returning to Haiti in early January for what was supposed to be a carefree retirement. Then the earthquake struck. I was asked to join the UN again, this time in Haiti, as Special Adviser to the Secretary-General's Special Representative there, Ambassador Edmond Mulet. I did not hesitate. After what had happened, could I be anywhere else?

So I was back to fourteen-hour days filled with grueling visits to relocation camps and destroyed schools. I drove to work through bumpy streets twisted by *bagay la*, "the thing." We refuse to name it "the earthquake," an absurd semantic shield against a possible return of the beast. I am now painfully aware that as a privileged survivor, I have the chance to play a role—even a modest one—in the ambitious national and international agenda to rebuild Haiti better. As a Haitian, I am part of that wounded land and can inject a different perspective in the decision-making process. As a long-time international civil servant, I have learned to cut through the paralyzing bureaucratic red tape that is too often part of working for the UN. The cataclysmic event I have lived through has forced so many of us to think "outside the tent."

At the International Donors' Conference "Towards a New Future for Haiti" held in New York on March 31, 2010, I was asked to be the spokesperson for "the voiceless" and to present the conclusions of a series of focus group discussions held with the displaced in the camps as well as with small farmers, market women, and tradespeople in the Haitian countryside. This appointment had an ironic aspect because I had spent the preceding thirty-four months as the Spokesperson for UN Secretary-General Ban Ki-moon and for the United Nations. Now for a privileged if short moment, I would be the spokesperson for the ordinary citizens of the country I call mine.

I was profoundly moved to be asked to lend a voice to those who had been isolated from the planning process and could not share their vision for rebuilding a more just and democratic Haiti. I felt privileged to relay their views on the priorities of decentralization and a sustainable agriculture as well as their demands for dignity, respect, and work beyond the handouts of emergency aid.

Two very personal reasons also motivated me to help transmit and amplify the voices of those most affected by the earthquake. The first reason had to do with one man: Jean Dominique, my companion of twenty-eight years. A radio journalist, he was called by many "the voice of the voiceless," the advocate of the *peyi andeyò*. In the early 1970s, he was the first to introduce Creole, the language of the majority, as the main language for news in a formerly French-speaking Haitian media. Above all, he was the one who dared, over and over, until he was assassinated in April 2000, to demand the participation of the poorest in the affairs of the state. Jean Dominique has remained such a beacon of our collective consciousness that, on January 13 on a Champs de Mars Square filled with survivors, I was not surprised when a desperate man, his hands raised to the skies, yelled to me, "Jando would know what to do." When I said, meekly, "Even Jean could not contain tectonic plates and the earth's movements!" I received a stern reply: "You don't know that, do you?" He was right; I don't.

The second personal reason to say yes to this project is my deep respect for Dr. Paul Farmer, Polo, our *ti doc,* who, beyond his role in public health policies and before that terrible January 12, has been a steady part of the twenty-year effort to listen, to hear and, in so many ways, to empower. It is said he has a Haitian soul. I know he does.

### Listening to the voices

The task seemed at first impossible: to reach out, in the five weeks before the March 31st International Donors' Conference on Haiti, beyond the silence of thousands of unmarked mass graves to the survivors, not only asking them for their own stories but also consulting them on the changes they wanted and their priorities for reconstruction.

Six partner organizations were involved in this exercise: the students of the Haitian Education Leadership Project (HELP); KOZEPEP, an umbrella group for several peasant associations throughout the country; Zanmi Lasante/Partners In Health, an organization that has been providing health care in rural Haiti for decades; ATD Quart Monde, an NGO that for the last twenty-five years has focused its work on the poorest in the slums of Port-au-Prince; the Office of the United Nations Special Envoy to Haiti; and the national officers of MINUSTAH (UN Stabilization Mission in Haiti). Working together and with the support of the United Nations development program, we conducted a series of focus groups in Haiti's ten *departments* (regions).

The objective was to capture the opinions and aspirations of Haitian citizens who are not members of organized civil society groups and, as such, would not be included in any consultation mechanisms conducted for the March 31 International Donors' Conference. This countrywide exercise did not purport to be a comprehensive opinion poll or a needs assessment. The time constraints did not allow for an exhaustive survey. But the responses we received from a fishing village in the Grande Anse or from the Jean Marie Vincent camp for the displaced in Port-au-Prince were amazingly similar in terms of the priorities expressed. Those consulted were sufficiently numerous and from sectors diverse enough to properly reflect the major concerns and needs shared by the Haitian people at large.

We were expecting reluctance, jaded responses, or even cynicism from the communities and individuals we were contacting. After all, although the freedom to express one's view had become a daily staple of our lives since the fall of the dictatorship in 1986, little had changed in the life of the majority of Haitians in the last twenty-five years. The decentralization featured in the Constitution adopted in 1987 had remained but a word. What had changed since the quake, however, as evident in so many of the focus groups, was the realization of the extent of the crisis. The roots of forty years of endemic problems were increasingly apparent not only to the intellectual or the economist or the social worker, but to the peasant in Papaye or Terrier Rouge and to the tent dweller in Port-au-Prince. Moreover, a new sense of urgency was felt, the need to use the terrible opportunity of that quake to finally make the changes we had dreamed of collectively thirty years ago: *chanje leta.*

What our more than four hundred facilitators recorded was the eagerness of those we contacted, in almost every community, to speak out and be heard, not only about what they had lived through and the daily difficulties they had been confronting since the quake, but above all about their views on the priorities for reconstructing the country, their country. Three weeks after the quake, no one could speak out. The few radio stations that relayed the voices of grassroots organizations were silent, except for some reporting on the conditions in the camps or the distribution of food aid. Many said that this was the first time since the quake that anyone was seeking their opinions. Some focus groups, originally limited to ten people, swelled to fifteen or eighteen participants. Gatherings in schools or cockfight arenas were at times difficult to harness because so many had so much to say.

### The focus groups

During the month of March 2010, 156 focus groups comprised of 1,750 Haitians—peasants, fishermen, market women, the jobless, traditional healers, teachers, camp dwellers, and students—living in all regions of the country, from Torbeck in the south to Terrier Rouge in the northeast, were brought together by two women at the UN, Nancy Dorsinville and Lizbeth Cullity. The groups were varied in composition and, given the purpose of the project—giving a voice to the voiceless—people in positions of authority or influence in the public sphere, such as senior civil servants and politicians, were not invited. They had other platforms from which to express their views. Although men were the majority, a few focus groups in Les Cayes and Aquin were exclusively women, which enabled them to feel that they could speak more freely.

### Fok sa change/*It has to change*

Most people referred to the January 12 earthquake as a life-shattering experience, materially and emotionally. The discussions revealed a high degree of stress and anxiety among the Haitians across the country, regardless of their gender, age, social status, or location at the time of the disaster. The effects of the trauma—even among those not directly affected by the earthquake—were evident as survivors eagerly relayed their stories. One told the harrowing tale of being buried alive in the rubble then extracted four days later; another remembered having to hold the hand of a sister being amputated of a crushed leg. Even a year later, excruciating memories linger. It was as if the quake happened yesterday.

Beyond the personal stories, one evident conclusion of the discussions was that Haiti needs to change profoundly and rapidly. With regard to reconstruction priorities, the answers in the focus groups were remarkably homogeneous. Many viewed the earthquake as a watershed and the beginning of a period of (re)construction in which all Haitians, rich and poor, could participate in their country's development. With this crisis came a deep sense of hope that such profound change is possible.

On an individual level, people wanted to be in control of their own future; they did not want to be dependent. They called for an end to discrimination, exclusion, and inequality. Another key finding, throughout the regions, was a crisis of confidence in the Haitian state, with perceptions of historical corruption, inaction, and official neglect.

During our focus group discussions, strong expectations were expressed that the international community would provide adequate support. Many wanted the reconstruction process to support Haiti by tackling preexisting structural problems such as an overpopulated capital, social inequalities, and an atrophied agricultural sector.

To the question, "Do you think Haiti can change for the better?" the answer was overwhelmingly "Yes. Haiti can and will change, and we want to be the actors of that change."

### A key word: participation

Throughout the different regions, the focus groups demanded an end to exclusion and for the participation of all, rich or poor, in the decision-making process. The exercise was an opportunity for people to express themselves, often for the first time, on issues of concern to their communities and to themselves as individual citizens.

Worried about being sidelined in the reconstruction process and also eager for jobs, citizens wanted to participate in setting priorities, on selecting projects adapted to the realities of each community, or on assessing tangible and measurable results. One group in Roseaux, a small town in the Grande Anse, insisted on the necessity that each community be consulted on its own priorities before a program is even conceived.

### One priority: decentralization

Most Haitians in the focus groups insisted on the decentralization and deconcentration of public services. Most people want job opportunities closer to home, no matter how remote their communities, and demanded a say in the development of their regions. The earthquake has shattered the image of Port-au-Prince as a place of opportunity, pointing to the need for a balanced and coherent development of the country, easier access to public services, and more job and educational opportunities outside the capital.

A very large majority of the Haitians we spoke to wanted to be able to live near their places of origin without having to relocate to the capital to study, make a living, or access public services. Many died or were maimed at the time of the quake because they came to the capital to study or simply apply for a passport. The point was painfully made by a mother who participated in a focus group discussion in Dame Marie. Her two children were attending schools in Port-au-Prince when the earthquake struck. They both came back to her with a limb amputated. Decentralization was widely seen as the remedy to the country's ills and to the unsustainable drift to urban areas.

### "Envestisman nan moun"/Investment in people

A clear majority of focus group participants, from both rural and urban areas, strongly believed in the critical need to "invest in people" —*envestisman nan moun*. They highlighted five key immediate priorities: education, the delivery of basic services to all, housing, support for agricultural production, and the building of communication infrastructures.

There seemed to be unanimity about the need to invest in human capital through education (including higher education) and training, at the local and regional levels. Haitians want more and better trained teachers, increased equality of access to education, and an efficient educational system. They want quality and standardized education for all children, with academic and vocational education available to all in both rural and urban areas. A focus group in Grande Anse, in Tozia, noted that they had no choice but to send their children to the city because their commune (district) has no secondary schools. A fisherwoman in Baudin, near Port-de-Paix, showed her calloused hands and said that the earthquake had taken away the hope she had pinned on her son's schooling. She had invested everything she had in his education, and now he was back from the capital, alive but with no prospects for the future.

As one of the participants in Grande Ravine, a poor neighborhood of Port-au-Prince, put it, *Yon timoun ki pa gen konesans, li pa gen anyen nan men li, li pas konsidere nan sosyete a.* "A child who is not educated has no tools for the future, and is not important in the society."

### Choosing where to live

From Limbe in the north to Cavaillon in the south, rural Haitians as well as city dwellers showed great attachment to their districts and neighborhoods. First and foremost, social ties are strong and many prefer to remain in their community whatever the obstacles. Focus group facilitators sought to understand the other incentives for people to stay in their current location, relocate, or move back to where they lived before the earthquake.

In the wake of the earthquake, thousands of people left their place of residence and moved into camps across the capital. Up to an estimated six hundred thousand initially returned to their regions of origin. Most people in the regions have relatives or friends who lived in the capital at the time of the earthquake, so people empathized with the victims and wanted to assist. But the effect of displacement weighed on host families and communities. Families often do not have the necessary capacity and space. Expanded households put pressure on limited resources, especially food. Suggestions as to how to meet these challenges varied among the focus groups: some wanted more food aid directed to the regions, while others called for an effort by the state to register and support the displaced, and even to help them relocate permanently outside Port-au-Prince.

## "Pou nou ka gran moun tèt nou"/*So we can be independent*

The Haitians we spoke to, including city-dwellers, stressed agricultural production as a top priority. Agriculture—perhaps more than any other sector—is considered essential to the country's wealth, and the prevailing sentiment is that the peasantry has always been neglected. Invariably, interlocutors made concrete demands for training, equipment, seeds, easier access to credit, and the introduction of modern agricultural techniques. Agriculture is also seen as a key source of employment: Many people said they would rather work on the land than seek informal jobs in the towns, from selling second-hand clothing in the streets to the "cash for work" menial jobs available since the quake.

All agreed that the country can and should become self-sufficient in food. During a focus group discussion in the city of Pétionville, a man, raising the issue of assistance after the quake, noted: *Pou nou granmoun tèt nou, fok nou ka bay tèt nou manje, kidonk si y ap ede nou tout bon fok yo envèsti nan agrikilti peyi a.* "For us to be independent adults, we must be able to feed ourselves; so if they really want to help us, they need to invest in agriculture."

### *A crisis of confidence*

We encountered a concern that the reconstruction may not adequately target and reach its intended beneficiaries. There was a general appeal for trustworthy authorities who would manage aid responsibly.

Discussions also revealed a deep and historic skepticism about the effectiveness of the state itself, its capability to articulate a vision and to bring about positive change. These perceptions of a state and a government absent or missing in action have replaced those that we encountered as journalists in the late eighties of a state viewed as predatory and oppressive.

Repeated demands were made for a responsible state. The general recognition was that public institutions, particularly the local government system, must be strengthened. Haitians insisted that the state should improve its capacity to respond to people's needs, which requires an administration staffed with competent civil servants. In some focus groups in the south, the inefficiency of the Haitian administration has created a distrust of the government and an identity crisis among Haitians. Focus group participants in the north (in Cap Haïtien, Limbe, Milo, and Grande Riviere du Nord) demanded a strong state that could effectively regulate the administration of the country.

During the two other crises that followed the earthquake this past year—the cholera outbreak and Hurricane Tomas—the government has tried to project an image of a caring and responsible state working through local authorities. How have the views we encountered last March changed? Our next focus groups, forming after more than a year of repeated crisis and the election of a new president and a new parliament, will certainly give us additional insights on the voiceless views of the state's responsibilities and their expectations of the new government.

### What aid?

In our exchanges on aid, the general conclusion was that responsible aid must reinforce Haiti's sovereignty. The overall purpose of reconstruction should be to enable the country to progress while avoiding aid dependency. Unsurprisingly, Haitians do not see their future as passive recipients of foreign aid. Several groups emphasized Haitian involvement in the reconstruction.

The demands are clear: The benefits of international aid must be shared equitably. The reconstruction of Haiti should also draw on Haitian resources and competencies. When I asked Nirline, a facilitators from ATD Quart Monde, what struck her the most from the discussions in the slum of Grande Ravine, she quoted a young man with no formal schooling speaking of what he would like to do in the future. He said confidently: Rebuild the national palace. *Nou wé Palé Nasyonal kraze. M ta renmen se pas engenye etrange ki ta rekonstwi l. M ta renmen ke se engenye Ayisyen ki ta jwenn travay sa a pou le yap gade sa, yo ta di se Ayisyen ki te rekonstwi l.* "We saw the National

Palace destroyed. I would like to see Haitian engineers rebuild it, not foreign engineers, so we can look at the Palace proudly in the future and say that Haitians built the National Palace." Many voices called for reconstruction to be designed to deliberately strengthen the capacities of Haitian civil servants, engineers, and other technical professions.

In Duchity, in the Grande Anse Department, many participants underlined the negative effect of aid on the production of small farmers. "Why can't the donors buy food from us and distribute that food to the affected regions?" one asked.

One key word came back over and over: respect. Haitians seek respect from the donors for those they are helping. Assistance, one focus group concluded, should be a joint decision between donors and aid recipients.

### Solidarity

When the focus groups met, more than two months after the January 12 earthquake, Haitians were still suffering from the psychological effect of the tragedy. The vast majority of people, even those outside the most affected areas of Miragoâne, Jacmel, and Port-au-Prince, suffered from post-traumatic symptoms such as stress, anxiety, and sleeplessness. Stress and anxiety were still evident a year after the quake, when, on January 12, 2011, several ceremonies and memorial gatherings marked the somber anniversary.

At the time we gathered our focus groups, three months after the quake, fear of another disaster was widespread. Many of those not physically affected by the quake continued to grieve for friends and relatives killed, particularly when bodies remained under rubble, and for those wounded or made homeless. This stress was compounded by feelings of frustration among the unemployed and a sense of pressure on local services caused by so many displaced people.

Adding to the stress generated by the catastrophe were concerns about its social and economic effects. In several departments, focus groups commented on the economic downturn that had coincided with the arrival of those fleeing the capital. Focus groups cited a general increase in prices, especially for basic goods, and the loss of re-mittances from relatives who used to live and work in the capital. They also mentioned an adverse effect on the *madan sara* who are key actors in the marketing system for agricultural products, after the country's main market—the Port-au-Prince metropolitan area—was disrupted.

Various focus groups reported that anxiety was heightened by security concerns. Residents in the metropolitan area reported an increase in robberies and assaults. They also expressed their fear of a return of prisoners who escaped from the national penitentiary and of renewed gang activities in their neighborhood. A year later, these fears have been exacerbated by a worsening security climate.

In these dire circumstances, the remarkable resilience shown by the focus group participants impressed many facilitators. Haitians have an obvious determination to come to terms with last January's devastation and to reconstruct their own lives. Many spoke of a profound sense of gratitude for having survived, and people of all beliefs have seen their religious faith strengthened.

In addition, many people reported a sense of renewed solidarity among Haitians. Participants proudly cited examples of young people rescuing victims from collapsed buildings with their bare hands or women sharing the little they had with other survivors.

The focus group participants also expressed a strong sense of attachment to their community and a desire to stick together, no matter what. In the Port-au-Prince metropolitan area in particular, where thousands have lost their homes and possessions, our discussions underlined the extent to which residents are attached to their own particular neighborhoods.

Despite the trauma and the losses, hope was alive even among the displaced.

### Dreaming of a new country...
An overwhelming majority of participants believe that Haiti can change for the better, but they insisted that this transformation implies a change of mentality at all levels of society. They envisage a complete transformation in the way individuals and institutions act,

through a new awakening, fostering a greater sense of civic responsibility and a new sense of unity.

They stressed the need to overcome social divisions and to join forces for a common purpose. In a Port-au-Prince focus group, one woman protested against existing inequalities in accessing education: *Pitit boujwa ak gran nèg yo al lekol e genyen yon metye, men pitit malere se pafwa yal lekòl e yo pa menm ka rantre nan inivèsite.* "The children of the bourgeois go to school and have a profession; the children of the poor seldom get to go to school and never get a chance to go to the university."

Participants felt the need to build a different country, less divided, where people are more equal. A participant in another Port-au-Prince focus group noted: *Depi tranbleman de tèa, tout moun siniste ke l te rich ke l te póv. Mwen ta renmen lè nap rebati peyi a, ke tout moun fè yon sèl san divizyon.* "Since the earthquake, we are all homeless, whether rich or poor. I would like to see the country rebuilt as one, without divisions."

One outcome of our collective quest to listen to the voices of those who are never heard was an uplifting sense of hope in the future. This was best put by a young woman in Port-au-Prince: *Menm si peyi a kraze li pap mouri.* "Even if the country has been destroyed, it will not die." The discussions in the Central Plateau—in Hinche, Papaye, Tomassique, and Cerca la Source—were animated and concluded with the participants declaring: *Haiti pap kraze.* "Haiti will not be destroyed." One positive side of the earthquake, according to the residents of Rue Alexandre, Bas-peu-de-chose, in Port-au-Prince, is that, today, solidarity, respect, and tolerance have become the "cements of communities everywhere," in the quake-affected neighborhood as they are in the *peyi andeyò.* Another positive aspect of the quake underlined by many of the focus groups is that they were finally being consulted on the future of their country.

All recognize that rebuilding Haiti will be long and difficult, but we Haitians are more used to marathons than sprints. Through coups d'état, hurricanes, and earthquakes, we have been rebuilding Haiti, seemingly from scratch, for two hundred years.

# GOUDOU GOUDOU

## NANCY DORSINVILLE

*O*n *January 12, 2010,* I traveled from New York to Port-au-Prince to attend a series of meetings. It was to be a twenty-four-hour, event-packed, whirlwind trip. Gessie Bellerive, Prime Minister Jean-Max Bellerive's sister, kindly came to the airport to have coffee with me as I waited for my luggage. Our mothers had been friends, in a different era. We now managed to intersect in the line of duty. Although it was to be a one-day trip, I had brought a full set of luggage. One always brings luggage when traveling to Haiti. Even before the earthquake, toiletries and other basic drugstore supplies were commodities much appreciated by family and friends. I always packed a generous array of them in my suitcases.

Everything was normal in Port-au-Prince City, or the Big Mango, as we like to say, comparing it to the Big Apple. On Wednesday, I was to return to the UN with the prime minister, who on Thursday was scheduled to address the International Financial Institutions (IFI) to follow up on the pledges they had made at a donors' conference in Washington, D.C., just months earlier, where "Haiti is open for business" had been the resounding mantra. For the first time in a long time, Haiti had a balanced budget, and things seemed promising for our impoverished country.

Eight of us from the UN were in the *salon diplomatique* (diplomatic lounge) at the airport in Port-au-Prince that day: two of my colleagues from the UN Office of the Special Envoy to Haiti were with me, and five Chinese peacekeepers from MINUSTAH (UN peacekeeping force in Haiti). The prime minister's sister, having worked at the UN in Geneva for many years, was reminiscing with my two co-workers. Meanwhile, I was mesmerized by my fellow travelers, the newly arrived peacekeepers from the Chinese Ministry of Public Security, who were being picked up by their counterparts already stationed in Haiti. I watched them greet each other with delight: They displayed a kind of synchronicity of movement that could have been choreographed. One of them had brought flowers, which she handed to the newcomers in an elegant, reverential manner. I later learned that the Chinese peacekeepers lived in a base where they cultivated a garden, and wondered if they had grown the welcoming bouquet.

Upon arriving in Port-au-Prince, I immediately went to a Global Fund meeting on AIDS, TB, and malaria. The meeting, concerning the future of the Global Fund's sponsorship of Haiti's national AIDS program, was critically important. Haiti's health officials were all present, from the health minister, along with his chief of staff and director general, to the head of the Haitian National Red Cross, the representative of the World Health Organization in Haiti, the operations director for Partners In Health, and the founding director of GHESKIO, the Haiti-based, leading research institute of the Caribbean region. Essentially, the entire cadre of high-level health officials in the country was in attendance. Generally, this type of meeting is held at the Montana Hotel, one of the best-known hotels in the country. But this time, the meeting was held at the Global Fund's CCM (Country Coordinating Mechanism) headquarters in Delmas 83, a suburb of Port-au-Prince.

As the prime minister presided over a heated debate between the country's leading health practitioners and policymakers, I began to feel the ground shaking and heard a cavernous noise engulfing the space. Given Haiti's history, the authorities present, and the nature of the meeting, I thought that I was hearing the sounds of another coup d'état. Although there had been infrequent, low-grade, isolated tremors over the years, the last earthquake in Haiti was more than a hundred years ago and had long been erased from our collective memory.

When the walls cracked open and parts of the ceiling began to fall on us, people started leaving the room. I instinctively crouched under the table. As a child, the nuns of my grammar school ordered us to do just that when there were politically motivated explosions. Almost everyone else had cleared the room when an international representative bent down under the table and urged me to come out. I made my way out of the room, through the crumbling stairs and into the courtyard. Outside, for the first time, I heard someone say: "It's an earthquake!" *How could this be?* I thought. *This is Haiti!*

We slowly moved from the courtyard to the street, where we had a better view of what we had escaped. The villa we had just occupied was leaning on one side; half of it, opposite where the meeting had been taking place, had fallen down. The large house next door had been flattened. Many of the health officials' cars had been destroyed by falling electric poles.

The streets began to fill with people, most covered with dust from the rubble, and many calling out to God. Some were screaming that it was the end of the world. Huge numbers of cars had accumulated on the roads, but many people were on foot, desperate to get home to their families. Within minutes of the quake, Haitians were working at removing their neighbors and loved ones from under the debris. Others were trying to bring injured people to safety or to some kind of health care. I witnessed spectacular displays of creativity; just about everything was used to carry the wounded: mattresses, planks of wood, doors that had been removed from their hinges, stretchers, *bourettes*, motorcycles, pickup trucks.

A storm raged inside my head: What is this? Where are these people coming from? Why are they covered in dust? Where are they going? I had been in Manhattan on 9/11, where the destruction had been contained. So in my mind, this earthquake, this foreign event that had occurred, was limited to one street or, at most, this neighborhood. I did not imagine that Port-au-Prince, our capital, had been destroyed, our cherished ministry of health and most of the other ministries along with it. A Durham University geophysics expert would subsequently assess the earthquake that shook Port-au-Prince and its surroundings to be "like thirty-five Hiroshima bomb

explosions hitting Haiti at once." But even before I heard that frightening comparison, my heart was being guided on the way of pro-
ceeding by the teachings of Father Pedro Arrupe, SJ, the medically
trained Jesuit priest who tended to Hiroshima's sick and dying.

As I stood there, trying to make sense of the inconceivable, Prime
Minister Bellerive came over and asked if I would go with him. I told
him that I would go to the General Hospital to help. Unaware of the
damage to the airport or the extent of the devastation throughout
the capital, I imagined that I could be useful at the outset and travel
home within a few days. I understood, however, that as a public servant, the prime minister could no longer travel to a UN meeting the
next day as originally planned.

Standing in the street with the astonished health team, I saw
schoolchildren, their colorful uniforms stained with blood, carrying
injured classmates on their backs. At times, several children worked
together to carry one who, having lost use of a limb, could not nego-
tiate the crowds. The traffic was growing. Drivers exchanged what
little information they had been able to gather from word of mouth
along the way: This street is blocked because all the houses are
down; that street is off limits because electric poles fell on cars in the
middle of the road; drivers are dead; that street is cracked open; people are trying to clear out that area. Everyone was outside, some
holding packages containing the few belongings they were able to
salvage. What would soon be dubbed *psychose béton* (psychosis, as in
phobia or fear of concrete) took hold of the population. Thus began
the massive exodus toward open spaces, which led to the proliferation across the capital of camps filled with destitute people.

After the earthquake, phones were not working. Even before the
quake, when they did work, the principal way of disseminating information in Haiti is through *tele-dyol* (*dyol* is the Creole word for
*mouth*). The radio broadcasts, for the few stations we were able to
tap, seemed to be on autopilot, with streaming music.

Bodies were everywhere. On the sidewalk, in the streets, protrud-
ing from the rubble, hanging out of cars, crushed under buildings,
suffocating inside crumbled homes. Dead people everywhere; everywhere.

Haitians have a profoundly extensive tradition of venerating the dead. In the days immediately following the catastrophe, many survivors could not locate their loved ones. People had been buried alive in their homes or places of work. The main morgue at the General Hospital was not working, and the morgues that are normally attached to funeral parlors were for the most part destroyed. In some neighborhoods, people sat in front of their destroyed homes, with their dead neatly wrapped, for the most part in pristine white sheets, by their side. They sat there as if waiting for something big to happen, even though the big event had already occurred.

Within a few more days, the stench of dead bodies was everywhere, and people walked the streets wearing masks. Those fortunate enough to have survived the earthquake wore an ashy cloak of fine white dust carried by the wind from the rubble. Word spread that putting toothpaste below one's nose would help cover the stench and help one breathe in the midst of the overwhelming dust. But though the dust settled everywhere, it did not obscure anything: not the excruciating pain, or the overpowering fear, or the deep gratitude for having survived. None of it could be hidden, not even by this ubiquitous, intrusive dust from the destruction.

In the days immediately following the earthquake, most UN staff stayed at the logistics base—log base, as we call it—the main UN peacekeepers' compound. We worked round the clock, doing both rescue and programmatic work and, when possible, finding a relatively quiet corner to sleep for a bit. UN employees went to dig under the rubble for their missing coworkers; they went on site to identify otherwise unrecognizable bodies. The head of the mission, Mr. Hedi Annabi, and the second in command, Mr. Luis Da Costa, were both acknowledged as missing and were believed to have died in the destroyed Christopher Hotel, which housed the MINUSTAH executive offices. When a computer was available and the Internet happened to work for a brief moment, people took turns sending reassuring messages to family around the world, as well as death notices to headquarters; every division lost workers. People who had been able to retrieve some clothing shared with others who had lost all. At log base, we were blessed to have electricity, potable water, and daily food rations of MREs (meals ready to eat, little packets of army combat food). Our community of grieving yet driven comrades was a resolute bunch of humanitarian workers from every continent. As someone pointed out, everyone spoke with an accent, but there was a common understanding born of shared traumatic experiences. Coworkers from different divisions, who may never have spoken to each other before, greeted each other as long lost friends. Discovering a familiar face among the survivors was electrifying.

Walking in log base one afternoon, foggy from sleep deprivation, I noticed an Asian man walking deliberately toward me. I made eye contact as he approached, an unspoken question stuck in my throat. He walked with purpose, yet his face was shrouded with grief. When he reached me, he simply put his head on my shoulder. He did so in a familiar way, as if he had rested his head on my shoulder many times before; he did it in a familial way—as if he, a Chinese man from a faraway land and I, a Haitian woman in her native land, were kinfolks. It was as though, immersed together in this tragedy, we had been compelled to know each other intimately and discovered that we were, in fact, the same. Existentially, we did know each other; our souls were united by sorrow.

As I hesitantly raised my hands to embrace him, I realized that he was one of the Chinese peacekeepers from the airport. I felt him heaving and heard his spasmodic breathing as he began to weep. In time, I learned that the Chinese peacekeepers had been in a meeting at the Christopher Hotel at the fatal moment. Their remains had been found that afternoon. They had journeyed all the way from China to die in Haiti, the country they had come to help, just hours after they had landed. *Requiescant in pace.* May they rest in peace.

In the days after the earthquake, nearly ten thousand families, approximately forty-eight thousand people, sought refuge in a vast, open space that had served as a military landing field. Having walked through this vast expanse of land, I slowly became aware that there was no curling smoke slowly climbing up to the heavens; there were no simmering pots. No one was cooking, anywhere in sight. No one had anything to cook; no one had anything to eat. This is how it began, before the shacks were built by people who needed shelter from the land that still rattled. Some fifty-odd aftershocks occurred in the weeks following the main event. At the time, we did not know that aftershocks were par for the course and would continue. Many of us did not even know that they were aftershocks. We thought, each time, that the worst was about to happen, that it would be the final blow.

The camp space seemed all the bigger because no structures were erected. I struggled to get my bearings: The sun was behind us, so we were facing north. Much was missing from the customary panorama. Except for the thousands of destitute families, nothing was there. The ground was barren. Even the gravel and the sticks that refugees eventually used to build had to be brought in. During those early days, small groups of people clustered around the modest bundles of belongings they had managed to salvage. Many stood, blank faced. Others sat on the ground or on whatever could serve as an impromptu resting device. Many were wounded and produced makeshift bandages from pieces of cloth they had scavenged from the rubble. Some were bleeding. Others had broken bones but were afraid to go to a medical station because word had gone out that people were getting amputations to prevent gangrene. Having lost their homes and their loved ones, many people chose to remain in the camps so as not to lose limbs. Here in the middle of nowhere, they were scared and suffering, but physically whole.

---

A Haitian doesn't just say: I went looking for my neighbor and knocked on his door. Instead, she mimics the sound of the action and says: I went looking for my neighbor and knocked on his door *kow, kow*. The folk art of effective storytelling in Haiti has one cardinal rule: The sound brings life to the story. If there is an accident on the road, a masterful narrator will not simply explain what occurred but will depict it in the culturally prescribed manner: The cobalt blue

2008 Toyota was approaching at full speed *voum* when the red- and yellow-colored *tap tap* abruptly made the curve *pheeew* and they collided *boom!* (Mass transportation across Haiti consists solely of a colorful fleet of mostly dilapidated trucks, adorned with vibrant naïve paintings, complemented by philosophical and biblical quotes. These trucks are called *tap taps* because of the noise they make while negotiating the country's many unpaved roads.) For the storyteller and her audience, sounds impart the nuanced details of the moment and not only enliven the account but render the story credible. Creole is not a tonal language, but it is hugely phonetic. Words don't stand alone but are reinforced by sound. Creole appropriates and conveys sounds in a powerfully onomatopoeic way.

When the earthquake occurred, Haitians used the descriptive term to convey what it was: *tranbleman tè,* or "earthquake." In the early days, they also called the earthquake *bagay la,* "that thing!" This vague, amorphous term struck me because it underscored that what had happened had no name and was so outside what we considered livable or bearable, that it could not be named. Yet, people had ascribed this un-namable thing, *bagay la,* anthropomorphic qualities: It had killed their loved ones, demolished their homes and often their businesses. Most of Haiti's population is Christian. In the Judeo-Christian tradition, to name something is to have power over it. Labeling the earthquake *bagay la* was for me indicative of the sense of collective powerlessness that people felt during the very first moments following the earthquake. Not being able to name or define what had happened, while recognizing the full force of its effects individually and collectively, bespoke the sense of utter despair and desolation that immediately gripped the survivors.

As people regained their center, in the chaotic aftermath of the earthquake, they slowly began to ascribe names to that terrifying noise, those tremors that shook the Mother of the nation, as we Haitians consider Port-au-Prince. It had to be named, and for the healing to begin, the name had to echo what shook our very core in those thirty-five infernal seconds. *Tranbleman tè* (earthquake), though descriptively correct, was not quite culturally accurate. *Bagay la* (that thing) was the ambiguous word expressing our post-traumatic stupor; it was merely an interim label. Creole is the language of our glory, the language of our fury; a vehicle to codify both our resistance, and resilience. As we began to awaken, the name for *bagay la* was coined, a neologism was created in accordance to Haitian norms and tradition: using the onomatopoeia *goudou goudou*. The disastrous event had been named. We, the people, were somehow, on our terms, regaining our bearings after the catastrophe. The first time I heard someone say *goudou goudou*, I shuddered. But then, I sighed. I understood. For me as a Haitian, this was the first step onto terra firma.

# MOTHERS AND
# DAUGHTERS OF HAITI

DIDI BERTRAND FARMER

## I. Rediscovering Haiti: December 2008–January 2009

Gripped by nostalgia or perhaps a strange premonition, I decided to bring my family to Haiti for the holidays back in 2009. For the first time, we did not stay in my hometown, Cange, where our work is based, but rather stayed in the capital city of my birth, Port-au-Prince. We visited many landmarks, including the National Palace, which we had never before taken the time to see. It was as if we had known that this might be our last chance to appreciate them before they were destroyed.

Political and familial circumstances had kept me away for a long time. I left Haiti for the first time in 1995 to pursue my studies in Europe. I was not ready to leave my homeland, but I had to take advantage of the opportunity available to me. In my heart, I never really left home; a profound love for my country remained with me. Each year, I would travel home for the long summer break and for the Christmas holiday. During my time away, I missed everything—the country's beauty, the sun, the beach, the warmth of the mountains, the landscape, the food, the music, my friends and family. I felt I needed to stay connected to my roots in Haiti to survive in Western culture, so I returned at every opportunity. Haiti's image abroad was never a positive one, but Haiti nonetheless remained my country, my home, and I remained fiercely devoted to it.

After completing my education, I returned to Haiti, determined to contribute to its renewal. But when an opportunity arose to move to Rwanda, I didn't hesitate. Despite the reservations some friends expressed about my living in a place with such a tragic history, I believed that I had something to learn from Rwanda. In September 2006, I moved there with my daughter Catherine—then only eight years old—to serve as the Director of Community Health for Inshuti Mu Buzima, Partners In Health's sister organization in Rwanda. After that our family grew by two more children, first with Elizabeth, a beautiful baby girl from our adopted home in Rwinkwavu, who joined our family at just one week old, and then with Charles Sebastian, who was born six months later. My family in Haiti often expressed regret that they did not have opportunities to become better acquainted with their grandchildren, nieces and nephew, and cousins. No matter how far away we are from our homeland, one's roots are one's roots—*lakay se lakay.*

Now at last I was bringing my family, as well as one of the young women helping us care for the children in Rwanda, to Haiti for a two-month stay. Close friends helped us to find a small apartment in the capital city, and I began to rediscover Port-au-Prince. We visited the Pantheon Museum and the Parc du Souvenir, went to the beach, spent time with family and friends, shopped for beautiful Haitian artwork, and enjoyed all the dishes that I had missed in Rwanda. At the end of our stay, we went to the northern city of Cap-Haïtien with my sister, her husband, and their sons, and an adopted Haitian daughter. We spent New Year's Eve there with friends. In Cap-Haïtien, I visited for the first time one of Haiti's historic sites, La Citadelle Laferriere, and also went to Labadie, the beautiful resort town that welcomes visitors from Caribbean cruises.

With my husband, "Dr. Paul," along, we certainly could not fail to pay a visit to the Cap-Haïtien Hospital, where we observed the hospital's staff struggling to provide high-quality health care to the people with the meager resources available to them. During the visit, we met a newborn boy who had been left for dead in a trash can in front of the main gate of the public hospital. The baby was found, rescued, and kept at the hospital to be treated for severe malnutrition. I was tempted to welcome him into our family, but we decided instead to pay for his care until he could be formally adopted by someone in his community.

At the end of the trip, as I packed my bags full of mementos from Haiti, I felt that I was bringing a little bit of home back with me. Little did I know that Haiti would follow me all the way back to Rwanda, that the baby boy we had just left would be only one of many children in danger whom we would be working to support from abroad, or that all the artwork and souvenirs I was carefully packing for friends and family would soon be auctioned to help pay for a desperate relief effort. Little did I know how narrowly my husband, children, and I were escaping disaster.

## II. Bringing Haiti to Rwanda: January 2010

We returned to Rwanda on, of all days, the 12th of January. We landed in Kigali at 7:55 P.M. after a two-day trip via Miami, New York City, and Brussels. By the time we cleared customs and arrived at our house, it was nearly 10 P.M. As the younger children prepared for bed, I e-mailed my family to let them know that we had reached Rwanda safely, and called some local friends, the Germain family, a Haitian couple with two children who also worked for international institutions in Rwanda. At 1 A.M., with everyone finally in bed, I turned off my cell phone and set my alarm clock for 6 in the morning. Catherine had already missed a week of classes, and we would need to get going early the next day to purchase her school supplies and get her to school.

The next day, after my morning prayer, I walked into the living room, turned on my cell phone, and discovered twenty missed calls from my Haitian friend Margalie. I wondered what could be wrong and became anxious that I had missed an opportunity to provide assistance to someone in trouble. I quickly dialed her number. She answered on the first ring, and asked if I had heard the news. "What news?" I asked. My heart started beating faster as I thought about my family in Haiti, my father. She replied, "*Nou pa gen peyi ankò, Ayiti kraze*": Our country is gone, Haiti is destroyed.

I could not speak. A few days previously, I had been there; my country had been standing on its feet. My friend was crying so hard that I could not understand her. I told her that I had to go, that we would talk later, and hung up the phone. Then I began shaking with grief. For a few hours, the world stopped. My daughter, who turned twelve that day, got neither a happy birthday wish nor a birthday party. Instead, she came home from school close to tears, asking, "What will happen to the children we met in Haiti? How will they go to school? How will this affect them?" I couldn't answer her. My heart was in pain. The torment had begun.

Words of sympathy were sent to me and my family by Rwandese friends and acquaintances: President and First Lady Kagame; members of the government; members of the different Ministries, especially the Ministry of Health; partners; members of our church; parents and teachers from our daughter's school; colleagues; other community members living in Kigali, Kayonza, Kirehe, and Burera. Phone calls and e-mails came in from around the world: sympathy and solidarity from Christine and Pat Murray from Zanmi Paris, Sylvie and Jamel, friends from Paris, my Danish classmate from grad school, Camilla, others from Holland, Senegal, Burkina, and Mali. Haiti was at the forefront in the news and the topic of every conversation. People came to us with expressions of compassion and empathy on their faces, though it was still difficult to control our grief.

I became panicked about the family and friends I had just seen in Haiti: my father and his second family, with their five children; my youngest sister, a nurse-anesthetist, and her husband, an obstetrician-gynecologist, and their young sons; the Lafontant family; members of the Zanmi Lasante administration; Loune; members of the local staff who came from Port-au-Prince; all the doctors that I have known for years. I was worried about Manmito, Tatie-Flore, Sindy, and their children Victoria, Cassandre, and Luidgi, who came to Haiti for the holidays. I was worried for my friend Zette; my classmates Yonide and her sister, my aunt Catherine and her daughter and grandchildren, my cousins Guy, Ricot, Kerline, and Baby and their mother Carole; my friends Nancy and Harry; our adopted daughter Natacha, who had started nursing school in Port-au-Prince; Clerveaux; all the PIH drivers;

all our friends and family... In that moment, all I could think about were the people dear to me and not about the bigger picture, the broader catastrophe and its effects on the country and people, which would soon consume every thought to come.

First, I tried calling Paul, still in Miami recovering from knee surgery, for news of the situation. Although he'd been calling every number he knew, he couldn't get through to Haiti and had almost no information regarding my family or colleagues from Zanmi Lasanté. But he believed that the UN headquarters had collapsed, killing the UN's country representative, whom I had met a couple of weeks earlier at a dinner hosted by the Prime Minister. He was sure that the Central Plateau, my home town, had been spared, but he was concerned about staff members, including our indefatigable Nancy Dorsinville, who had flown to Haiti the same day for a meeting with one of our partners in Port-au-Prince. None of my phone calls to the country went through, either.

On January 13, the news was full of images of death in the capital city. All main federal buildings, including the National Palace, had collapsed. Just days before, with my children, I had taken pictures in front of the Palace, which had been beautifully decorated for the holiday season. Now the caption to these photos reads, "Palace, *before* the quake." It is the event that has split our lives in two; everything is now *before* or *after*, every small memento, every vacation, every family photo.

For me, the tragedy that hit Haiti on January 12 has changed everything. After the tragedy, my two young nephews, one eleven months and the other two-and-a-half, joined my family in Rwanda. Their father was injured in the quake, and the family lost everything they worked hard to build over the years. All over the world, Haitian families have welcomed or adopted Haitian children and sheltered them through these difficult days; but the difficult days haven't ended yet, it seems. More than a year later, Ricky Ryan and Richard Jaden are still living with us in Rwanda, missed terribly by their parents.

Catherine too was deeply affected. Literally overnight, she went from a relatively happy and carefree eleven-year-old to a deeply concerned twelve-year-old with a mission. Catherine did everything she could in those months after the quake to help our relief effort. She mobilized friends, Rwandese and Haitians, in building donation boxes out of cardboard and decorating them with brightly-colored flowers and hopeful inscriptions. "Kigali Stand Up with Haiti!" the boxes said; Catherine seemed to take this on as a personal motto. She spoke of the injustices of a world in which she could go to school, sleep with a roof over her head, eat three meals a day, and enjoy the love and attention of her two parents, while children in Haiti were being herded into camps and orphanages, enduring terrible hardship and with uncertain futures. Catherine didn't limit this talk to home or to school—she spoke of Haiti to anyone who would listen.

It is largely because of my daughters, I believe, that I have been so affected by the plight of young girls in post-quake Haiti, who suffer more cruelty and injustice than even Catherine could possibly imagine. Whenever I hear of the plight of a young girl in a place such as Camp Parc Jean-Marie Vincent or Carradeux, I can't help but think of my own family and the terrible nightmare of trying to raise a daughter under such wretched and dangerous conditions. These thoughts—and images of my own daughters' faces peering out from under a tent somewhere in Port-au-Prince—haunt me. But they also motivate me to keep pushing, keep working for a better future for women and girls in Haiti.

Immediately post-quake, however, our focus was not on the future but rather on helping our countrymen survive in the terrible and desperate present. The day after the earthquake, the small Haitian community in Rwanda—six Haitians and two adopted friends of Haiti—met at my home to see how we could raise funds to support relief and rebuilding efforts after the earthquake. We launched a six-month long "KIGALI STANDS UP FOR HAITI" campaign. With support from other Partners In Health staffers based in Rwanda, we organized a number of fundraising events, starting with a cocktail party at Heaven Restaurant, continuing with a Haitian brunch at Republika Restaurant, and ending with an Ethiopian and Eritrean dinner buffet at Lalibela Restaurant. The support of our Ethiopian and Eritrean friends and colleagues in Kigali was a particularly valued resource; they quickly mobilized their extensive expatriate community to fundraise, host events, and generally aid our efforts. The earthquake was a call to action for a diverse group of expatriates and Rwandans alike, who came together in a remarkable show of solidarity for the sake of Haiti.

Catherine's school, Green Hills Academy, launched the first student-run fundraising campaign. Churches, schools, and radio stations invited us to deliver speeches and promote our relief efforts. Radio stations supported fundraising for several months with an ongoing radio campaign. The Anglican Church of St. Etienne immediately wrote a check, organized prayer sessions, and offered their kind friendship and support to our grieving family. Private businesses gave whatever they could, from cash and in-kind donations to services and logistical support. Donations of plane tickets, handicrafts, hotel rooms, electronics, gift certificates, and more were raffled or auctioned to raise funds. Staff of Inshuti Mu Buzima, PIH's sister organization in Rwanda, pledged 10 percent of their salaries to Haiti. These are just a few examples of those in Kigali who have joined us in standing up for Haiti—there are so many more. From this campaign, we raised well over $30,000, a significant contribution for a small country known best for its own struggles to overcome one of the world's worst humanitarian crises of the past two decades.

My family has reason to be grateful to Rwanda, our adopted country, both for the government's support of Haiti's government and for the generosity and commitment of the many individuals who helped us raise money and awareness, as well as our shattered spirits. Only days after the quake, the government gave a generous donation to Partners In Health's relief efforts. The message accompanying their donation revealed an incredible solidarity between the countries. Haiti is truly blessed to count Rwanda among its friends.

### III. The Plight of Women and Girls in Haiti: June 2010

In June I returned to Haiti for the first time since the tragedy. It was extremely hard to land in Port-au-Prince and see with my own eyes what I had watched on TV. At first, I feared my reaction. From the plane, approaching Port-au-Prince, I could see the masses of shelters and tents stretching to the horizon and could not stop my tears.

Then the passenger sitting next to me asked whether it was my first time back since the "event." She shared her own story of survival, as did everyone else that I met on my short visit home. Being in my destroyed country helped me to mourn.

A few months after that, I returned again, this time to witness firsthand the situation of women and girls living in some of the thirteen hundred spontaneous settlements in and around Port-au-Prince. My work with Partners In Health in Rwanda, initially focused on assisting their government in the development of its national community health program, had more recently involved working with women's organizations there to address the needs of vulnerable women and girls at the community level. I hoped that my visits to the camps in urban Haiti would allow me to identify areas of possible Rwandan-Haitian collaboration.

Images of the camps, at the time home to 1.3 million people, were by then familiar to the outside world: sprawling landscapes of makeshift tents where food, water, and sanitation are in short supply. Less evident in those media images was the struggle of women and girls amongst the desperation and violence, and the shadow crisis emerging from that: a wave of forced pregnancies resulting from the rape of young girls, unprotected behind the thin walls of what were supposed to be temporary shelters.

The situation of women in Haiti has always been precarious, but on this trip I found thousands of women in the camps on the brink of survival. Access to the most basic human needs of food, water, proper shelter, and education are severely limited for everyone, but girls and women face an added dilemma: satisfying those basic needs often places them at high risk of sexual violence and exploitation.

In the overcrowded camp in Parc Jean-Marie Vincent, I met ten-year-old Virginie. The day after the earthquake that left her father dead, she had moved here with her mother and four siblings to the settlement at the outskirts of downtown Port-au-Prince. Virginie's mother had sought work in town, lugging produce for market women, to provide food for her children, forcing her to leave Virginie responsible for her younger siblings. In her mother's absence, Virginie was repeatedly raped. The improvised house of sticks and other scavenged materials she lived in provided little protection from the men who prey on young girls. Speaking with Virginie, I thought again of my own daughters, and the heartbreaking decision her mother was forced to make between physical and social vulnerability—between hunger and safety.

Sexual assault and rape had been common in pre-earthquake Haiti—a fact that had led us years before to conduct our own ethnographic studies of "forced sex" in the rural countryside—but the social structures of family and community had provided some protection for women and girls. The collapse of Haiti's social infrastructure in the January 12 earthquake also destroyed these physical and social safeguards against sexual violence.

As vulnerable as Virginie was within her family's shelter, she and other girls are at even greater risk when they venture to the bathroom—little more than a crude dark closet with a hole in the ground, where they squat in darkness. These primitive latrines are also often far away from "home." Many girls described being followed and attacked on the way to the toilets. While police may patrol some camps during the day, and citizen brigades have formed in some camps to escort women and girls to both latrines and cooking areas after dark, armed men continue to prey upon them.

Shortly before my visit, the women's committee of Parc Jean-Marie Vincent had identified Virginie's family as being among the most vulnerable in the settlement. Fabiola Coqmard, Partners In Health's Women's Health Coordinator, began to address the family's most immediate needs, first by providing a proper tent. Recently, PIH has helped Virginie's family to relocate to a less populous camp, where Virginie can attend school, and helped her mother start a small income-generating activity to enable her to both work and remain with her children in the camp.

When I spoke to Virginie, I asked her what she wanted for her future. She said that she would like to go to school and become a nurse so that she could repay her mother for her hard work caring for the family. Although our immediate efforts can provide some protection for Virginie and her family, her future, and that of all Haiti's young girls, depends on a broader investment in their education and empowerment. This means ready access to school and a decent shot at a decent job when their education is complete.

The frequent sexual assaults, combined with inhumane living conditions, have led to an epidemic of unplanned pregnancies in adolescent girls and women. The medical coordinator for Partners In Health expects hundreds of pregnancies in the Park Jean-Marie Vincent camp alone if conditions don't improve—and the number is likely to climb even higher in coming months. Many women will deliver their children in the shelters of bedsheets and rubbish that make up their temporary homes. When twenty-eight-year-old Martine gave birth to a child in the camp, she had nowhere to place the newborn but in a bowl of dirty towels. With only bedsheets and linens as cover, the future of Martine's newborn and others born in the camp is bleak.

I left the camp with a renewed dedication to increasing awareness of the day-to-day atrocities that women and girls are facing in Haiti. Right now, food, water, and shelter are critically needed and in short supply. But if we address these basic needs while neglecting the education and empowerment of women, we will continue to leave them and their daughters vulnerable to rape and the prospect of bearing children of rape for years to come.

In Haiti, women are the centerpost—the *potomitan*—of our families and society. The reconstruction of Haiti will succeed only if we strengthen its centerpost by educating and empowering our country's women and girls. The impact of women's empowerment and leadership can be seen firsthand in Rwanda, where it has been key in transforming a country devastated by one of the worst tragedies to afflict humankind into one progressively more able to ensure access to social services for its population. Rwanda still confronts many challenges to achieving its ambitious goals for recovery and rebuilding, but its emergence as a model for all of Africa provides a vision of what is possible for Haiti after the earthquake.

## IV. Lessons from Rwanda: March 2011

In less than thirty seconds, in an unprecedented cataclysm, our public and private infrastructure vanished; our friends, family, and children disappeared; places and things firmly inscribed in our memories were destroyed. The earthquake created a rupture, and, just possibly, a new chance to become one people and one nation. It should be a chance for profound transformation and the beginning of the construction of a New Haiti where all Haitians, rich and poor, educated and illiterate, from public and private sectors, can participate in their country's development. Naysayers will claim that this hope is naïve or misguided, that Haiti's government is too weak, its people too poor, the damage too grave. To these people I say only one word: Rwanda.

I knew when I moved here in 2006 that I had a lot to learn from Rwanda, but I could not have expected just how valuable these lessons would prove to be in Haiti. In March 2011, just over a year after the quake, a Rwandan colleague of mine put it this way: "Rwanda and Haiti, they are the same. People lost family members. They lost husbands. They lost wives. They lost children. People's homes were destroyed and everything they owned was taken away from them. And afterward, people had to keep on living." My colleague is a warm and generous woman with a ready smile and an indefatigable spirit. Even after her husband, a Tutsi, was killed by a neighbor during the genocide, she took in six Hutu orphans to live alongside her own five children, and has supported all of them ever since. When I asked her how she kept on living in the wake of so much loss, she responded simply: "I worked." And she smiled as she said it.

My colleague attributes her resiliency partially to the ethic of hard work and self-reliance promoted by the post-genocide government's "public awareness" campaigns. But she also cites its sensitivity to gender issues and the importance of female empowerment in allowing women like her to gain access to the cash economy, to keep their children—and, in many cases, their neighbors' children—clothed, fed, and in school, and to find new meaning in a life which, for many, was suddenly absent of the husbands, fathers, sons, and brothers they used to love and care for.

As of 1994, 70 percent of Rwanda's population was female. It was largely on the backs of these women—victims of rape and physical violence, wives abandoned by husbands imprisoned or fleeing imprisonment, women who had lost family members, friends, neighbors, lovers, children—that Rwanda was rebuilt. And as Paul often likes to say, it was built back better. In Haiti, we often wax poetic about the role of women as the centerpost of the nation, but Rwanda has actually put this idea into practice, with an emphasis on female leadership, economic empowerment, and education.

In Rwanda, leadership quotas and an emphasis on female involvement in both community and national-level decision-making has formalized women's role in good governance. A minimum of 30 percent of government seats are reserved for women, though this quota is regularly surpassed. The 2008 elections broke the world record for highest percentage of female representation in Parliament, at 56.2 percent. Even at the village level, generous quotas are set for female representation in local leadership positions, and efforts are made to include women in community forums, planning meetings, focus groups, and other venues. Finally, a Ministry of Gender and Family Promotion was created to help coordinate local, decentralized efforts within a national agenda for gender equality. This agenda has become a central project not only of good governance in Rwanda but of Rwandan society as a whole, with even banks and other private businesses setting high standards for female representation in the workforce.

Women are being empowered in Rwanda politically and economically. They are organized into associations and cooperatives and are offered mutual support and solidarity while seeking access to the cash economy, and banks that would otherwise be unwilling to take a risk on, say, a loan to a banana seller in Ruhengeri, are happy to help agricultural cooperatives raise capital. It is generally accepted that these women's cooperatives are secure investments because experience has proven them to be among the most reliable in terms of repayment. And as many proponents of microfinance have noted, women are more likely to invest in household maintenance and human resources such as health care and education, pushing the country's development agenda forward in the process. As part of its Vision 2020 plan, Rwanda now aims to qualify as a middle-income country within the next decade, thanks in no small part to the solidarity and entrepreneurship of its working women.

Rwanda's investment in its youth is also paying off. For boys and girls alike, educational opportunities offer promise for a better future. Educational associations at the university level seek to harness the brainpower of young scholars to focus on national development challenges and solutions. And admissions quotas at these universities ensure that women's voices are included in these associations.

Rwanda has drawn on its rich cultural heritage by adapting its traditional practices to respond to modern challenges. The *Itorero Imbangukiragutabara*, Kinyarwanda for National and Traditional Academy, was traditionally used to educate youth about Rwandan culture. In 2007, Rwanda revived the practice of *Itorero* as a forum for promoting unity and other positive values, such as living peacefully with others in a spirit of respect, integrity, solidarity, and tolerance. Organized as month-long civic education programs for Rwandan youth, *Itorero* engages the Rwandan people to participate in the country's development strategies.

Central to the *Itorero* is the message that Rwandans of all ages, sexes, and social classes—from community health workers to teachers, university professors, students, and ordinary citizens—contribute to the development of their country. A lesson that we as Haitians can draw from this approach is that we must not wait passively for governments or NGOs to provide solutions to our problems, but must actively partake in the reconstruction process.

The great strides that Rwanda has made over the past seventeen years offer not only hope but also a way forward for countries struggling to rebuild in a post-disaster context. For our friends in Rwanda in the mid-1990s, this progress was perhaps unimaginable, following unprecedented destruction and terror. For Haitians, it offers one blueprint for the type of transformation we seek in the wake of our own tragedy.

With the support of President Kagame, and the remarkable teams in the Ministries of Health, Education, Foreign Affairs, and Local Government, the Haitian community in Rwanda established a Haiti-Rwanda Commission to disseminate lessons from Rwanda's experience in Haiti's rebuilding process and foster cooperation around challenges common to both countries. In my role as its Chairwoman,

I am charged with facilitating exchanges between my colleagues in Rwanda who have been at the forefront of the country's renaissance and my fellow Haitians who seek to draw both hope and pragmatic policy approaches from their progress. In the last several months, we have initiated a series of projects to bring together both the leadership and people of both countries.

A focus of my efforts as chair of this Commission has been on the youth, which represent Haiti's best hope for a brighter future. At the Commission's request, the Government of Rwanda offered full-tuition scholarships at the National University of Rwanda for five Haitian students whose studies were disrupted by the earthquake. These students, who we hope will be the first of many to study in Rwanda, not only will have access to an undergraduate education but will return with the skills and commitment to rebuilding our country. Rwanda's was not merely a gesture of solidarity but also a measure of the progress that was possible.

This nascent cooperation has given birth to a much more ambitious initiative to bring students to institutions of higher education across the African continent for undergraduate studies. Building on the South-South Cooperation, we have been working to secure opportunities for Haitian students in other countries in the region. Lesotho, for example, has already made a similar pledge following my visit to Maseru. Other nations will surely follow. Our mission is twofold: contributing to the development of a new generation of leaders in the country while addressing the educational crisis created by the earthquake. The Commission has set the goal of bringing two hundred students to study at institutions of higher education in Africa in 2012. It's an ambitious goal, but my work in Rwanda, and my visits to other countries in the region, have convinced me that such exchanges will help young Haitians learn about alternative models of recovery and also allow them to serve as living links between our wounded country and the continent that also calls us home.

# HUMANITARIAN AID, IMPARTIALITY, AND DIRTY BOOTS

LOUISE C. IVERS, MD, MPH, DTM&H

*On Saturday, January 16, 2010,* I stood battle-weary on the tarmac at Port-au-Prince airport. A huge Canadian Airlines aircraft had just landed, bringing tons of supplies and a medical team. Scores of small private aircraft also dotted the tarmac. Military airplanes roared into position, and men and women in combat fatigues walked with a mission across the runway. Behind us, hundreds of Haitians and foreign nationals were lined up in the shadow of the fractured airport terminal building, waiting for a flight out.

The previous four days had been some of the hardest of my life. I had seen the city that I called home flattened. I had witnessed unimaginable pain and loss. Working in a makeshift clinic at the United Nations logistics base, I had seen some of the best and worst of humanity. Now, waiting for a ride home, I felt that the airport, my airport, was being invaded. Newcomers descended the steps of high-class private jets sporting "Earthquake 2010" t-shirts hot off the presses. Stethoscopes at the ready, boxes of granola bars in the backpacks, they posed for team pictures. It was a civilian and a military invasion, a "save Haiti" invasion.

I am a doctor—an internist, an infectious disease and tropical medicine specialist, and a public health practitioner. I have spent the last seven years working in Haiti with Partners In Health, caring for patients and trying, with the support of a large Haitian team, to address some of the underlying causes of disease amongst the poverty-stricken. When the earthquake struck on January 12, 2010, I was in a meeting with my colleague Kim Cullen and members of the World Food Program in Port-au-Prince. We had been planning a research project to document the effects of food assistance on the rural poor living with HIV. The area where we met, in the foothills of Petionville, was later documented to have experienced some of the most severe shaking during the earthquake. Kim and I spent the night on the driveway of the WFP building, setting up a makeshift first aid hospital.

That night was hellish. As scenes of devastation unfolded in the streets around us, a small group of us worked as a team—going outside the gates to help where possible, lifting rubble, carrying the injured inside the gates, comforting children who had been separated from their families. Some sat glued to the spot, paralyzed by fear as hundreds of aftershocks threatened to topple the already damaged buildings beside us. Others leapt to help in any way they could. An administrator became comforter of the dying; a researcher held the hand of a small child separated from his family; my driver, Médé, used his car jack to free trapped limbs; Kim became a first-class nursing assistant. We witnessed injuries that no one should have to suffer, deaths that were senseless, pain that must have been unbearable but was borne. As helicopters flew overhead, the driveway became a temporary refuge—survivors huddled together, seeking solace from one another. A couple sat cradling their adult son, rocking him back and forth, even though he had already bled to death from a leg injury.

During the night, a certain kind of order was established in the driveway. A few individuals in particular were calm and decisive in the face of the chaos; I later learned that they were ex-servicemen in the British Armed Forces. Kim and I triaged patients with red stickers from research supplies salvaged from our car, which was buried beneath the wall of a nearby house.

Few things are more desperate for a physician than the knowledge that a medical problem is curable, treatable, or manageable with the right assortment of basic medical supplies only to have none of them: a tighter tourniquet, a pain medication, sterile water. A driveway and a first aid kit are not meant to treat mass casualties. When a handful of Argentine soldiers from MINUSTAH arrived to take some of the injured to medical care, we felt as though our work had not been totally in vain. The soldiers appeared to me to be almost heaven-sent. Where the injured would be moved, I did not know. But moving patients seemed to offer the only possibility of surgery or proper wound care. Given what I later discovered about the state of the city's hospitals post-earthquake, however, moving these five or six injured was unlikely to have made much difference to their lives. Most hospitals lacked even the basics.

The driveway where we worked was part of the UN headquarters collection of buildings, and many of us worried that when vehicles came to move UN staff, Haitian nationals might be left behind. We were promised by those in authority that everyone on the driveway would be brought to the same place. So, when trucks arrived the next morning and UN peacekeeping (MINUSTAH) soldiers entered the building compound to escort us out, we packed up our medical kits. The injured, all but one of them Haitian, filled every empty spot on the benches of the trucks. Sitting side by side with them were disheveled international UN staff, many of whose colleagues and friends were missing and suspected dead. Having carefully watched out for us during the evening, our colleagues from the UN ensured us that Kim, Médé, and I were included in the group of evacuees.

I waited to be sure that none of the patients on stretchers were forgotten. A man with crushed feet, who had pulled on my shirt, begging for help every time I passed by the previous night, looked me in the eye as I climbed up to the last seat in one of the trucks. A MINUSTAH soldier, weary-eyed, clearly pained by what I knew to be the loss of his colleagues just 100 meters away at the UN headquarters office, took time to reassure me that he would take responsibility for this man being moved. He urged me to take my seat. I sat beside a short, dark-skinned soldier who closed up the truck and tapped his long gun on the back to signal that we could move off.

The white canvas truck made its way through the battered streets of Port-au-Prince while pedestrians handed us their injured. "He's a police officer" (a young man with a serious head injury). "She was at the General Hospital" (a small child with burns to her face). Somehow, we became a lifeline for Haitians. Getting in the truck meant getting care—or at least the hope of getting care. We moved at a snail's pace down the rubble-filled streets. Block after block revealed familiar landscapes gone. Streams of people walked with determination—to find their families, to check on their homes, to search for the missing. Cries of pain and wails of despair filled the air.

Our convoy of trucks loaded up more and more of the injured. The Haitian sun gave no reprieve. A mother sat facing the street on one of the army cots that we had placed in the space between the benches of the truckbed. As she held her child, she also tried to comfort the stranger on the cot. The man had a head injury and struggled to move around, confused and bewildered. I believed that his injury was life-threatening. The UN soldier took his plastic water bottle and cut it to make a drinking cup for the infant. Later he gave up his seat as another injured person was handed in to us. Then he found a position that would block the sun from the child's face, relieving the mother of at least that job. Together we found some cloth, and seeing me struggle to tear it, he put away his gun and cut the cloth into sections that we handed around to protect against the heavy dust that burnt our eyes and our lungs.

At that time, as a survivor of the earthquake and as a doctor with a nongovernmental organization, I was glad that MINUSTAH was there. If it weren't for the soldiers, how would I have left the grounds of the building, unfamiliar as I was with all but the main roads of Port-au-Prince? How would these patients have received care? I felt a sense of safety somehow and comfort in the fact that we were en route to what I believed would be medical refuge for these patients.

Moments later, reality struck. My truck, having somehow become separated from the others during the drive through the city, came to a stop in front of the Argentine military hospital facing the UN logistics base. A female soldier at the gate was denying us entry. Knowing that I was the only doctor, the blue-helmeted soldiers in the front of the truck gestured for me to get out, and so I did, accompanied by my new shade-providing comrade. The soldier at the gate spoke neither French nor Haitian Kreyol, the two national languages of Haiti. My Spanish being limited, I spoke in English. She gesticulated wildly that we could not enter. I stood just inside the gates, outraged that a UN truck could not enter a UN hospital. I tried to explain that the acting head of the UN in Haiti had guaranteed that we could be brought to a hospital.

"No Haitian nationals can be taken care of here; we are full," a male in uniform lied. Behind him, scores of mattresses were piled one on top of the other, and a medical team stood anxiously by, waiting for patients, their mandate to care for UN staff members, not Haitian civilians. When my Sri Lankan escort interrupted and said "Sir, she was told that she could bring patients here," he was given a fierce look. When he continued. "Excuse me sir, permission to speak," he was again reprimanded. After four or five more minutes of pleading, then pointing out angrily that they didn't have any patients in their wards, and then asking him to call his boss, all to no avail, we turned around and boarded the truck.

I cursed the hospital as we backed up noisily and headed toward the UN logistics base across the street, where the other trucks must have gone. We were easily granted access but were told that there was no hospital—just a makeshift clinic under semipermanent tents. Here I spent the next three days working almost nonstop with other volunteers, trying, again with almost no supplies, to provide some kind of semblance of medical care to the seriously injured. Many volunteers worked around the clock; some were UN staff assigned to other things but helping here anyway. A British ex–Royal Air Force engineer kept up my spirits. We lifted and moved patients, found them food and water, set up our open air operating room, and transferred hundreds of the most seriously injured to vehicles for the airport and evacuation to Martinique, Dominican Republic, Miami, Canada—anywhere with a functional operating room was a better option.

Now here I stood on the airport runway, ready to escape briefly from the crumbling city, the terrifying aftershocks, and the stench of death. Although my Partners In Health colleagues had arrived to help and urged me to take a break, I was overcome with the feeling that I was abandoning them.

One close colleague stepped off the private plane on which I would later that day hitch a ride home. We hugged. I was relieved to know that reinforcements were arriving. My voice was hoarse with dust as I shouted instructions over the roar of jets, struggling to transfer ninety-six hours of information in five minutes. Spotting U.S. soldiers in uniform, my colleague asked: "Have there been any episodes of violence yet?" What kind of violence did he mean? "The soldiers against the Haitians," he said.

I was frustrated by this immediate negativity. It was not the first time since the earthquake that I'd felt this way. Days earlier, sitting in a corner of the temporary UN office where we had found an Internet connection, another much admired colleague and I had a tense exchange after she described the United States as "occupying Haiti again." She had seen U.S. soldiers prevent Haitians from entering the General Hospital to search for relatives. Through my lens, exhausted, having witnessed firsthand the scale of the devastation and desperate for the sight of those who could really help, both colleagues' characterization of U.S. action seemed too negative, compounding my feelings that nothing would work, and that we should expect only the worst. Their interpretation didn't acknowledge the possibility that great power could be used for good.

Certainly not everyone in Partners In Health agrees on the issue of military involvement in humanitarian activities. Most of my colleagues had not yet worked in a disaster situation where military assets might be necessary. My days in the crisis offered context in which to view this situation. The comments of both colleagues were founded in a healthy suspicion based on Haiti's history with militaries, the U.S. military in particular, and on our own organization's experiences in Haiti.

Partners In Health in Haiti began in 1983, twenty-five years into the brutal dictatorship of the Duvalier family, and witnessed a violent Haitian military rule from 1991–1994, before the Haitian army was demobilized in 1995 by President Aristide. Older Haitians remember still the U.S. military occupation of 1915–1934. Even beyond this legacy, most civilians have just cause for skepticism and distrust at the sight of foreign armed forces on their soil.

Unlike some aid organizations, PIH/ZL (Partners In Health/Zanmi Lasante) has no strict doctrine regarding collaboration or interactions with military on professional or social levels, although written policy prohibits weapons inside our vehicles and clinics. In general, our aim is to forge partnerships with other groups, recognizing the complex set of experiences and skills that in collaboration will provide sustained improvement in conditions for the people in the areas in which we work. During my tenure in Haiti, we have used a commonsense approach to military collaborations. When UN forces arrived to stabilize the country after President Aristide's departure in 2004, PIH had both planned and unplanned interactions with MINUSTAH by virtue of their three bases near us in the Central Plateau and Artibonite departments.

My perception of MINUSTAH in rural Haiti before the earthquake, influenced by the opinions of my Haitian neighbors and coworkers, had been one of the heavily armed, resource-intense activities that seemed to have little apparent relevance to the day-to-day needs of the largely peasant farmer population. For these predominantly peaceful, highly rural parts of the country, the struggle of day-to-day survival in the face of severe poverty and serious food insecurity was greater than the largely urban issues of kidnappings, gang violence, and common crime. The inequity of a $601.58 million budget for stabilization in a place with such pressing development needs was flagrant. In 2008, many of our neighbors, the rural poor, questioned the effectiveness of MINUSTAH when the response to a series of four tropical storm and hurricane force rains was slow and inadequate despite the fact that MINUSTAH had resources that could have been faster mobilized to help. In post-hurricane Gonaïves on September 6, 2008, the same day that UN and other sources reported that "access to

Gonaïves remains virtually impossible," a PIH four-wheel drive vehicle traveled the road to the flooded city to transport supplies. The trip was repeated the next day, uneventfully.

We did have some positive interactions with MINUSTAH, including help transporting an X-ray machine one day while we were stuck in the road. Some volunteers from the forces participated during their free time in our community activities, but other community activities promised by the local battalions of MINUSTAH, such as repairing the latrines in a primary school, were not fulfilled. The breadth of PIH's collaboration with MINUSTAH expanded positively and significantly in 2009, when a Brazilian military MINUSTAH engineering core participated in the design and construction of a bridge, donating bridge parts to the government of Haiti.

Waiting on the runway that day, I considered the kindness of the MINUSTAH soldier who had accompanied us from the driveway, and the pain on the face of his commander who had been attempting to rescue colleagues at the nearby UN headquarters. However, in the context of this massive disaster, it was not just my personal perspective on MINUSTAH that was important. All humanitarians had a right to think cautiously about a military presence and to wonder in what context they would act.

I returned to Haiti four days after that initial departure and quickly got back to the tasks at hand, working frantically with a team of colleagues on a series of new projects: providing assistance at the general hospital and developing healthcare services at some of the spontaneous settlement camps. Things remained chaotic, but we were slowly getting our own communications lines in order and assigning each team member a specific task. Our interface with the U.S. military was now an almost everyday occurrence. The USNS Comfort, a U.S. Navy medical treatment vessel, arrived the same day that I returned. Docking two miles off the coast of Haiti, it served as a much-needed tertiary referral hospital for the most severely injured. A Brigham and Women's Hospital junior doctor, one of our residents in Global Health Equity, arrived to join our team. Handing him a cell phone, I asked him if he would manage our patient transfers. "Do you need me to call you about them?" he asked. "Only if you need my help," I replied. Days later, I overheard him calling out GPS coordinates for a helicopter landing zone near our own main hospital in Cange. Despite this being his first working trip to Haiti and with almost no Creole or French skills, he not only had quickly started coordinating our own transfers of patients, but had also figured out how to leverage the goodwill and determination of the U.S. military stationed at the General Hospital and was organizing military helicopter flights for evacuations. At the General Hospital, all but one of our staff reported positive experiences with the U.S. military, describing their willingness on an individual level to do whatever they could and attempts to make their own "big machine" of an organization flex to accommodate the shifting humanitarian needs.

Military involvement in humanitarian activities has become increasingly common since the end of the cold war. Nonmilitary humanitarian actors (typically aid agencies and nongovernmental organizations but also others) must fulfill their role to decrease human suffering by providing services with impartiality. In situations of conflict or violence, association or perception of an association with any one side can prevent those who want to help from gaining access to victims and can also endanger staff. One set of guidelines* for interactions of nonmilitary agencies with military agencies in conflict notes: "The most important distinction to be drawn is whether the military group with which humanitarians are interacting is, has become, or is perceived to be a party to the conflict or not."† Association with military, even if the particular task of the military at that time is to provide support or to reduce human suffering, can have serious consequences for aid organizations.

---

*IASC Principles on Military-Civilian Relations, January 1995; "Guiding and Operating Principles for the Use of Civil and Military Defense Assets in Support of Humanitarian Operations" (Task Force Report), September 2005. "Civil-Military Relationship in Complex Emergencies—An IASC Reference Paper," June 2004; Civil-Military Guidelines and References for Complex Emergencies, OCHA, 2008; Guidelines on the Use of Foreign Military and Civil Defense Assets in Disaster Relief—"Oslo Guidelines," Rev. 1.1, November 2007.

†"Civil-Military Relationship in Complex Emergencies—An IASC Reference Paper," Office of Humanitarian Coordination, United Nations, 2004, http://ocha -gwapps1.unog.ch/w/lib.nsf/db900SID/DPAL-62GCWL?OpenDocument 2011).

In post-earthquake Haiti, the U.S. military mission was officially humanitarian. Reflecting President Obama's "whole of government response" to the crisis,* the U.S. military worked under the direction of the U.S. Agency for International Development (USAID). The choice of military actors to assist in humanitarian assistance was controversial, but in pragmatic terms, the budget, human resources, and logistics assets of the U.S. military are well beyond those of USAID. At the height of the U.S. military footprint, some twenty-two thousand troops were in Haiti or offshore providing assistance, compared to some hundreds of USAID civilian workers—many of whom were seconded from other nations' programs.

At the time of the earthquake, the deputy commander of U.S. Southern Command had been in Haiti. I believe that his personal determination to relieve human suffering set the conditions for his command of Joint Task Force Haiti. For the most part, the troops that he led displayed respect and diligence in their pursuit of supporting the victims of the earthquake. He and his team became a familiar site at a huge temporary settlement camp in Port-au-Prince where my Haitian colleagues and I spent many hours and days during the subsequent months. Haitian community leaders, themselves survivors living in the settlement camp with almost fifty thousand other people, from whom I regularly take my cues, were and are avid fans of the assistance from U.S. military. One day, several of them called me aside and said with glee about the U.S. troopers: *Gade Doktè Louise— bòt yo sal.* "Look, Dr. Louise: They got their boots dirty." So often, people offering help (so-called humanitarian actors included) are not willing to get into the grimy part of the work.

Political and military motivation should be separate from humanitarian assistance. By definition, humanitarianism requires impartiality, which is not possible if aid is delivered as a tool to sway opinions, to win support, or to advance one ideology over another. As an organization that partners first and foremost with the poor,

---

*The White House, "United States Government Haiti Earthquake Disaster Response Update 1/21/10," http://www.whitehouse.gov/the-press-office/united-states-government-haiti-earthquake-disaster-response-update-12110 (accessed March 28, 2011).

PIH looks to those we serve for legitimacy and also to determine what is in their best interest. Paul Farmer wrote in 2003:

> NGOs must, therefore, take great care in attending to their mission of service to the afflicted; because this is the only way they can truly represent the needs of the victims, and avoid common mistakes and historical irresponsibility. It is when we ignore legitimacy in our pursuit of "effective" developmental models, or when we ignore problems that don't fit our own conceptions of what is wrong or how to fix it, that NGOs find themselves complicit in the violence they mean to stop or, at the very least, allay.
>
> Pragmatic solidarity is what allows us to be discerning in which partnerships benefit our patients, and which ones may harm them.*

In truth, no one group or individual has a monopoly on humanitarian actions or goals. The sheer devastation of the earthquake, the flattening of infrastructure, logistics capacity, and medical care, and the loss of key leaders in governmental and nongovernmental sectors required a huge, multifaceted effort. In the face of such catastrophe, we could not afford to ignore military assets. If military cannot by definition be humanitarian actors, they can surely accomplish humanitarian tasks. In Haiti in those first weeks and months, we needed and I welcomed all who came with a humanitarian task in mind, a determination to help achieve the common objective of saving lives and reducing suffering, and a willingness to get their boots dirty.

---

*Nicole Gastineau Campos and Paul Farmer, "Partners: Discernment and Humanitarian Efforts in Settings of Violence." *Journal of Law, Medicine & Ethics* 31 (2003): 506–515.

# LOPITAL JENERAL STRUGGLES TO SURVIVE

EVAN LYON

*Dedicated to Dr. Alix Lassegue, Ms. Marlaine Thompson,*
*and the heroic staff of l'Hôpital Université d'Etat d'Haïti*

*T*he Haitian State University Hospital, *l'Hôpital Université*
*d'Etat d'Haïti* (HUEH), is known in Port-au-Prince and beyond as The General Hospital, *Lopital Jeneral*. It is the largest
public hospital in Haiti and the nation's most important medical institution. The national medical and nursing schools occupy the same
campus, with roots reaching back to the era immediately following
Haiti's independence in the first years of the nineteenth century. Until 2002, when the initial class of physicians graduated from Haiti's
first private medical school, Notre Dame University, the State University was one of very few providers of physician education in Haiti.
Generations of Haitian medical professionals proudly claim HUEH as
their alma mater despite the fragile infrastructures of the hospital
and university, which have weathered many storms, including political change, military unrest, rapid urbanization, hurricanes, and
continuous financial stress.

*Lopital Jeneral* is often the only facility available in the nation for
medical specialty referral and care. It is also, sadly, a hospital of final
resort for the destitute sick and dying. Among the rich and the poor,
the general consensus is that anyone with means would seek care at

another center before going there. HUEH is at once a proud national teaching hospital, an essential referral hospital, and a physically and financially poor facility where clinicians struggle to provide quality compassionate care under crippling conditions. Those who work in Haiti have long been witness to this struggle. The devastating earthquake that rocked Haiti on January 12, 2010, revealed the conditions at the hospital to a worldwide audience.

Everyone has seen photographs of the crumbled domes of the previously grand National Palace. *Lopital Jeneral* sits one block behind the National Palace. At the moment of the earthquake, two-thirds of the hospital was destroyed. The surgical hospital, emergency room, and main operating suites were rendered unusable; all pediatric facilities and half of the internal medicine wards were destroyed; the lab and its equipment were reduced to rubble; and the chronically understocked pharmacy was left in shambles. The State University School of Nursing collapsed while the second-year students sat in a lecture, killing nearly the entire class, along with several of their professors. Perhaps 125 to 150 people died in this one building alone.

On the night of January 12, the HUEH campus was rent by the cries of the hurt and dying—and filling rapidly with more casualties from the disaster. A courageous few staff tended to the injured with flashlights and the few materials they could salvage.

As the sun rose on the morning of the 13th, the extent of the devastation to the campus became clearer. The structural damage, itself immense, paled in light of the human suffering that flooded the hospital as patients—first tens and then hundreds—arrived, searching, too often in vain, for care.

Although many of the hospital staff were now homeless, a brave number of them, as well as Haitian friends and volunteers, came immediately to the hospital to offer their assistance, displaying the same bravery it takes to run toward a burning building. The first foreign assistance workers from the International Medical Corps (IMC), a United States-based nonprofit humanitarian organization, arrived within twenty-four hours to find a devastated campus and very few staff members able to work. By the second and third days, more outside assistance arrived to support the Haitian staff and the IMC in triaging patients, prioritizing the hundreds in need of urgent surgery, and providing first aid and medical treatment as materials allowed. Teams from NGOs around the world, including the International Red Cross, Medécins du Monde, Swiss Humanitarian Aid, Medécins Sans Frontières, and a number of smaller organizations such as Partners In Health/Zanmi Lasante (PIH/ZL), quickly followed. In those first few days, much of the effort was simply stopping the bleeding and attending to the dying.

At the moment the earthquake struck, I was in a clinic caring for people living with HIV in Montgomery, Alabama—applying skills I had learned in Haiti to aid another poor community. During that first night, like everyone connected to Haiti, I did not sleep. It was nearly impossible to gather news from loved ones in Haiti, or much information at all.

A year-long volunteer posting, a few blocks from HUEH, had introduced me to Haiti in 1996. Until I moved to Alabama in 2009, my work centered on Haiti—as a teacher, as a community health volunteer and human rights advocate, and as a physician. When the earthquake struck, I felt, like so many others, that I had no choice but to return there. At Partners In Health's direction, I went to HUEH to volunteer as a doctor—and more important, as part of a team working as a bridge between the Haitian public health system, HUEH leadership, and the many international volunteer relief workers.

When I arrived at HUEH with colleagues from PIH, on the fourth day after the catastrophe, approximately fifteen hundred sick and injured people were spread around the grounds of the hospital, seeking shade or creating shelter from salvaged materials. Many had nothing more than a cloth sheet for cover. A small, newer building at the top of the sprawling campus that had not been seriously damaged by the earthquake was quickly converted into basic operating rooms. Narcotic pain medicines were in very short supply and available only during surgery, with perhaps one dose following. There was no oxygen, making inhaled gas general anesthesia impossible. Operating time was limited by daylight, though teams pushed into the night wearing headlamps. Conditions were clean but far from sterile. Basic surgical supplies were limited, to say nothing of the simple but specialized hardware needed to mend a broken bone. Our surgical teams were forced to resort to a hardware store hacksaw for amputation: a tragic and lasting image of what patients faced in Port-au-Prince's largest hospital.

By the fourth day, more than one thousand patients had been identified as needing major surgery, including amputation, bone repair, and cleaning of dead and infected tissue. That day, we performed between thirty and forty procedures. It took eight days to obtain the antitetanus vaccine we needed. The clinical teams watched helplessly as deadly cases of tetanus and gangrene accumulated day upon day, affecting tens of victims at a time. Unknown numbers of patients who died from infection, blood loss, and simpler medical illnesses might have survived if the hospital had withstood the earthquake.

Even if the hospital campus had been built to withstand an earthquake of this magnitude—as it would have been in a nation not beset by centuries of underdevelopment—and even if the necessary supplies had been available, HUEH would not have been able to function in those first weeks without its staff. As the largest public hospital in Haiti, HUEH employs more than two thousand people. Every single employee was affected by the disaster. Many died. Many more were rendered instantly homeless, tending to basic needs and to injured family and friends with whatever materials they could find. Nearly everyone suffered severe psychological trauma. As is the case throughout Haiti, and especially in the public sector, General Hospital had too few medical professionals even before the earthquake. Senior faculty at HUEH are paid about one-tenth of what they could earn in a private clinic. The situation is even worse for clinical nurses and nurse educators, the vast majority of whom are required to work more than one job to make ends meet. The hospital's cardiology department was relatively strong before the earthquake, with six practicing and teaching faculty. One cardiologist died in the disaster; two others will not return. The entire internal medicine faculty was reduced to fifteen individuals.

The General Hospital also houses the central morgue for the city of Port-au-Prince. Despite the lack of electricity on the campus and the resulting lack of refrigeration, the morgue was the natural place to gather the majority of the casualties that occurred on January 12, 2010, at 4:53 P.M. and in the hours, days, and weeks that followed. No one who worked there will ever forget the image of the dead, stacked and overflowing around the morgue. Nor can we forget the sight of loaders working around the clock to move those who had died to mass graves in dump trunks, their headlights illuminating a scene of unspeakable horror and sadness. The pavement around the morgue remained slick with bodily fluids for several weeks. The smell of dying was everywhere and unrelenting.

In the first days after the earthquake, many remarked how peaceful the streets of Port-au-Prince seemed, even as open spaces were being claimed as camps for the displaced. The darkness and silence of the capital was broken only by the candles or cooking fires of the homeless and the hushed sounds of crying, conversations, and prayer. Dozens of Zanmi Lasante (Partners In Health) doctors and nurses, as well as a few foreign volunteers, circulated throughout Port-au-Prince until 2 and 3 each morning, moving supplies, transporting the wounded, and organizing to provide assistance wherever a foothold could be found. We never worried about our safety on or off the HUEH campus in the two weeks after the disaster.

In stark contrast to the reality in the capital, media outlets around the world began reporting on increasing insecurity and the threat to foreign aid workers in Port-au-Prince. We witnessed hundreds of calm and organized aid shipments and read in the press about unruly crowds and near riots. One breathless article reported that the doors of the national penitentiary had been thrown open, allowing four thousand dangerous prisoners to run amok in the streets. In reality, prisoners had escaped, but with pretrial detention rates of 80 percent, four out of five prisoners in Haiti have merely been accused of a crime. This majority had not yet come before a judge for trial, acquittal, or conviction. Legal scholars in Haiti and the United States estimate that there were no more than three hundred to four hundred dangerous criminals among the escapees. Nonetheless, a compelling and alarming narrative was set in motion.

Superficial intelligence gathering and reporting had tragic consequences for the disaster response efforts at General Hospital and many facilities throughout Port-au-Prince. An already weak supply chain—including a partially destroyed, single-runway airport and devastated machinery at Port-au-Prince's only deepwater port—was further throttled by rumors of danger in the streets. Supplies stopped arriving inside the disaster zone due to these false rumors. Lifesaving medicines, surgical supplies, food, and water collected on the tarmac and in warehouses as patients died in unsupplied hospitals.

Within two weeks of the disaster, a number of volunteer aid workers arrived in the town of Milot, more than 150 miles and six hours from Port-au-Prince. The undamaged *Hôpital Sacré Coeur* addressed all the surgical patients near Milot within forty-eight hours, and relief workers were left idle for days. Everyone was safe, but there were no patients. Without false concerns about security in Port-au-Prince, perhaps these volunteers could have been where they were most needed. With a narrow window in which to address life-threatening injuries immediately after the disaster, lives were lost because of this kind of missed chance.

---

By the time eight weeks had passed since the disaster, the majority of foreign aid organizations had left the HUEH campus. Two organizations—the International Medical Corps and ZL/PIH—continued to provide volunteer clinicians to attempt to meet the hospital's needs. More than a dozen other voluntary organizations assisted with safe water, sanitation, logistics, and supplies. For four months, the emergency department was housed in a series of tents near the entrance of the hospital, an extremely challenging setting for intensive care.

Even as a majority of the wards were housed in crowded and impossibly hot tents, clinical rounds by Haitian and visiting physicians resumed. Along with the routine staff, medical and surgical residents returned to work. By May 2010, a new class of Haitian interns had begun their training and nursing students were back to their studies under tents pitched in a gravel field where their school once stood.

In the months after the earthquake, substantial promises were made about rebuilding the physical infrastructure of General Hospital but progress has been very slow. On February 17, 2010, Nicolas Sarkozy became the first French president to visit its long-independent former slave colony. President Sarkozy toured Port-au-Prince with President René Preval and promised 207 million euros in aid, including the cancellation of 56 million euros in Haitian debt held by France. France and the United States have promised to provide equal co-funding totalling $50 million to go to rebuilding efforts at HUEH. As of this writing, no reconstruction of HUEH has begun under this support, although a feasibility study has been launched.

Unfortunately, this deferred promise to Haiti is but the latest in a centuries-old series. Haiti's history of poverty, environmental destruction, and political chaos, often sown outside its borders, has been discussed elsewhere in this book. Recently, increasing international debt and the austerity of "structural adjustment" has further diminished an impoverished public sector. Basic political, civil, social, and economic rights, including the right to health, cannot be assured by the weakened state. The public sector lacks both the physical and social environment required to create good health for its citizens and adequate health care resources for illness prevention and treatment.

In the popular media, and even in much of the technical and scholarly reporting on Haiti, it has been noted far too frequently that this island nation is "no stranger to suffering." This is a fact, but it is rarely given a full context. Unlike the facts of nature—the unrelenting shifts of the earth's crust or the seasonal Atlantic storm circulations that yearly threaten the region—this fact can be changed. The disaster on January 12, 2010, was an *unnatural* disaster at the dangerous intersection of a natural trigger (the magnitude 7.0 earthquake centered 13 km below the Carrefour neighborhood of Port-au-Prince) and an absolutely *unnatural* vulnerability created in Haiti by centuries of political, economic, environmental, and social forces.

Seismologists frequently write: "Earthquakes don't kill people. Buildings kill people." The earth's movements are not the basic pathophysiology (the unique, disease-defining characteristic) of "earthquake illness." Earthquake illness is a disease of social construction, its severity determined more by the capability of buildings to withstand seismic activity than by the intensity of a tremor. The capability to respond as emergency and health care workers depends, as we've seen tragically in Haiti, almost entirely on how physical and human infrastructure fare on shaking ground.

On February 27, 2010, a magnitude 8.8 earthquake, one of the most powerful recorded in human history, occurred off the coast of Chile. It is dangerous to compare tragedies such as the earthquakes that occurred in Chile and Haiti, but a number of differences are striking. The earthquake in Chile was five hundred times more forceful than the disaster in Haiti, yet best estimates suggest that nearly three hundred thousand people died in Haiti while fewer than six hundred died in Chile. Fewer buildings fell and fewer people died.

It is our responsibility as human beings and as those who care about the present and future of Haiti, not to forget that manmade conditions allowed this unnatural disaster to take such a devastating toll. These conditions took more than two hundred years to create; they could be reversed in much less time. But unless our historic memory is long enough and our analysis of the tragedy is deep enough, efforts to respond—however generous—will be insufficient. If suffering from earthquakes is a disease of social determination, most meaningfully inflected by poverty, than to prevent the next January 12 we must change the social context in which people live.

The international humanitarian response to the earthquake in Haiti, while inadequate to the continuing needs of the Haitian people, seems nearly as unprecedented as the disaster. The generosity, attention, and love shown to Haiti in the weeks and months following the earthquake was humbling and inspiring. Yet for Haitians and those in solidarity with the nation, the speed at which Haiti faded from the headlines was frightening. Without serious and coordinated efforts to address the root conditions that caused the unspeakable suffering beginning on January 12, 2010, another disaster like this will assault Haiti. The trigger may be rain or a microbe; it may be continued deforestation or a malnourished body; it could be another earthquake. In the fall of 2010, we saw tremendous, unnecessary suffering and death from cholera—a disease that has not affected Haiti for at least one hundred years. But if the structural and social conditions for Haitians do not change, the question is not whether another tragedy will occur but when.

No successful strategy for creating lasting, positive change is simple. But in terms of public health, some directions are clear: investment must be made in the public sector, including the rebuilding of a better General Hospital and sustained investment in the material and human resources needed to provide health care for all Haitians. From the perspective of the National University, this investment must include improved and continuing education.

If nursing students at HUEH were able to recommit themselves to their studies—just four months after losing their classmates, under tents covering the patch of rubble where their school once stood—the very least we can do as an international community is to assure that a similar tragedy won't visit Haiti again.

# DOCTORS IN TENTS

## DR. DUBIQUE KOBEL

*O**n the 12th of January,* I was working at the health center where my wife, Nadège, had a job. She was ill that day, so I was filling in for her. After work, I went straight home to study for my board exam in community medicine, which was scheduled for the following day.

When I got home, Nadège was in the dining room with her mother and our baby girl, Annabelle. I ate and was going to our room to take a bath when suddenly the ground tilted. Having lived through several earthquakes in Cuba, I realized what was happening. I made my way to the dining room and saw Nadège's mother, with Anna in her arms, crying out "Jesus, Jesus." She shouted at Nadège to pray with her. Nadège's little brother was chanting psalms. I told them all to take shelter with me at the edge of the room. As we stood there, I remembered that the night before, from about 11 P.M. to midnight, the dogs had been barking a lot and running in every direction.

We lived in a house with two levels, and usually we heard a crowd upstairs, creating lots of noise. But that day the house was eerily silent. When the shaking subsided a bit, we made it to the stairs and got out of the house. Around us, we saw multistory houses collapsed on themselves. Even then we didn't understand the magnitude of the disaster. At some point, we realized that people were dusty with sand and cement, some were rolling around on the ground, some were screaming, and others were covered with blood. We began to understand the gravity of the situation.

I turned to look toward the side of the nearby hills, where buildings were toppling like dominoes, each collapsing into the next. A cloud of white dust rose into the sky, mingled with the cries and screams of the wounded.

We decided to head toward Pont Rouge, where my mother lived. I needed news of her, at any cost. Along the way, I came upon James, an old friend from Cuba. His arm had been broken. My shock gave him the impression that I was laughing, and he said: "Kobel, there's an earthquake and you're laughing." I told him what I had lived through and where we were going.

On our way to Pont Rouge, we saw fallen towers, collapsed houses and public buildings, and smashed cars. Motorcyclists were carrying the injured, and people were screaming and running in all directions. Anxiety and uncertainty were writ on every face, as those who survived tried to find out the fate of their missing families and loved ones.

At Pont Rouge, neighbors told me that my father's house had collapsed and that my mother and brothers were at Parc Jean-Marie Vincent. I went there to search for them. As the evening's shadows began to fall, it was hard to see, and I called out my mother's and my brothers' names. Someone told me where to find them, and we joined one of my sister's-in-law, the wife of my brother Wendy, and my four-month-old nephew, along with other children and women. At least four women gave birth in the camp that night.

Then I went to Christ the King in Delmas 3 to inquire about my father and my other brothers. My pilgrimage continued back to Pont Rouge to reassure my mother about the fate of my father. I walked to Petionville to check on another loved one. The entire journey, I saw many dead lying on the road and on the sidewalks. Beside the Church Altagrace in Delmas, I greeted an old friend, a priest, praying with a large gathering of the faithful. We talked a bit, and I continued on my way. It was risky to travel on foot because of the live wires on downed electrical towers and the continuing tremors. Luckily, the people I had gone to see were unharmed.

Around one o'clock in the morning, I returned to our house,

which looked as though it had been made of cardboard. I ran inside and took a few suitcases, some milk for Annabelle, and a lamp. Back outside, I saw that the devastation blocked my previous route. I found another way back to my family and arrived at Parc Jean-Marie Vincent about 2:30 A.M.

The next day, we had to find something to eat and drink. We had nothing but what I took from the house, and had lost our bearings. The park was like a public canteen, with people sharing what little they had with one another. A strong wind began to blow, and people began to scream and run, fearing a tsunami in the wake of the earthquake. During the panic, we were separated for a few hours before being reunited back at the Parc.

We had to keep Annabelle in our arms all day long. Exhausted, my mother-in-law was inspired to make a makeshift bed for the baby consisting of a plastic tub, some cloths, and a mosquito net. The corpses rotting in the streets attracted swarms of flies, which covered Annabelle's net and also found their way inside it. She was still covered with dust, and had to be changed often. While we were in the park, she caught conjunctivitis twice.

We spent our days on the street in Charlotin and evenings at the Parc Jean-Marie Vincent. I was always worried because the situation in the park was intolerable. People had nowhere to put their waste and were burning their trash so the air smelled foul. However, we thought it best to stay put at the park because all the movements from place to place were not good for Annabelle. We needed some stability, so we tolerated the presence of flies on everything we touched and people fighting all day long, some even throwing stones. Finally, portable toilets were installed, but the smell was even worse when they drained. My mother-in-law did everything in her power to protect Annabelle from the stench, putting cologne on her face and body. We ultimately spent five months living in those conditions.

Although we were refugees in the park, we saw that the people there needed care and understood that it was our job as physicians to take care of them. We couldn't remain indifferent to their suffering. Word that doctors were working in the camp spread quickly, and wounded people started arriving from every direction.

As graduation gifts, in Cuba, we had each received a kit including stitching materials, so we started to operate. Cases beyond our competence and equipment we referred to Centre Ste Catherine in Cité Soleil, where a Cuban surgeon was operating. The days passed thus. Nadège's younger brother paid for us to travel to the pharmacy to buy some medicine, and we did the best we could in those unsustainable, unhygienic conditions.

At the end of January, we met Dr. Lambert, Pierre-Paul, and Maxo from Zanmi Lasante, Partners In Health. They were planning to visit Caradeux, Dadadou, and Plant 2004. I told them about our work at the park, the number of refugees there, and the conditions, and then I asked them to visit. We had never been visited by a government representative, although I had met a foreign journalist and a Haitian journalist in the Parc. The Sisters of Charity, dressed in blue, arrived but left after a short while because they didn't work in the health sector.

The doctors from Zanmi Lasante did come, and they stayed to serve the people living in Parc Jean-Marie Vincent. We joined their team, initially as volunteers. As funds were raised, we were hired and have been part of the Zanmi Lasante team ever since. They have supported us and allowed us to continue our work up to this very moment.

For the country of Haiti, the earthquake of January 12 was a fatal blow. For me, it was an unforgettable experience. I grew up, matured, and realized what life is, real life. The earthquake changed my way of seeing and understanding things and marked me indelibly. Nothing surprises me now.

So much has been destroyed that only traces of our old life remain in our new one. When we first began to offer care to patients in Parc Jean-Marie Vincent, Nadège and I used a table and chairs that I retrieved from our home—these are now part of the furniture at Clinic Zanmi Lasante.

# THOSE WHO SURVIVED

## NAOMI ROSENBERG

*W*hen the earthquake hit Haiti on January 12, 2010, Seleine Gay, a twenty-seven-year-old mother of three, was selling juice underneath a local hospital in Port-au-Prince. She managed to squirm out from under two stories of fallen concrete, her leg destroyed, and hobble to the closest hospital. For days she lay there with only a bit of gauze wrapped around her rotting leg and no medication for the pain. Her husband and children were not allowed in the hospital due to the crowds and chaos. Seleine gave birth to her first child in her early teens and, before the earthquake, was making just enough money each day to find some food and water for her family. For five days she lay still, stared at the ceiling, and prayed.

On Saturday, January 16, several doctors came by. Seleine heard a man say that she would surely die by morning. A few hours later, with no time to say goodbye to her family, she was evacuated from Port-au-Prince in the middle of the night. She arrived in Philadelphia, a city she would know, for months, only through the narrow windows of the hospital.

Seleine had not been to school in Haiti and could not read or write. She was given consent forms and heard discussions of a do not resuscitate order; these were foreign to her, but she learned how to mark an X when handed a pen. Her lower leg had to be amputated the day she arrived, surgeons sparing her knee and thigh in a BKA (below the knee) procedure. They tried to comfort her by cheerfully telling her that some people "still play tennis" with a BKA and prosthetic device.

In the days following her operation, Seleine was lively, confident, and efficient. She fed and bathed herself before dressing and carefully massaged the stump she referred to as "her baby." Nurses and doctors trailed in and out of her room. Visitors from a nearby church and Haitians living in Philadelphia came to offer support.

Two weeks after her arrival, however, Seleine began to not eat or sleep. When she asked her husband, still in Haiti, about their children, he told her he had sent them away. For days she couldn't find them as they were shuffled from relative to relative. One of every twenty calls she made to Haiti would be answered, only to be disconnected after a few seconds. Her amputation led to several infections, and Seleine did not understand the operations that were necessary in their wake. Every setback made her feel like she was failing her assignment to recover. She lay still, stared at the ceiling, and prayed.

Each of the patients who survived the earthquake and came to Philadelphia for treatment has a harrowing, tragic and important story. It is impossible to tell each of those stories here, but I can share a bit more of Seleine's story. I hope the others' stories will also be told one day.

On Tuesday, January 12th, as the world learned of the hundreds of thousands injured by the earthquake, countless surgical, medical, and supply teams began preparing to deploy to Haiti. Those working in Port-au-Prince, however, quickly realized that it would be days before visiting surgeons could begin operating in makeshift field hospitals set up throughout the city. One walk among the thousands lying injured in General Hospital also made it clear that many would not survive to see the arrival of those teams.

On Friday, January 15, Dr. Joia Mukherjee, Medical Director of Partners In Health, suggested that PIH consider evacuating some of the injured for surgical care. For years, PIH had been operating a

Right to Health Care (RTHC) program, which brings patients to the United States and elsewhere when care is not available in their home countries. Many RTHC patients require cardiac surgery; occasionally we provide chemotherapy or surgical intervention for young cancer patients easily treated with the tools of modern medicine. PIH triages these patients, lines up institutions willing to donate treatment, shepherds families through the arduous passport and visa processes, and then addresses the need for clothes, food, and other supplies upon the patients' arrival. A PIH staff member stays with patients and their families through tests, operations, and appointments, careful to understand the treatment so that he or she can offer comprehensive and meaningful guidance and support during a tremendously difficult time. When patients are ready to leave the hospital, we also place them in a home and assist throughout the outpatient treatment while preparing them to return to their home country with whatever follow-up care is necessary.

Described this way, the process sounds tidy, but it never is. For a young rural Haitian, often ill for years, leaving the countryside for potentially lifesaving treatment can be a harrowing experience. The abrupt transition from illness to health and from rural Haiti to the cutting edge of modern scientific research and medicine can be both lifesaving and brutal. Whenever our staff picks up a patient arriving in Boston, usually in the middle of the night due to flight schedules, and whisks him or her to the hospital emergency room, we find ourselves face-to-face with the gross inequities that cause many to suffer greatly from treatable, preventable illness and injury.

After Dr. Mukherjee's January 15 request that we look into evacuation for the injured, the RTHC team set to work. I immediately contacted my home institution, the Hospital of the University of Pennsylvania (HUP), while others went to our contacts at hospitals in Boston to see what they would be willing to do. Dr. Richard Shannon, Chair of Internal Medicine at HUP, responded within the hour. "I have contacted the CEO of HUP. Let's do it." Without a doubt, this quick response made possible the days and weeks of work that would follow. With HUP's guarantee of free care for the injured regardless of their ability to pay (often the most difficult piece to put into place in the pre-earthquake era), we could approach the many United States government institutions responsible for immigration and say confidently that transport and treatment for the dying had already been arranged. We would simply need permission to leave Haiti and enter the United States. However, obtaining these permissions was not a simple matter in a place where the nucleus of government and the majority of government facilities had been destroyed. Our contacts in the embassies, immigration offices, and airport in Haiti were no longer available. The city of Port-au-Prince was in chaos, and the air traffic control tower was out of commission. The United States military was taking over the airport, and getting a landing slot in Haiti became a Herculean task.

Vanessa Kerry, a doctor who has worked with PIH for many years, and her father, Senator John Kerry, stepped in to help immediately. Dr. Kerry made contact with USAID and others to help pave the way for the necessary permissions. Senator Kerry, as head of the Foreign Relations Committee, had taken a leadership role in congressional efforts following the earthquake, and a member of his staff guided us in requesting the appropriate permissions to proceed with evacuations. Tremendous efforts were made by those in the network of government agencies tasked with various Haiti assignments to get us landing slots and alert Homeland Security to our arrival. Given the life-or-death urgency of getting some patients to the hospital, we were able to get permission for some of them to go through customs without passports and photo identification—patients' copies of which had been destroyed in the earthquake, and the original documents destroyed along with Haiti's National Archives—in time to save their lives.

A medical evacuation company donated its plane and crew for what would become our first post-earthquake evacuation. The pilot and plane nurses were far more than a flight crew. One in-flight nurse had served in the U.S. Army and would later prove a strong advocate and a whatever-it-takes friend as conditions in Port-au-Prince made it difficult to land, load patients, and take off in the time needed to give them the best chance of survival.

At 8:05 P.M., as the plane took off from Fort Lauderdale, three PIH doctors—Evan Lyon, Joia Mukherjee, and Louise Ivers—were in

Port-au-Prince, making their way to the damaged General Hospital, where many patients had gathered. People later asked, "How was that one group chosen?" The patients would likely tell you, "Only God knows. Obviously God has a plan for my life." But we used the principles of the Right to Health Care program, which prioritizes patients who would die without care, who could not be treated in their own country, and whose lives could be saved with a relatively straightforward intervention readily available in the United States. Hundreds if not thousands of people fit that description that night in Port-au-Prince. Our doctors had to choose five: the plane could carry four patients who could sit and one who could lie flat. In the end, our doctors chose Seleine Gay; a four-year-old boy, Given Dorsinde Denera; Given's father Marcel Denera; a twenty-one-year-old orphan, Rose Sherline Pluviose; and a thirty-three-year-old mother of three, Berlyne Bernard. With little discussion, our patients were brought out of the hospital into an ambulance and jostled through Port-au-Prince to a plane waiting on the runway at the airport.

Upon arrival in Philadelphia, U.S. Customs and Border Protection opened the door to the tiny plane, and the patients were loaded on board an ambulance, smelling of urine and blood and dying flesh. The immigration intake process was mercifully quick. By 5:55 A.M. on Sunday, January 17, the group was traveling to Hospital of the University of Pennsylvania and Children's Hospital of Philadelphia (CHOP), where teams in both hospitals worked tirelessly to save the patients' lives.

The weeks of surgeries, tests, procedures, and appointments that followed are difficult to chronicle. All three adult women required amputations—two upon arrival and one a few days later after a brief attempt to save her foot. The wounds were gangrenous; after each woman's initial operation, doctors would need, again and again, to "revise the stump," each time taking off a bit more bone to stay ahead of infection. It is difficult to know what each person was feeling during that time. I spent the days racing back and forth among the women, who were dignified and gracious under the most difficult of circumstances. It was a lengthy stay: Seleine and Rose Sherline remained in the hospital until February 23, Berlyne was discharged on March 4, and Given left the hospital during the last week of March.

By September 2010, nine months after the earthquake, twenty-one people had been evacuated from Haiti to Philadelphia in the care of Partners In Health. Thirteen of them had been hours away from death. Our patients and their guardians ranged in age from two months to fifty years. Their education, socioeconomic status, and life experiences are as varied as those of any twenty-one strangers plucked out of a disaster anywhere in the world. Now, in many ways, this community of circumstance has become a family. Ricot Noel, who arrived in April, now says "We live like brothers and sisters. If one of us is sad, thinking about what happened, we can know. We just know."

Many times, the Haitians in Philadelphia referenced January 12 as "the day I died." Sometimes they also referenced January 17 or January 31 as "the day God saved me." Today they are all recovering. The tools and comforts of modern medicine have been made available with great success. They are healing from injuries and illnesses that threatened to take their lives within twenty-four to forty-eight hours had they not been evacuated from Haiti. And yet the complexity of survival in United States is overwhelming. Among just this one group in Philadelphia, the list of losses is long: five limbs, the ability to walk, a wife, a mother, seven neighbors, nine houses, two businesses, possessions too numerous to count. These patients were uprooted and dislocated from their families, from a language they understand, from their country full of people with a common experience and grief. They are still trying to make sense of what happened to them.

It is the central work of any doctor to help the patient in front of her. The tension between serving those in front of you and seeking to reduce the risk of their ending up in front of you, as Paul Farmer has described, keeps many of us up at night. We try hard to plan our next moves thoughtfully and delineate in our mind's eyes the communities we serve and the institutions we choose to align ourselves with. At times, the possibility of erasing the ever-widening gap between the world's rich and poor becomes reality in the experience of one small group of individuals. In this case, institutions answered the call and a community came together to heal the sick and comfort the suffering.

---

How do we care for the sick and injured after they are here? What are the responsibilities of those who bring them? How far should we go to make them healthy? The Partners In Health model emphasizes the concept of accompaniment, be it for patients in Haiti's rural Central Plateau or Boston's chronic disease clinic. A community health worker is hired and trained to deliver medications each day, as needed, and to return to the hospital with a checklist of deliveries and any relevant medical information they've collected while visiting their patients. *Accompagnateurs*, as we call those community health workers, have been the backbone of twenty years of work in rural Haiti, constantly teaching one another and the newer teams in Rwanda, Malawi, and Lesotho the best ways to provide high-level care under difficult physical, economic, cultural, and geographical conditions.

In Philadelphia, our program remains true to form. During the initial weeks, I spent hundreds of hours in the hospital talking to doctors, joining patients for various tests and procedures, helping them make phone calls home, and trying to provide consistency in lives that had been torn apart. A call to all PIH donors and supporters drew enormous response. We needed for these families anything and everything one might need in daily life—the basics of food, shelter, clothes, and transportation. Our patients arrived with literally the clothes on their backs—some without even shoes. A local contractor put together a team of men who spent twenty hours a day rebuilding a house that had been donated for the patients to live in. The contractor remembered the earthquake in Mexico City, near the city of his birth, and quickly learned how to make the house handicap-accessible and otherwise ease group living for the Haitians. Local donors visited the hospital with fresh fruit and supplies from their own homes, and they continued to help with rides, with outings in an effort to make the days more fun, and by paying for any number of things. We simply could not have cared for these patients as we did without the network of generous and compassionate people that PIH has built throughout the country.

As the patients grew stronger and were able to leave the hospital, we moved them into the house and hired three Haitian home health aides to help with bandage changes, to supervise medications, to cook and clean, and to navigate the washing machine, grocery store, and bus system. As the months passed, we had become a family. We spend many nights eating together and many weekends in one another's homes celebrating birthdays and anniversaries or simply passing the time. When there was a death in my own family last year, my Haitian family attended the funeral. They wouldn't have it any other way.

It is hard to know what will come next for these families. Some were given an "indefinite" stamp to stay in the United States. Others were granted two years. Some will be healthy enough by then that they could go back to Haiti. Two of the children will need years of follow-up that would be best provided in a country with abundant tertiary care. But physicians in Haiti would certainly do their best with physical therapy and additional surgeries if necessary.

As an organization, we are facing difficult decisions about the future of these patients. PIH brings patients here for treatment and, when that treatment is complete, helps them get home—healthy and often with social supports such as school fees, a new house, and clothes for the other children in the family. This "turnover" allows us to continue bringing new patients to the United States for care while spending the bulk of our resources in the countries in which we work. Should these cases be any different? We grapple with the ways in which we could continue to provide support. PIH often struggles with how to allocate money between needs in Haiti and organizational or patient needs in the United States. These patients are no exception. As difficult decisions arise, we do our best to make them mindfully. And I watch carefully to see how Sherline negotiates difficult terrain in her wheelchair, knowing that sidewalk quality on a Philadelphia street is light-years away from the roads and rocky terrain of rural or even urban Haiti.

In August, I spent a week with my family in the Outer Banks in North Carolina, a spot we visit each year. It is a sacred time away from the daily grind of work and school. This year, three of the children from Haiti—Given, Bettina, and Lolo—came with me. I hoped to give their parents a break for the first time in six months, and to give the kids a chance to leave the house and experience a week at the beach. When we arrived, the kids eyed my family and our surroundings with suspicion and wonder. They stayed close those first few hours, clinging to me and refusing even to go to the bathroom by themselves. By the end of the week, the kids were playing in the sand with my young cousins while I read upstairs. They were willing to interrupt their time outdoors only to yell "cornflakes please" to the closest adult and then sprint into the house in their wet bathing suits for a quick refueling.

Given sprinted in his walking cast and tenderly put sunscreen on his mountain of scar tissue. Bettina waited twice a day for her medications. The kids wanted to shower multiple times each day, marveling and giggling at the free-flowing warm water and the fact that they weren't in Haiti anymore; there weren't hundreds of others waiting, jostling, and yelling for them to hurry up so others could share in the limited resource. Lolo, the fifteen-month-old who had lost his mother in the earthquake, had nightmares, screaming and inconsolable at 3 A.M. The four of us shared a king-size bed decorated with a seashell comforter.

Nine months after the earthquake, we reviewed the numbers: more than two hundred thousand dead; more than twenty thousand amputations; a million injured; more than a million homeless. Enormous effort has gone into saving the lives of the small number of people who arrived in Philadelphia. In this we see both the mission of Partners In Health and, more generally, the heart of medicine. Although we are always allocating limited resources based on the greatest good for the greatest number, we never consider a single effort to be "a drop in the bucket" or energy wasted. If we did, our organization would have stopped the moment we were spending ten thousand dollars to treat a single AIDS patient in rural Haiti or in our first effort to make life-saving chemotherapy available to a young woman afflicted by breast cancer there. Now we are proud to say that both treatments, both tools of modern medicine widely accessible in the "developed" world, are available to patients in Haiti. Moreover, their use is no longer truly extraordinary or expensive there. We, the world's wealthy, must have the courage to dream big for the communities we serve and to take on the challenge of turning high hopes into reality. Today, in early 2011, it is devastating to realize that "dreaming big" for families in Haiti may consist of clean water for a household wracked by cholera, or a new home for a family living under a tarp in Port-au-Prince. But the patients here in Philadelphia are living testimony to what is not only possible but *required* if we are to fulfill our mission of providing comprehensive, high-quality health care to the destitute sick.

I am proud to declare that these twenty-one lives are worth extraordinary effort. Some people have asked: "Couldn't you have used that money to help even more people in Haiti?" Medicine cannot stop to argue when there is a patient suffering on the ground. The great joy of a life in medicine is that ability and that mandate: to do whatever it takes for the patient in front of you. No matter how deep the tragedy, or how expansive, we continue our work—one patient at a time.

# FIRST WE NEED TAXIS

## TIMOTHY T. SCHWARTZ

*hat do they do?* I am in Léogâne, epicenter of the earthquake, ten days after it struck. I am addressing the question to Joseph (not his real name).

Few people on earth could be better qualified to answer the question. Joseph is an American foreign service officer who has spent his thirty-two-year career in some of the poorest, disaster-wrenched countries on earth: Congo, Rwanda, Nigeria, Angola, Sudan, and now, for the past four years, Haiti.

The people I am asking him about are two officials from DART, the United States Disaster Assistance Response Team. Who could be more qualified to organize logistics than an organization with a name like that? They are some forty feet away, doing the same thing that Joseph already did: interviewing a pair of paramedics from the United States.

The paramedics are two among hundreds of people who got tired of seeing the thousands of untreated Haitians on television, packed into clinics, sitting in streets and empty lots waiting for medical attention. And so they got off their couches, bought plane tickets, and came to Haiti to do something about it. For three days, they have been treating hundreds of patients a day.

The DART officers are scribbling in notebooks; the paramedics are talking and surely saying the same things they said to me and Joseph. Next, the DART officers will interview the Cuban doctors and a half dozen German paramedics from another independent aid agency, all of whom Joseph and a series of other officials—Canadian, U.S. Navy, UN—have interviewed, and all of whom are tired of being asked the same questions—most importantly, "What can we do to help you?"—and receiving no help in return.

"I don't know what the hell they do," Joseph replies, squinting at them. "They usually don't even leave the office."

After the DART officers have visited all the other doctors and paramedics, Joseph and I are huddled with them. Joseph has introduced me, explaining that I am an anthropologist who has worked in Haiti for the past twenty years and that I have volunteered. The two DART officers, a man and a woman in their mid-thirties, are stone-faced. As we talk, I am imagining that, after ten days of rescue chaos, this is finally the beginning of a coordinated aid effort. These people, I am thinking, are the real thing. They're feeling out the zone, taking notes, and in another couple days, the United States will come in here and put everything in order.

For the sake of efficiency, I volunteer to visit all the other aid agencies in town and gather information. The DART officers think that would be a big help. They can go on to the next town with Joseph; I will stay here and get the data. This way they can maximize their time out here in the field. It's agreed.

Léogâne is a small town, covering less than a square mile. And it's starting to fill up with NGOs and medical agencies.

Daphne Mervil, a student at Léogâne Université Episcopal d'Haïti nursing school, tells me, "Within hours after the earthquake struck, we had more than five hundred injured people." The nursing students and their two instructors did the best they could to care for the injured. They stacked the dead behind the building and laid the wounded back out in the field. The first doctor, an American, arrived Friday, three days after the earthquake. But significant help did not begin arriving until the following Monday, seven days after the quake, when Joseph and I visited the first time. Now the help seems massive.

I am standing next to a large Canadian flag listening to the public relations representative of a Canadian field hospital. They have twenty beds, meds, and can see two hundred patients per day. Next, I am with the director of the Medécins Sans Frontières (MSF). Around us men are carrying poles. A bed goes by. Tents are going up. I'm jotting it all down. Lists of doctors, psychologists, surgeons, nurses.

In all, eight medical groups and twenty-eight aid organizations are in Léogâne. All but the Cubans, who were here when the earthquake struck, have arrived in the past couple days. In a few more days, about the time most of the field hospitals get finished, the flow of gangrenous survivors will abruptly abate. Those that didn't get help will be dead. Some of those who did will be missing limbs. A lucky minority will have been treated and returned to a relatively normal, if traumatized, life. Then a new avalanche of patients will begin, what the doctors call primary care patients, the many Haitians who were already suffering from chronic diseases, worms, and infections before the earthquake. They will come to take advantage of the opportunity to get high-quality medical care, for Léogâne is turning into a massive hospital.

But for now, hundreds of wounded are pouring in and Léogâne has all these organizations with different capacities and supplies. The Spanish Red Cross has water makers. The Austrian Red Cross has latrines and pumps. The French at MSF have meds and a laboratory for blood work. The Japanese are the only ones with an X-ray machine, but the Germans are bringing another. The Cubans have four surgery rooms, twenty general practitioners, and five orthopedic surgeons. Heart to Heart at the Nazarene Church has pharmaceuticals, vaccines, and disposable medical supplies; and on and on.

---

"Wait! Can you take a baby back to Port-au-Prince with you?" a German paramedic asks. The baby, he explains, has a hematoma on its head and is in critical condition. "If it does not get to the children's hospital, it will die."

I don't want to take a baby with a busted skullcap twenty miles back to the city, through congested streets, battle my way into a hospital crowded with earthquake survivors, and then try to find a doctor to take the baby from me. I am trying to be a journalist here, and now I have this little volunteer job for DART. I am on a motorcycle, which means I really cannot take the baby. But what do you do?

"I will find someone to take the baby," I tell the paramedic and get on my motorcycle.

It can't be difficult. All these aid agencies plus the U.S. Marines, the Canadian Navy, the Canadian Army, Chilean, Nepalese, and Brazilian soldiers, and the UN World Food Programme. They are camped all over the place, in closed and guarded compounds, and they all have vehicles. I crank the bike. I try the Marines first.

"I don't think it's going to happen, sir." I am standing in a field where U.S. marine helicopters have been landing and taking off all day, talking to a marine who's guarding the launchpad. "You guys can't airlift the baby out with you? It's only this big." I hold my hands out. He looks like the classic bad-ass marine. Blond, tough, cradling a machine gun, mouth full of chewing tobacco. "It seems like it would be the perfect system," I say, trying not to seem aggressive. "You guys could just take injured people back to Port-au-Prince with you when you go."

His eyes light up, "That's what I've been saying: evacuate people in helicopters."

"Well, why the hell won't they do it?"

"Hey man," he spits a large black mouth full of tobacco juice into the dirt, "I just work here."

———

I am at the entrance to the Canadian army compound asking another heavily armed soldier if his people can help the baby, when two white American men and a Haitian-American man jog over, dressed in fresh surgery garb. They pass right by me and talk to the Canadian guards, explaining that they are a group of five orthopedic surgeons. Do the guards know of any hospitals where they can do surgery? As the guards tell them about different hospitals, the doctors are shaking their heads and growing more frustrated. They have been to all those hospitals and they won't do. They lack supplies or already have too many doctors. Defeated, the doctors begin to walk away. I hear one say, "Let's go back to Port-au-Prince."

"Wait!"

The doctors stop. "Can you take a baby with you?" I ask.

"Oh, no, no, no." says the Haitian-American doctor.

I can't believe it. "What the hell do you mean, 'no?'" I want to unload this moral burden. "The baby is dying."

"Where's the baby?" He asks.

"Follow me."

We arrive in the compound, me on my motorcycle, the doctors following in a battered sedan. When they get out of the car and realize that the surrounding tents are field hospitals, the doctors brighten. "Are they doing surgery in there?" a young American doctor asks me, ducking into the nearest tent to check it out.

Meanwhile, the other four doctors cluster around the baby, which is nestled in its mother's arms, mouth in a kind of scowl close to her breast. The baby's eyes are closed, the sockets sunken and dark. The hematoma, a squishy baseball-sized glob, is off one side of its head. When one doctor pokes at it, the baby's scowl tightens into a grimace. The mother appears about to cry.

The doctor goes into diagnostic mode, "There is nerve reaction."

"Yes." The other doctors nod their heads.

Then the four doctors, standing around the seated mother and baby, launch into a brisk discussion. They use medical jargon, nod a lot, and in less than sixty seconds reach a conclusion. They break. Two of the doctors duck into the surgery tent where their colleague had gone earlier, another heads for the car, and the last one, the Haitian-American, remains. "The baby," he addresses me directly, "is not *dying*," and he then drives his point home, "as you said."

He is off the hook.

"The baby should have an X-ray," he continues, aiming the directive right at me. "When you are finished with that, get the number of the X-ray. Tomorrow, when I come back through here, I will take a look at it."

Even if I could take the baby for an X-ray and keep track of the mother, I know that I will never see this doctor again. Indeed, Léogâne will probably never see this doctor again.

The other doctors come out of the surgery tent shaking their heads and talking about the lack of equipment. They cannot work here. Defeated, they head for the car, all five of them.

"Wait!"

They stop.

"Can't you take the baby?" I ask.

"No, no, no." They all get into the car.

I am pushing it, I know. Five doctors, surgeons no less, in the wake of the most destructive earthquake in the history of the Western hemisphere. But then, the X-ray machine is on the other side of town, miles away at the Japanese field hospital. I can't carry the baby on my motorcycle.

"Not even to the X-ray machine?" I ask, but none of the doctors are even looking at me now. They are climbing into the car, closing the doors.

———

When the earthquake struck, I was in the Dominican Republic. I drove to Haiti with Ben, a retired special forces army major. We drove through the night, down dark and deserted Dominican roads, and arrived in Port-au-Prince with the rising sun. We had come to help.

I've spent a large chunk of the past twenty years living and working in Haiti as part of the aid industry. Like so many people who've worked here, a sense of frustration and failure haunts me. I've watched the country sink ever deeper into a quagmire of misery and despair while I've accomplished nothing tangible to stop the process; indeed, occasionally I have earned a respectable salary or, by Haitian standards, a fortune. Now with the earthquake, the tasks at hand are obvious. Thousands of injured and homeless people need immediate help, no question about it. No need to sit down and write a proposal or a plan; no time for meetings or evaluations. It's just a matter of doing something, fast. So we came to help, to pull people from the rubble, to carry people to hospitals.

That first day we helped the Embassy and USAID officials evacuate. We carried their luggage. Then we stood there in the Embassy parking lot, watching as the American officials pulled out, a long line of black SUVs, headed to the airport. "As an American," Ben said to me as we stood there, "I find this a little embarrassing."

The second day, desperate to participate, Ben and I hauled around a team of rescuers in my truck. But we didn't feel like we helped. Their supervisors, who were orchestrating our movements over a radio, kept directing us to the same four high-profile sites, sealed off compounds where we would join dozens of other rescue teams, and where we did nothing, absolutely nothing. We sat there. It was wrecking our nerves.

Like the doctors who couldn't be bothered with the baby, we wanted to do the things we felt we could do best. We imagined ourselves translating for doctors, carrying the wounded, fetching supplies. So we abandoned the rescue crews and spent the morning of the third day trying to attach ourselves to a medical team. The only medical team we found was an air force team in the U.S. Embassy, but they were not authorized to leave the compound. They had been there for almost two days but had not performed any surgery because they had no medical supplies. Not medics ourselves, we went to the airport to try to fetch their medical supplies. But we had to have security clearance. So we attached ourselves to an 82nd airborne unit. We were supposed to act as translators, fly in on the helicopters with the troops, talk to the crowds through bullhorns, coax them back as the soldiers delivered food and water. But instead, we wound up sitting around for six hours with fifty soldiers and a crew from *60 Minutes,* doing nothing.

Frustrated, Ben got on a boat and sailed for the Bahamas. I went home, back to the Dominican Republic for a few days. I thought that when I came back there would be some organization; that someone would have taken control of the logistics. Then I could find a place where people could make the most use the skills I have to offer.

When I got back, a new trend had taken hold. Armed security guards and soldiers barred access to most compounds: the Embassy, the airport. Offers to help aid agencies came back null. I settled into being a journalist. And that's what I was doing when I volunteered for DART and the problem with the baby came up.

—————

The baby was only a single incident. While I was going around to the different hospitals gathering information for DART, other doctors and paramedics had stopped me. First someone wanted hypertension medicine for a woman with preeclampsia. Then a person wanted me to lead a team of surgeons to another hospital where they had facilities to work on a patient suffering a particularly complex wound. Finally I realize that this is an opportunity.

Haiti has all this equipment and capacity but it's scattered all over and no one knows what is where. Perhaps more important than anything else, the Japanese have the only X-ray machine in Léogâne, but it is on the far side of town. But where I am, the doctors are amputating limbs because of infection and are trying to evaluate the degree of damage before they do so. If only they could get to that X-ray machine. The solution is easy: They need a vehicle to ferry people back and forth.

I realize that at this point we don't need more doctors, and we may not even need more equipment or medicines. What we need is communication and transportation between the organizations that are here. I go around with the bright new idea: "We can pay a taxi to haul patients to the X-ray machine."

Everyone, Germans, Cubans, Dominicans, even the Canadian director of the field hospital thinks it's a great idea. But no one has funds on hand to pay for it. So I go out and with my last $20, a lot of promises, and arguing, and putting the moral burden on someone else—in this case Haitians—I hire a taxi. As we are pulling into the compound, I see a helicopter lifting off. "Okay," I ask one of the German paramedics, "where's the baby?"

"In that helicopter," he says pointing to the sky. "We are sending it to Port-au-Prince to be flown to Miami."

"What?"

"Yah," he says, in a heavy German accent, "it will die soon if we don't."

I am at a compound called New Missions talking to Boga, a Haitian man who says that he is in charge of regional NGO coordination. I think Boga might have something wrong with him. Who stands around in the middle of an earthquake saying they are coordinating, though it is clearly evident that in the ten days since the earthquake he has not coordinated a damn thing?

I introduce Boga to ten motorcycle taxi drivers—all of whom he already knows by name—and explain that they are here to run errands and transport medicines, messages, and people between the different hospitals. "If the doctors need anything, you send these guys." Then, getting a little ahead of myself, I tell him that DART will help us coordinate. Boga is delighted. I introduce him to the driver of the van I hired the day before, put him in charge, and then head back to Port-au-Prince where I can report to DART and start working on pulling together the coordination effort.

On my way home, riding my 400 Suzuki, I calculate the tasks that have to be accomplished. I will begin by circulating a text message explaining that this is a coordination of aid efforts to best manage the resources and not duplicate efforts. I will explain that everyone should direct requests for airlifts to DART. DART will surely set up a switchboard where doctors, paramedics, and other aid workers can direct requests so that we don't inundate one another with e-mails. It's a no-brainer.

On the median that divides the road are makeshift tents of sticks and deteriorated plywood boards with bedsheets hung over them for cover. My phone starts buzzing. It's the director of MSF hospital in Léogâne, and he needs to evacuate someone. I call Joseph, who is with the DART guys. They make some calls and then Joseph tells me everything is taken care of. I feel good because things are happening. Taxis, evacuations. I'm helping.

When I get back to Port-au-Prince I text DART but get no response. In the morning, still no response. I head back to Léogâne.

The first thing I see when I get to the mission compound is our taxi van pulling out of the compound, headed for the X-ray machine. It is full of wounded and bandaged people. A leg wrapped in fresh white plaster sticks out a back window. The side door is open and I can see people sitting on one another's laps. Despite all the inertia and my ineffectiveness that first week, I now have something to contribute.

But who is going to pay for this? There's plenty of money. Wyclef Jean and Hollywood just collected sixty million dollars. The UN released some thirty-six million. The European Union gave an enormous sum. Obama released one hundred million. My friends and family have been calling, asking which organizations to send money to. All I need is $300 per day.

I go back on the road, back to the city, to find money. I pass an aid vehicle. No one but the driver is inside. A line of colorful buses and trucks comes down the highway, their roofs piled high with furniture. People are fleeing the city, leaving crumbled homes and dead family and friends behind. As I travel down the asphalt edge of an earthquake-cracked stretch of road, I see a piece of plywood propped in the middle of the road, scrawled with the words, "Help us. We are people too." It occurs to me that the sixteen-mile stretch between Léogâne and Port-au-Prince, an area punctuated with collapsed buildings, has not a single field hospital. They're all in Léogâne.

All I need is $300 per day. That's less than the per diem for UN employees. Any one of the rescue workers is making twice that. It's just a matter of explaining the situation to the right person.

"No problem." The guy is telling me on the phone.

Bingo!

"I am the country director," he explains, "I will authorize three weeks' pay for the taxis."

I was speaking to Randy Wortenson, the U.S. director of World Wide Village, an organization that is in the process of erecting one of the largest medical facilities in Léogâne. He's glad to help. "That's what we're here for."

I explain to a group of the paramedics and doctors that I have talked to their head guy, Randy Wortensen, and that we have an okay for them to pay. "You don't have to take my word for it," I tell them, "he'll be calling you."

"Man, that's great," A big muscular American guy named Shane shakes my hand. "This is exactly what we need," Shane is saying, "We got guys coming out of here with busted femurs and they lay out there by the gate for days. No way home."

Now aid workers and surgeons are asking if we can get other stuff, such as supplies and transport to the airport. Boga and Shane are already coordinating the taxis. A surgeon explains that he has a woman who he needs to evacuate because he doesn't have the equipment to operate. "She is going to lose her leg," he tells me. Then he tells me about the supplies he needs and asks if I could talk to the DART guys about having the surgeon come down to look through what they have. Of course I can! The DART guys sent me over here. And this is important.

Shane and the surgeon walk us partway to the gate. One of them introduces me to the guards there: "He's going to be coming in and out." The guards smile and nod. The three Haitian motorcycle taxi drivers who have been following us around stand at the gate beaming. The sense of mission is thick, and everyone knows their part.

Just then, one of the American aid workers runs up behind me. "Chris needs to talk to you." I return to where I was not two minutes before, but something is different. The surgeons and Shane have scattered. A handsome thirtysomething doctor named Chris is telling me, "I misunderstood what you were saying. We don't need anything."

"What?"

"Yeah, we have everything we need."

"What about the taxis?"

"We have five vehicles." He is taking the blood pressure of a Haitian man. "They are all out in the rural areas right now, scouring for patients."

I don't have time to figure this out, not at the moment. "What about the surgeon and the surgical equipment he asked for?"

"I am in charge here," Chris snaps, "not him."

I leave. Dejected.

———

I've tried to find the money but I can't. I called and e-mailed Randy but he didn't respond. The Germans said, "We have no money." The Canadians told me, "We pay for our own taxis." DART at USAID never responded to my messages. I don't even know if they received the information I collected for them.

Now I am sitting with Joseph asking him what the hell I am going to do. Like many people in USAID, Joseph started in the Peace Corps. He set out to do compassionate, good things for people, but after thirty-two years he's been tempered by the reality of the bureaucracy and geopolitics. In recent years, an institutional division has come up between his bosses at the State Department and their confidence in USAID. USAID, of which DART is a part, has come under heavy fire. They've been blamed for undermining the Haitian economy, for failing to create effective development, and for failing to make NGOs accountable. Then, in the past year, before the earthquake, a switch in politics has left the USAID high command sitting in the cold, under a continuing resolution, meaning without money to do anything but keep things going. Meanwhile, the U.S. State Department has been rewriting our policy toward Haiti, with little input from the experts in the field.

"They're all managing up," Joseph tells me. "Writing briefs for the bosses in Washington. No one has time to focus on the guys below them, the ones who are actually out here doing the work." I've been hearing about USAID getting sidelined since we first became friends. Joseph's brow narrows. "The vultures are circling. They're picking our bones."

We're two weeks after the earthquake, and every night is the same. More stories of ineptitude, failure, fear, aid-lock at the airport.

Joseph is one of the most seasoned officers in USAID, and he can't get money for taxis. USAID actually has a taxi service contract in place but we've been unable to access it.

"Look," he stands up. "Here," pulls his wallet out of his back pocket and starts counting off twenties until fifteen of them are on the table. "You understand my dilemma. I usually program millions of dollars, but I can't pay for two weeks of taxis."

———————

The next morning, I get to New Missions in Léogâne to pay off the taxis. I get off my bike. One of the motorcycle taxis pulls up next to me; the driver wants to collect his pay. A Cuban doctor comes out and starts hollering at him. She wants to know where the hell he has been, why he is shirking his job when they have patients here, dying, patients that need to be transported to the X-ray machine. They need medicine from MSF. I intercede. "No one is paying him."

She stops and looks at me blankly, "Oh," she says and walks off.

I go into the medical tent, and see an attractive young woman with a freshly bandaged stump at the end of her arm. They've just cut off her hand. She is sitting there, on the end of the bed, listening to the doctor's advice as if they just removed a mole. No tears, no hysteria. She nods and asks the medic a question in broken French.

On the other bed a man is snoring. He inhales loudly, his whole body shaking. I've never seen anyone sleeping so hard. It's the first time I've seen someone in a coma.

I always come into this tent. I like the medics. They are not complicated like the doctors. They are always courteous— and all business. They work constantly, on some days treating more than two hundred people. I feel badly that I can't help them. Every time I've been here I have asked what they need. Every time I've relayed the message to officials at DART or the Embassy. And every time I've come back empty-handed.

I go out the backside of the tent. A small black truck, with rusted metal sides wired to the frame, is parked in the courtyard. Two men standing next to it are engaged in earnest discussion. They need to evacuate the man in a coma, but they are afraid that the ride might kill him. I call the number of the ambulance service that Joseph gave me, the one that USAID, through OIM, has a contract with. Sure, they'll come. But they don't know when they can get here, and we must have six patients to pick up, and we need to transport them ourselves to a pickup point some six miles from here.

I find the van and we send the man in a coma to Port-au-Prince. Then I find the motorcycle taxis and tell them to keep working; we have money coming. They believe me. After all, they think I'm with DART.

I go out back, to a field behind the building, and sit down in the grass where no one can see me. I bury my head my hands. Now I get it. Before I arrived ten days ago, Boga was here, in his own country, trying to help. When the organizations finally started arriving, he greeted everyone and did whatever he could to assist them. How frustrating it must be for him, knowing that he could do something if the foreigners who came to help—the doctors, paramedics, aid workers, and DART officials—would just make use of him. They didn't. They were too new, too poorly organized, too confined in their rules, and too captured in their own bureaucratic trap to do the obvious.

---

It is now January 26, two weeks after the earthquake. OCHA, the United Nations coordinating body, has arrived and set up a tent in Léogâne. Everyone is there: representatives from the Canadians, Japanese, French, Spanish, Austrians, Germans. The Dominican doctor is there. Chris from World Wide Village is there, lying on the grass at the entrance to the tent. A woman is explaining the coordination process. There are three important items. "First we need taxis to run between the different hospitals..."

If there was a happy ending, for me, it was this: A donor sent $2,500 to pay for the taxis.

# THE OFFICIAL

## JENNIE WEISS BLOCK, O.P.

*L*eslie Voltaire was in New York, just about to leave the United Nations Office of the Special Envoy for Haiti shortly after 6 P.M., when he got word of the earthquake. The director of the National Library of Haiti called from Port-au-Prince. "This is hell. Bad things are happening. I cannot call your wife, I cannot call your family, but everybody is panicking. I saw my house trembling and I saw a lot of dust in the sky." Leslie begged her to go to his house about a mile away, but she could not leave her children and feared that the roads would be impassable.

Leslie and I are colleagues at the UN, where I work as Paul Farmer's chief of staff. As envoy to the secretary-general of the UN, Leslie Voltaire serves as our first and primary link with the Haitian government. Born in Haiti in 1949, Leslie earned his architecture degree at the University of Mexico and was a Fulbright Scholar at Cornell for a master's degree in urban planning. He has served in every Haitian administration since 1990 in many different capacities, including minister of education, director of urban planning, and chief of staff to President Aristide, making him a politically savvy expert on Haitian history and governance.

After receiving the news of the earthquake, Leslie began frantically calling Haiti, to no avail. He went to the Haitian Mission Office at the UN, desperate for information about his family and his country. As CNN began showing horrible images and the news carried stories of thousands upon thousands dead, he feared and imagined the worst: his family was crushed to death in the rubble of their home. Finally, late in the afternoon the next day, he got a message from someone who had talked to his wife, Carole. She was alive and at home with two of his three children, but their eighteen-year-old son, Luigi, was missing. Carole was terrified. Luigi had been with a friend, and they had plans to go to a new restaurant for dinner. Carole made her way to the restaurant and saw that it had collapsed. She spent that night filled with dread. Luigi finally got in touch with her the next day, but Carole wasn't able to reach Leslie and let him know that Luigi was alive for another thirty-six hours.

Leslie was getting many calls from people all over the United States and Canada asking for information about their families in Haiti. Because he held a high-level official government position, they assumed he would have information. This was far from the case; like everyone else, he was hearing the news as it slowly trickled in. He got word that his mother, who lives in the mountains, was alive, but the rest of the news he received was terrible. Many friends were dead or missing.

Leslie told me of the death of his close friend and business partner, Phillippe Dewiz, a Belgian engineer and infrastructure expert. "President Préval had nominated him as my partner, to help me in my mission. I was supposed to go with him to a meeting at the MINUSTAH headquarters at the Christopher Hotel, but instead, I was called to New York. Otherwise, I would have died with him there." About a hundred of our UN colleagues died at the Christopher, including the secretary-general's representative and head of the UN Mission in Haiti, Hédi Annabi, and his deputy, Luis DaCosta. In the coming months, there would be almost daily memorial services at the UN Headquarters in New York.

Getting in and out of Haiti for the first few months after the earthquake was very difficult. The airport had been taken over by the U.S. military, the daily volume of flights was tripled, and landing slots were hard to come by. It would be more than a month until commercial flights would resume, and the only way in and out was on a private plane. About three days after the earthquake, Leslie called me, trying desperately to find a ride to Haiti. We arranged for him to travel with Paul out of Miami. At Miami International Airport, I gave Leslie two duffel bags containing tents for his family, chocolate for his wife, baby clothes for President Préval's three-month-old grandchild, and supplies such as masks and pharmaceutical products.

When Leslie landed in Port-au-Prince, darkness covered the city. The ride to his house took twice as long as usual. There he found a large group of people seeking refuge with his family. No one would enter the house; they were frightened that the house would collapse, especially with the many strong aftershocks occurring day after day. They had been sleeping outdoors in the garden and in the car. Carole was adamant: "You cannot go into the house." Although Leslie had designed and built their home and felt sure it was safe, he kept redoing the calculus in his head, recounting how the structure was built and how many rebars he had used. Leslie's family members counted among the very lucky: They had water from a rain collecting system and food from a friend who owned a restaurant.

Early the next day, Leslie asked a friend to drive him around Port-au-Prince. "It was a shock," he said. "It's not the same thing when you see it on the TV as when you see it in 3D. The smell was overwhelming even though I was wearing my mask. All my references were gone. The most shocking thing was to see my school, where I spent fourteen years, down." He went immediately to the government palace, which had relocated to a police station next to the airport, to see what he could do. Ministers were arriving on motorcycles, and he asked them to tell him what happened on the first days. Their losses were staggering. One minister lost both of his sons. Another both of his parents.

Leslie was worried about President Préval. Reports on TV said Préval was "not showing up and there was no government." Leslie found President Préval at the police station. He no longer had a home or an office. Many members of his administration were dead, injured, or distraught over the deaths of family members. They had no way to communicate with each other or the outside world. The supermarket had collapsed, and food and water were scarce. The banks were closed; there was no money. The radio stations were down. President Préval had to decide what to do with the tens of thousands of bodies piling up on the street. He ultimately made the decision to bury the bodies of the Haitian dead in mass graves without identification, forgoing the burial rituals of the community. Excruciating as his decision was, the stench was overwhelming and rescuing those trapped in collapsed buildings and caring for the living had to be given a priority. "The trucks were full, and going on and on and on and on," Leslie remembered, "and the only thing you could think is, 'What about my friend? What about my sister?' Days were spent just counting victims and seeing who was alive."

In the midst of this chaos, President Préval nevertheless immediately organized a reconstruction task force. Leslie joined the task force and gathered as many architects and engineers as he could find to brainstorm about what could be done. He worked closely with NGOs and the UN shelter cluster to find tents and tarps to offer even the most basic shelter to the 1.5 million people living outside. Leslie made multiple visits to resettlement camps. "I sometimes talk to people in the camps about their futures. I'm trying to tell them that they will be better, knowing that it can be better. But I don't see the resources, and when you are under a tent, you don't understand the notion of patience."

In Leslie's view, Haiti was the least organized country in the hemisphere before the earthquake. An estimated 250,000 residences and 30,000 commercial buildings were destroyed by the quake. The majority of municipal buildings were severely damaged or ruined, including the Presidential Palace, the National Assembly, City Hall, and the main jail. Half the primary and secondary schools were destroyed, along with the three main universities. Leslie estimates that only 5 percent of the buildings in Haiti are built by professionals; the rest are self-constructed. And these self-constructed structures came tumbling down in a matter of minutes, killing more than a quarter of a million people, and injuring and maiming countless others.

Complicated reasons exist for Haiti's incapability to build and maintain adequate systems of infrastructure. To begin with, countries with extreme poverty are always marked by a lack of infrastructure.

Two aspects of infrastructure development are particularly relevant to Haiti's situation: historicity and interdependence. Haiti's slave revolution in 1804 set the country on a course like no other. Since that time, political violence and the resulting instability have plagued Haiti, creating less than ideal circumstances for infrastructure building. Because systems are constructed over generations and tend to evolve and improve over time, Haiti's changing paradigms for governance and management have repeatedly interrupted or ruptured the development of infrastructure. Leslie explains, "When we had a colonial society, there was one set of infrastructure. Then we had a rupture, [which] destroyed everything: the institutional, the physical, and the economic platform of that colonial society. So it reinvented a new society of free slaves, and reorganized the country around a few cities with the vast majority of people liv[ing] in the countryside without infrastructure."

Leslie claims that the Haitian mindset militates against the concept of interdependence. "Haitians will do everything to avoid being controlled or dominated, even when you are an equal partner." Given Haiti's history of slavery and radical oppression by numerous forces, it is easy to understand this way of thinking, although it is not necessarily helpful in building the interdependent relationships that are so common and useful in the global world. This thinking forges what Leslie calls "intentional isolation." He believes this attitude is slowly changing. In the last twenty years, Haiti has developed a new openness to entering into "globalization and international relations with other countries." Leslie believes that to enter into "the capitalist world, we need to be self-sufficient in food and energy, at least, with strong exportation. For these things to happen, Haiti needs institutional and physical infrastructure."

A far greater aspect of the tragedy than the problem of failed infrastructure was the loss of thousands upon thousands of Haitian students who died at schools and universities. "Because the earthquake struck in the afternoon," Leslie says, "a lot of schools and universities were filled with students; the losses of these young people were great. At a school where I taught, six hundred students died." When the seminary fell, all the seminarians in Haiti died. The loss of the national treasure of an entire generation of Haiti's best and brightest is a loss that cannot be measured or replaced. The school system, Leslie argues, must be the first priority when rebuilding infrastructure.

———

Today, Port-au-Prince is an urban disaster. Close to three million people are crowded into a city without even basic services such as water, sanitation, and transportation. Devoid of any city planning, commercial and residential are intermingled in a patchwork of confusion.

Shortly after the earthquake, Leslie approached Elizabeth Plater-Zyberk, Dean of the School of Architecture at the University of Miami, who is internationally known as one of the founders of the New Urbanism movement. Together, working with a team of Haitian and American architects, they came up with a bold and ambitious reconstruction plan for Haiti. The plan redistributes large parts of the population of Port-au-Prince to smaller Haitian cities and organized rural communities, many of them a safe distance from areas most vulnerable to natural disasters.

One of the goals supported in the plan for Haiti's development is to restore a population balance to the country by building up other cities and creating sustainable agricultural villages in rural areas. The relocation of schools, hospitals, and industry will develop what Leslie calls "magnets of attraction" based on job opportunities and educational and social services. The plan also includes a reimagined Port-au-Prince, with zoning segregating residential from commercial activities in the dense parts of downtown and strict building regulations for earthquake-resistant construction. The new city layout also calls for the development of various kinds of public spaces—parks, squares, markets, exchange centers—including a beautiful historic district.

An article calling the plan "lucid and surprisingly convincing" appeared in the *New York Times* on March 31, 2010, sparking enormous interest. "I thought nobody would see it because it was published in the Art and Design section. *Everybody* read it. I got calls from all over the world inviting me to come and share Haiti's plans. So many people want to help." Since that time, Leslie has criss-crossed the United States and the Caribbean sharing the vision for a new Haiti. "I'm interpreting the Haitian plan and have illustrated it in drawings and renderings so I can explain to the people what is happening."

This is surely not the first plan for Haiti's renewal. Leslie showed me the presentation that he uses in his speaking engagements, which places intricate drawings of a master plan for the city of Port-au-Prince prepared in 1785 alongside the renderings by the University of Miami in 2010. Success is by no means guaranteed and depends on economic, social, and institutional rebuilding. Continued international goodwill, the difficult process of consensus building, the real possibility of another natural disaster during the next hurricane season, and competing priorities all affect the process. And as Leslie well knows, "it takes time to build. The decision-making process is very intricate, very difficult to do . . . there is a difference between decision-making and decision-taking."

The reconstruction process has indeed proven to be difficult. As I finish this chapter, a year after the earthquake, progress has been painstakingly slow, life in Haiti remains unbearably hard, and those who work untiringly for Haiti's recovery are deeply frustrated. The massive needs of more than a million people in tents, the rebuilding of physical and institutional infrastructure, and the negotiation of a complex political landscape are overwhelming challenges. But Leslie remains dedicated to his country, and all of us working for Haiti forge on. Even disinterested observers cannot help but root for Haiti. Even skeptics cannot help but be impressed by the fortitude and grace with which the Haitian people are bearing up. They are a strong lot. Leslie says it best. "We are warriors. It's in our DNA."

# BUILDING BACK BETTER

### JÉHANE SEDKY

*I*n May 2009, President Bill Clinton was appointed the UN Special Envoy for Haiti. His passion for Haiti, dating to his post-honeymoon visit to the island nation, was well-known. He had been deeply engaged with Haiti while President of the United States and had launched a development program for Haiti at the Clinton Global Initiative.* He had been successful as UN Secretary-General Kofi Annan's Special Envoy for Tsunami Recovery in 2005 and 2006. Now Annan's successor, Ban Ki-Moon, looked to President Clinton for his unmatched convening power.

Ban recognized that progress was being made in Haiti and believed that a focused effort could result in further success for the country. The UN peacekeeping operation that had been deployed in Haiti since 2004 had dramatically reduced the levels of violence in the country; reported kidnappings had declined from an average of thirty per month in the first half of 2008 to fewer than eight per month in the first half of 2009.† However, the UN recognized that what Haiti needed most was private sector investments, which UN officials and peacekeepers had little expertise in attracting.

---

*Established in 2005 by President Bill Clinton, the Clinton Global Initiative (CGI) convenes global leaders to devise and implement innovative solutions to some of the world's most pressing challenges.

†Report of the Secretary-General's on the UN Stabilization Mission in Haiti (MINUSTAH), September 18, 2009.

I had worked for President Clinton in his capacity as UN Special Envoy for Tsunami Recovery. Trained in human rights law, with a focus on women and children, I have spent the majority of my UN career at UNICEF. Although I have seen firsthand what organizations such as UNICEF can do at the country level to improve the lives of communities, I also know the limits of UN agencies' mandates and capabilities. With President Clinton in the lead, however, I sensed that the UN had a unique opportunity to create positive momentum in Haiti.

I was the first one recruited to serve President Clinton in his capacity as UN Special Envoy for Haiti in June 2009. By early August, his team consisted of five staff members. We were thrilled to learn that Dr. Paul Farmer would soon be appointed President Clinton's deputy. Both Farmer and President Clinton had agreed to lead the UN effort for a salary of one dollar a year. Their mission was to build on the success of UN peacekeepers in establishing stability and seize the political moment to jump-start international investment and strengthen the government's capability to deliver social services to its people.

During President Clinton's first visit to Haiti for the UN in June 2009, he met a twenty-seven-year-old Haitian who ran a fuel briquette project. The program processes household waste into briquettes in an environmentally responsible as well as a less-expensive alternative to wood-based charcoal that people can use for heat and cooking. The president immediately saw the environmental value of the program and its potential to reduce community violence through youth employment. He was also determined to support this young entrepreneur who had successfully run the project in one of the poorest neighborhoods in Port-au-Prince. After watching a group of young Haitians sorting garbage to make the briquettes, President Clinton told us that he would help make this small project an example of "building back better," an expression he had coined while working in the countries affected by the tsunami.

During another visit to Haiti in October 2009, President Clinton met Valentin Abe, a Cote d'Ivorian who had studied in the United States before moving to Haiti, where he created Caribbean Harvest, a fish farm run on solar energy. When President Clinton visited the small farm outside Port-au-Prince, he was captivated by Valentin's ingenuity and commitment to helping the poor. Valentin's fish farm teaches local farmers to grow fish and then farms out fingerlings to families who raise the fish in cages in nearby ponds. (The cages are privately owned and each family is responsible for their investment.) After the growing cycle, Caribbean Harvest collects the fish and transports them to Port-au-Prince for sale; the profits are shared evenly between Caribbean Harvest and the farmers.

It's difficult to imagine now, post-earthquake, how optimistic we were in the fall of 2009. Our UN office strategized around two central concepts. First, the country's future had to be guided by the Haitian people. And second, we would position Haiti not as a lost cause but as a country primed to make a huge leap forward. Our objectives: facilitate job creation through private sector investments; secure donor disbursements; support hurricane preparedness across the country; and promote coordination of the estimated ten thousand not-for-profits working in Haiti. Both Paul Farmer and President Clinton often reminded us that "in its two hundred years of independence, Haiti has never had a fair chance." We were determined to use the extraordinary momentum created by our bosses to turn the tide and put an end to unfulfilled pledges to the island nation.

From day one, President Clinton made it his responsibility to hold donors accountable to their pledges. Equally important, the mission of the UN office was driven by support for Haiti's own vision for its recovery, not the international community's. Paul Farmer calls this approach "accompaniment." It means that any intervention in Haiti must be built on the premise that Haitians will lead. We would work with the Haitian government, support efforts to recruit and train Haitians whenever possible, and advocate that a greater portion of aid funding be channeled to direct budget support for the government.

During their October 2009 visit to Haiti, President Clinton and Dr. Farmer attended a high-level private sector meeting organized by the

Inter-American Development Bank in Port-au-Prince. President Clinton was the keynote speaker. His attendance at the meeting helped to draw an estimated five hundred investors to Haiti, most of whom had never set foot on the island. The conference began with then-Prime Minister Michèle Pierre-Louis announcing: "Haiti is open for business." A survey conducted by the Inter-American Development Bank on the heels of the conference revealed that 97 percent of the participants expressed an increased level of interest in investing in Haiti.

Back in New York, our small team was working closely with the Inter-American Development Bank to compile the first comprehensive, dynamic, web-based directory of not-for-profits working in Haiti. More not-for-profits per capita are in Haiti than in any other country except for India, and coordination among them is woefully lacking.

By December 2009, momentum was building. For the first time, the tone of the international media coverage on Haiti was hopeful. Meanwhile, private investors were showing interest in committing to Haiti. An estimated thirty-five thousand short-term jobs were created nationwide between March and September 2009.*

Just before Christmas, Paul Farmer convened a meeting with the staff. Each technical expert had to present his or her 2010 plan and provide strategic advice on how the UN office should fill in existing gaps and accompany the government of Haiti on its path towards recovery. Paul was focused on hurricane preparedness. He was visibly worried about the next cyclone season. Our disaster expert, a staff member from the UN, said: "Paul, the next disaster will most likely be an earthquake or a tsunami."

At 5:02 P.M. on January 12, 2010, I was at my desk in the Office of the Special Envoy in New York, preparing for a meeting with philanthropists and private sector investors the next day. My colleagues

*Report of the Secretary-General on the UN Stabilization Mission in Haiti (MINUSTAH), September 18, 2009.

Nancy Dorsinville, John Harding, and Ricardo Sanchez were on assignment in Port-au-Prince. As I worked on a briefing note, I received a "red earthquake alert" by an e-mail message, part of a natural disaster alert system to which I'd been subscribed since the tsunami. A 7.0 earthquake had occurred in Port-au-Prince. I immediately e-mailed and texted Nancy, John, and Ricardo: "Are you okay?" Nothing. Within minutes, my New York colleagues were in my office. We were in a state of shock. Was Paul Farmer in Haiti? No. He had just left a week before. Had anyone heard from Nancy, John, and Ricardo? No news.

Each hour brought worse news. We sat in the UN's Situation Center, listening to live updates by satellite phone from the top UN officer, Brazilian Commander Carlos Alberto dos Santos Cruz. Cruz's voice was controlled but shaken as he recounted what he saw: The UN compound, holding approximately two hundred staff members, had collapsed. Both the head of the mission, Hédi Annabi, and his deputy, Luiz Carlos Da Costa, had been in a meeting with a Chinese delegation on the sixth floor of the UN compound when the earthquake struck. That meant that our colleagues—their chiefs of staff, administrative assistants, and special assistants—were also in the meeting with the Chinese. As we were absorbing this update, we learned that another UN building had collapsed. So too had the National Palace and the Hotel Montana.

The next day, President Clinton addressed the United Nations General Assembly. He conveyed determination to support the Haitians as they recovered from the worst natural disaster in the region's history, and he set out the foundations of his "building back better" approach. As he stood there, with Paul Farmer at his side, in front of 192 delegations and countless media and UN staff, we had a momentary sense that we could pull through this, that Haiti would get back on its feet.

President Clinton continued to use the term "building back better," and it took on a more profound meaning. The phrase was about not rebuilding to pre-earthquake standards but using the disaster as an opportunity to define and support a sustainable vision for Haiti. Haitians must be in charge of their own destiny. International organizations and not-for-profits must coordinate their efforts and strengthen Haiti's government and local institutions instead of implementing programs that have unintended negative consequences (such as food aid leading to the destruction of the Haitian agriculture sector).*

At the time of this writing, we can point to a few initiatives led by the Office of the Special Envoy and aimed at laying the foundation for Haiti's long-term recovery.

### Tracking international assistance

On March 31, 2010, the government of Haiti, the United Nations, and the U.S. government cohosted the International Donors' Conference Towards a New Future for Haiti in New York. This conference culminated in $6.2 billion in pledges for 2010–2011. The Office of the Special Envoy (OSE), together with the government of Haiti and the United Nations Development Programme, supported the conference by launching online, real-time tracking of donor pledges. These efforts made the conference one of the most transparent of its kind, and built upon advances made by the Office of the Special Envoy in tracking the April 2009 Washington, D.C., conference pledges to Haiti.†

The tracking of international assistance was part of the Office of the Special Envoy's original, pre-earthquake mandate. President Clinton was determined to ensure that the funding for Haiti's recovery would be transparent and that donors would be held accountable for the pledges they had made. Before the earthquake, the Office of the Special Envoy was the only entity tracking overall aid to Haiti, and the only one with credible information on the April 2009 Washington donor conference pledges. Between December 2009 and January 2010, due in large part to the work of the Special

---

*Decades of inexpensive food imports (coupled with food aid from well-meaning nonprofits) have destroyed local agriculture in Haiti.

†In 2009, the OSE tracked more than US $1.7 billion in pledges of aid, including US $479 million from the April 2009 donors' conference in Washington, D.C.

Envoy, Washington conference disbursements increased from 12 to 30 percent.

## Changing the way not-for-profits work in Haiti

Any thoughtful analysis of the work of the not-for-profit community in Haiti before the earthquake will reveal that although intentions were usually good, the results of the work often did little to make lasting change in Haiti or, in many cases, to even help Haitians. This lack of long-lasting effect has many explanations. The work of not-for-profits was uncoordinated and did little to reinforce the priorities of the Haitian government. International NGOs expended great effort determining ways to address problems they saw, but often they did not include Haitians in meaningful ways as they developed those plans.

International NGOs are accountable to their international donors—not to the disenfranchised communities they are trying to serve. They often deliver goods and services but less often pay local salaries. As a result, NGOs have created a culture of dependency rather than self-sufficiency. Many years of effort by NGOs has served to only weaken the already weak government, which did not, even before the earthquake, have the resources to pay its employees. As a result, public health and education officials are paid intermittently, hospitals lack basic medicines and supplies, and schools are 90 percent privately owned and unregulated.

Some NGOs have sought to break this pattern. After weeks of quiet advocacy from President Clinton and Paul Farmer, Gail McGovern, CEO of the American Red Cross, committed $3.8 million to strengthen the Hôpital Université d'État l'Haïti (HUEH). In addition, the Red Cross provided a $500,000 grant for hospital equipment and an additional $2 million was approved for support to the hospital. Paul Farmer helped the government of Haiti meet the conditions set by the American Red Cross so that they could discharge their responsibilities to their donors and stakeholders. This was the first time the American Red Cross has provided direct budget support to a government. Imagine if we could replicate this model in the education sector or throughout the social sectors.

## *Increasing the level of commitment to budget support*

A little more than two hundred years ago, Haiti produced three-quarters of the world's sugar. Yet despite this wealth in natural resources, the island nation is now the poorest in the Western hemisphere. This is largely due to its history, fraught with donor governments undermining its capacity to thrive. Promises were broken, debt was imposed, dictatorships were supported, and natural resources were depleted.

Since the earthquake, donor disbursements to Haiti have been consistent and debt forgiveness has been forthcoming. The donor community is committed to supporting Haiti. But will it be willing to invest directly in the government? Or will it continue to channel the majority of its funding through the not-for-profit community? Without a solid commitment to budget support—and without the capability to control the monies flowing in and the capacity to strengthen its own public institutions—Haiti will never fully recover.

This is why, in all its advocacy with donors, multilateral institutions, nongovernmental organizations, and foundation partners, the Office of the Special Envoy has promoted investment in budget support for the government of Haiti. This advocacy effort, and President Clinton's personal engagement with donors, has as of December 2010 helped mobilize US $226.7 million in new commitments to budget support following the earthquake, in addition to $122.4 million in existing commitments.* Although this figure represents a small percentage of the total contributions to Haiti from the pledges made at the New York conference ($5.6 billion for 2010–2011), it is an important step in the right direction.

---

*Donors disbursed a total of $189 million was disbursed to the Government of Haiti and an additional $45 million through the Haiti Reconstruction Fund in the 2010 calendar year from the pledges made at the New York donors conference. The International Monetary Fund reports that during the Government of Haiti's fiscal year 2010 (1 October 2009–30 September 2010) donors committed $250 million in budget support to the Government of Haiti, of which $225 million was disbursed to the government.

As this book goes to press, I am struck by how heartbreaking the last few months have been for those of us who care about Haiti. Recovery has been slow, rubble still fills the streets of Port-au-Prince, and hundreds of thousands of people still live in camps. The spread of cholera has exacerbated an already dire situation.

Yet, pockets of hope exist. The government of Finland, for example, announced a 700,000 euro contribution to teacher salaries. This contribution is significant because it represents a shift in priorities; rarely do donors provide budget support in the form of salaries.

What will Haiti look like in ten years if we truly commit to "building back better"? Although we are humbled by the question and realistic about what can be achieved, our vision for "building back better" includes a robust public sector (especially in health and education), investment in job creation, food security, safe housing for all Haitians, and a truly participatory recovery process, where Haitians from all walks of life are consulted in a meaningful way. This vision for Haiti, although it is one we believe in and strive for, is far from reality today. A week before Christmas 2010, our team met with Paul Farmer for dinner. While we discussed the cholera epidemic and the disputed first round of presidential elections, some of us found it difficult to remain optimistic about the possibility of "building back better" in Haiti. Paul was quick to remind us of Haiti's history of struggle, the fighting spirit of Haitians, and the need for perspective in our analysis. "You must not think of where Haiti will be in two years but where it will be in one hundred years, and how what we do today will help Haiti in the long run," he said.

Whether displayed in the streets of Port-au-Prince or in the camps, the resilience of the Haitian people is resounding. Haitians are survivors. The twenty-seven-year-old Haitian whom President Clinton met on his first visit as Special Envoy is now selling his briquettes to the UN, which is using them to warm meals for school children. The plastics and metals that cannot be used in briquette production are sold to recycling companies at market value. And the consumers of the briquettes pay 78 percent of the price of a comparable amount of charcoal.* Meanwhile, since meeting President Clinton, fish farm owner Valentin Abe was among those voted the hundred most influential people in the world for 2010 by *Time* magazine.

Although these compelling stories of "building back better" have received significant media attention, we cannot forget the hundreds of thousands of other Haitians who quietly face their predicament with determination and fortitude.

The truth is that "building back better" is not easy. The process takes time and involves setbacks and frustration. Impatience is growing. Earthquake survivors are still living in tents while cholera has gripped the nation, killing tens of thousands. But a natural disaster is not a moment; it's a tragedy that unfolds over many months. It took seven years for Japan to rebuild after the 1995 Kobe earthquake. In the United States, those still displaced by Hurricane Katrina provide a stark reminder of how even the richest nations take years to recover from a natural disaster. The extent of the damage caused by the recent 9.0 earthquake and tsunami in Japan is still unclear. Yet in Haiti, in less than thirty minutes, an estimated 222,570 people died and an additional 300,572 were injured. This natural disaster may be the worst in recent history. The challenges ahead seem daunting, but we cannot escape one truth: The survivors of the quake deserve to have their country rebuilt as they dream it to be, not as it once was.

---

*More information on the UN briquette program at http://www.haitispecialenvoy .org/press/celebrating-earth-day (accessed April 22, 2010).

# NOTES

## Chapter 1

1. R. Yates. "Universal health care and the removal of user fees." *Lancet* 373 (2009): 2078–2081.

2. Such anxieties were warranted: there were at least fifty-two aftershocks of magnitude 4.5 or greater in the two weeks after the quake. See Mike Melia, Jonathan Katz, and Michelle Faul. *As Haiti Mourns, Quake Survivor Found in Rubble.* Associated Press: January 24, 2010. Available: http://savannahnow.com/latest-news/2010-01-24/haiti-mourns-quake-survivor-found-rubble (accessed April 15, 2011).

3. See Rudy Roberts. "Responding in a Crisis: The Role of National and International Health Workers—Lessons from Haiti." Merlin: London (August 2010).

4. Mobile Army surgical hospital (MASH) units are field-ready medical tents containing emergency medical equipment, oxygen, electrical generators, and other supplies; they are deployed by the military during disasters and other medical emergencies. Many of us hoped that MASH units might be leveraged to strengthen health systems in disaster zones, leaving behind more robust surgical capacity.

5. For more details about the USNS *Comfort*, see http://www.navy.mil/search/display.asp?story_id=50653 (accessed April 15, 2011).

6. In her chapter, "Humanitarian Aid, Impartiality, and Dirty Boots," Louise Ivers considers the role of the U.S. military in the immediate earthquake response in more detail. For coverage in the media, see "Haiti Earthquake: Confusion at Airport Hampers Aid Effort." *Telegraph:* January 18, 2010. Available: http://www.telegraph.co.uk/news/worldnews/centralamericaandthecaribbean/haiti/7016051/Haiti-earthquake-confusion-at-airport-hampers-aid-effort.html (accessed April 15, 2011).

7. Cange is a former squatter settlement in central Haiti where Partners In Health first began working about twenty-five year ago. In a previous book, in keeping with conventions in anthropology, I changed the name to "Do Kay" in writing about its early history. See Paul Farmer. *AIDS and Accusation: Haiti and the Geography of Blame.* (Berkeley: University of California Press, 1992). Chapter 3, "January 12 and the Aftermath," considers its role in the aftermath of the earthquake as a referral facility for overcrowded urban hospitals and clinics that encountered the

brunt of the patient load. Cange took in hundreds of quake victims in need of surgery, and later, rehabilitation.

8. Some have argued persuasively that palliation of pain ought to be considered a basic human right; this young woman's story, and the stories of so many quake victims we've seen in the last year, renders vivid the need for such an entitlement. See, for example, J. Stjernswärd et al. "The Public Health Strategy for Palliative Care." *Journal of Pain and Symptom Management* 33 (May 2007): 486–493; E. L. Krakauer et al. "Opioid Inaccessibility and Its Human Consequences: Reports from the Field." *Journal of Pain and Palliative Care Pharmacotherapy* 24 (2010): 239–243; F. Brennan. "Palliative Care as an International Human Right." *Journal of Pain and Symptom Management* 33 (May 2007): 494–499.

9. The devastation caused by the earthquake led many to think about what theologians call theodicy: how to explain the existence of grotesque suffering while still believing in goodness and dignity. In speaking about the Haitian earthquake, how could this level of extreme suffering be explained or justified among a people who had already suffered so much? There was no shortage of commentary on this score. Pat Robertson, a Southern Baptist televangelist, offered the following explanation: Haitians "were under the heel of the French, you know Napoleon the 3rd and whatever, and they got together and swore a pact to the Devil." (See "Pat Robertson Blames Earthquake on Pact Haitians Made with Satan." *ABC News:* January 12, 2010. Available: http://blogs.abcnews.com/politicalpunch/2010/01/pat-robertson-blames-earthquake-on-pact-haitians-made-with-satan.html). (I was in Haiti at this time, and didn't even note his comment but had the great privilege of working with Operation Blessing International, a humanitarian organization associated with Robertson. As much as I disagree with his theodicy, all I can say is that this organization was one of the very finest, and best led, we worked with in the year after the quake.) As noted, another more humble sort of theodicy comes from medicine: the January 12 earthquake as an "acute-on-chronic" event. This temblor wreaked havoc because adverse social conditions and extreme ecological fragility primed Port-au-Prince for massive loss of life and destruction when the ground began shaking on January 12. This topic will be explored throughout this book.

10. For more discussion on the provision of surgical care in Haiti (and reflection on the harmful consequences of a fee-for-service health care financing model in the context of care there), see L. C. Ivers et al. "Increasing Access to Surgical Services for the Poor in Rural Haiti: Surgery as a Public Good for Public Health." *World Journal of Surgery* 32, no. 4 (2008): 537–542.

## Chapter 2

1. Haiti-Katrina parallels are discussed in a short essay, "From Gonaïves to New Orleans" (available: http://www.pih.org/news/entry/from-gonaives-to-new-orleans/, accessed April 15, 2011). It highlights the social forces that influence disasters natural and unnatural: "Disasters are never wholly and purely 'natural,' as the residents of New Orleans and dismayed onlookers have discovered. How can we pretend that racism, a social disaster, played no role in the aftermath of Kat-

rina? . . . There are many reasons Jeanne, a slow-moving tropical storm with relatively low wind speeds, caused such devastation in a country it never even crossed, and those reasons are social. And just as those left behind in New Orleans had to suffer humiliation and uncertainty, in spite of the valiant efforts of many (including some of our own supporters), so too did Jeanne's survivors." As the huge toll taken in Haiti by Jeanne came to light, journalists arrived to cover the story and, again, the story will sound familiar to those following Katrina. CNN reported that UN peacekeepers, in place since the violent overthrow of Haiti's elected government, "fired into the air to keep a hungry crowd at bay" and "fired smoke grenades as crowds of Haitian flood victims tried to break into a food distribution site." The relief workers themselves, it seems, were in need of relief: "As they waited for days, one woman yelled at a Red Cross worker on the balcony of City Hall, 'Help me. I'm hungry.' The Red Cross volunteer yelled back, 'I'm hungry, too.'" It's no wonder that New Orleans' and Haiti's disasters sound similar.

Many Americans have forgotten that the Louisiana Purchase was the direct result of Napoleon's defeat at the hands of the Haitians in 1804. Haitian President Jean-Bertrand Aristide, in exile in South Africa, made reference to this history in a condolence note made public recently: "The connection [between Haiti and Louisiana] . . . finds new root in a shared human suffering caused by this week's catastrophic storm and ensuing floods." Others have explored the extent to which no disaster is simply "natural." See, for example, Neil Smith, "There's No Such Thing as a Natural Disaster." *Social Science Research Council*, June 2006 (available: http://understandingkatrina.ssrc.org/ accessed April 15, 2011) and E. Klinenberg. "Denaturalizing Disaster: A Social Autopsy of the 1995 Chicago Heat Wave." *Theory and Society* 28 (April 1999): 239–295. Two of my former students are now publishing a moving account of an unnatural disaster—the collapse of a dam in Gujarat, India that leveled the city of Morbi in 1979. See Utpal Sandesara and Thomas Wooten. *No One Had a Tongue to Speak.* (New York: Prometheus Books, 2011).

2. For example, see P. Farmer et al. "The dilemma of MDRTB in the global era." *International Journal of Tuberculosis and Lung Disease* 2, 11 (1998): 869–876; P. Farmer. *Infections and Inequalities: The Modern Plagues* (Berkeley: University of California Press, 1999), especially chapters 7–9, pp. 184–261.

3. My colleagues and I have explored these and other epidemics in several studies in books, including *The Global Impact of Drug-Resistant Tuberculosis* (Harvard Medical School/Open Society Institute, 1999), Paul Farmer. *Pathologies of Power: Health, Human Rights, and the New War of the Poor* (Berkeley: University of California Press, 2005); Farmer, *Infections and Inequalities.*

4. S. S. Shin et al. "Treatment Outcomes in an Integrated Civilian and Prison MDR-TB Treatment Program in Russia." *International Journal of Tuberculosis and Lung Disease* 10 (2006): 402–408.

5. P. Farmer et al. "Community-based Approaches to HIV Treatment in Resource-poor Settings." *Lancet* 358 (2001): 404–409.

6. Sachs is an outspoken champion of poverty reduction. In *The End of Poverty: Economic Possibilities for Our Time* (New York: Penguin, 2005), he argues that a series of "traps" linked to poverty keep poor people from amassing enough capital to

save and invest; they are thereby unable to reach the first rung of development. We're working with an economist, Matt Bonds, who has been helping us study the impact of efforts to spring poverty traps in rural Rwanda. See, for example, M. Plucinski, C. N. Ngonghala, and M. H. Bonds. "Stochasticity and Safety Nets Imply Lower Barriers for Breaking Disease-Driven Poverty Traps." *Journal of the Royal Society Interface:* under revision (2011); and M. H. Bonds, D. C. Keenan, P. Rohani, and J. D. Sachs. "Poverty Trap Formed by the Ecology of Infectious Diseases." *Proceedings of the Royal Society, Series B* 277 (2010): 1185–1192. [Royal Society, Series B 277.] See also Sachs' book *Common Wealth: Economics for a Crowded Planet* (New York: Penguin, 2008), which considers the growing risks caused by global forces such as climate change, population growth, and poverty. What were once issues of moral concern now pose immediate security threats, Sachs argues. "When a country is too poor to provide its people with basic necessities such as health care," he writes, "and when the underlying ecology makes agriculture difficult without fertilizer and irrigation, any change can push society off the edge and into outright desperation. ... Something as simple as bad rains can trigger internal conflicts when a society is living on the edge of survival." (Sachs, 2008, pp. 278–279.)

7. See "Consensus Statement on Antiretroviral Treatment for AIDS in Poor Countries." March 2001. Available: http://www.cid.harvard.edu/cidinthenews/pr/ consensus_aids_therapy.pdf (accessed April 15, 2011).

8. D. Walton et al. "Integrated HIV Prevention and Care Strengthens Primary Health Care: Lessons from Rural Haiti." *Journal of Public Health Policy* 25, no. 2 (2004): 137–158.

9. For more on the collaborations that led to the foundation of l'Université de la Foundation Aristide, see "A New Generation of Doctors." *Partners In Health Bulletin* (Summer 2003). Available: http://parthealth.3cdn.net/77b68edofa3597528f_ qpm6b5bie.pdf (accessed April 15, 2011). It's my hope that we will be able to revive this effort in the future because the need has never been greater than now.

10. See, for example, P. Farmer. "Political Violence and Public Health in Haiti." *New England Journal of Medicine* 350 (2004): 1483–1486; Farmer. *Pathologies of Power,* especially "Preface to the Paperback Edition," p. xxi; Paul Farmer. *The Uses of Haiti* (Monroe, ME: Common Courage Press, 2006), p. 376.

11. Cyril Mychalejko. "Lawlessness, Kidnappings, and Murder in Haiti." *Upside Down World:* July 26, 2006. Available: http://upsidedownworld.org/main/news -briefs-archives-68/372-lawlessness-kidnappings-and-murder-in-haiti (accessed April 15, 2011).

12. Azadeh Ansari and Reynolds Wolf. "An Unusually Destructive Hurricane Season Ends." *CNN:* December 1, 2008. Available: http://www.cnn.com/2008/U.S./ 11/30/hurricane.season.ends/index.html (accessed April 15, 2011); Matthew Weaver. "Hurricane Ike Forces Mass Evacuation in Cuba." *Guardian* (September 9, 2008). Available: http://www.guardian.co.uk/world/2008/sep/09/cuba.cuba (accessed April 15, 2011).

13. The transcript of the letter is available online at http://www.pih.org/news/ entry/i-have-never-seen-anything-as-painful-paul-farmer-writes.

14. See Chapter 3 "January 12 and the Aftermath," note 2 and also p. 55.

15. P. Farmer. *AIDS and Accusation: Haiti and the Geography of Blame* (Berkeley: University of California Press, 1992), pp. 186–190.

16. Galeano notes that real coffee plantation wages in Haiti ranged from $.07 to $.15 a day. See Eduardo Galeano. *Open Veins of Latin America: Five Centuries of the Pillage of a Continent* (London: Monthly Review Press, 1971), p. 98. Since 2006, the Préval administration raised the minimum wage in nongarment sectors to $5 per day (eight hours). For clothes to be exported to the United States, however, workers can be paid about $3 per day. Both the $3 and $5 rate have triggered outrage—from opposite positions—within Haiti and without. See, for example, Robert Naiman. "Haitian Garment Workers Should Get at Least $5 a Day." *Huffington Post* (February 23, 2010). Available: http://www.huffingtonpost.com/robert-naiman/haitian-garment-workers-s_b_473262.html (accessed April 15, 2011). The story is so old that I was able to write a well-honed (but less well-researched) article about the topic in 1988: "Blood, Sweat, and Baseballs: Haiti in the West Atlantic System." *Dialectical Anthropology* 13, no. 1 (1988): 83–99.

17. See Chapter 6 "From Relief to Reconstruction," p. 152.

18. Paul Farmer. "Haiti's unnatural disaster." *The Nation:* September 17, 2008. Available: http://www.thenation.com/article/haitis-unnatural-disaster (accessed April 15, 2011).

19. See, for example, James Smith. "Public Health Crusader Could Join Obama Team." *Boston Globe* (May 14, 2009). Available: http://www.boston.com/news/politics/politicalintelligence/2009/05/public_health_c.html (accessed April 15, 2011).

20. Trenton Daniel. "UN's Deputy Special Envoy to Haiti Wraps up First Trip." *Miami Herald:* September 9, 2010. Available: http://missionmanna.wordpress.com/2009/09 (accessed April 15, 2011). I didn't use my special red UN passport often after this trip because when I returned to Miami, the immigration official who scanned the passport was unimpressed. When he swiped it, the officer gave me a quizzical look. "What does it say?," I asked. "Nationality invalid," he replied.

21. Some with disaster management experience include victims' sentiments (including complaint) in their analysis and strategy. "Do not underestimate the emotion that confronts innocent victims of any disaster . . . You have to deal with those," said Kenneth Feinberg after the BP oil spill in the summer of 2010. See Martha Moore. "Man at Helm of Oil Fund Master of Mediation." *USA Today:* June 27, 2010. Available: http://www.usatoday.com/news/nation/2010-06-27-Feinberg_N.htm. Some of Feinberg's success in guiding policy after the spill, including legal settlements such as the 9/11 Compensation Fund and the BP Fund, comes from the attention paid to the ire that victims feel when forces beyond their control deprive them of compensation and resolution. A failure to honor such sentiments tends to weaken legal resolutions.

22. The point was made by Mildred Aristide in her excellent book on the topic, *L'Enfant En Domesticité en Haïti: Produit d'un Fossé Historique* (Port-au-Prince, Haiti: Imprimerie H. Deschamps, 2003), pp. 89–90: "It is clear that Haiti's rural development and the faltering road to a national public education system have been and remain at the center of the propagation of child domestic service in the country. This explains why the prototypical image of a child in domestic service is one

of a child from the impoverished countryside seeking an education, working in the city."

23. Timothy T. Schwartz. *Travesty in Haiti: A True Account of Christian Missions, Orphanages, Food Aid, Fraud and Drug Trafficking* (Self-published, 2008), p. 66.

24. For more information on the construction of the bridge to Boucan Carré, see Partners In Health's September 2009 online bulletin, available: http://www.pih.org/pages/pih-e-bulletin-2009-09 (accessed April 15, 2011). Also see a short documentary clip in which Dr. Louise Ivers discusses the importance of the bridge, available here: http://www.pih.org/pages/service/ (accessed April 15, 2011).

25. Ophelia Dahl. "Thomas J. White Symposium 2009 Remarks." October 3, 2009.

26. The hatchery had been designed by charismatic and talented Ivoirien agronomist Valentin Abe, whose work is mentioned in Jéhane Sedky's essay "Building Back Better."

27. The baby was named Rolando in honor of our guest.

28. For more about the conference, along with a critique of donor activity in Haiti, see Robert Maguire's briefing for the United States Institute for Peace (Special Report 232, September 2009). Available: http://www.usip.org/files/resources/haiti_after_donors_conference.pdf (accessed April 15, 2011). "The state's lack of capacity to render public services," Maguire argues, "has resulted in the virtual absence of the government as a positive presence in citizen's lives, thus stoking citizen frustration and weakening the democratic process. Donor support of nonstate entities has created an environment that lacks coherence, particularly in support of national development plans."

29. Kathie Klarreich. "Haiti's Working Better." *Miami Herald*: December 8, 2009. Available: http://www.haitiinnovation.org/en/2009/12/09/haitis-working-better-piti-piti (accessed April 15, 2011).

30. See, for example, J. Frenk et al. "Comprehensive Reform to Improve Health System Performance in Mexico." *Lancet* 368 (October 2006): 1524–1534; J. Frenk "Bridging the Divide: Global Lessons from Evidence-Based Health Policy in Mexico." *Lancet* 368 (2006): 954–961.

31. Bolduc survived the August 19, 2003, truck bombing of the UN headquarters in Baghdad. The explosion killed seventeen UN staff, including Sergio Vieira de Mello, the chief envoy to Iraq, and injured more than one hundred others. "Truck Bomb Kills Chief U.N. Envoy to Iraq." *CNN* (August 20, 2003). Available: http://edition.cnn.com/2003/WORLD/meast/08/19/sprj.irq.main/index.html. See also Samantha Power's stirring book on this topic, *Chasing the Flame: Sergio Vieira de Mello and the Fight to Save the World* (New York: Penguin, 2008), which explores the perils, moral and logistic, of such missions.

### Chapter 3

1. David Halberstam. *The Best and the Brightest* (New York: Ballantine Books, 1992).

2. The church-run Collège La Promesse in Pétionville collapsed on November 7,

2008, killing ninety-two students and teachers and injuring one hundred fifty or more. Like most buildings in Port-au-Prince, the school had been self-built by the property owner without the help of engineers or any sort of building code. See "Death Toll Rises to 92 in School Collapse in Haiti." *New York Times* (November 8, 2008). Available: http://www.nytimes.com/2008/11/09/world/americas/09haiti. html (accessed April 15, 2011).

3. Pierre-Louis was voted out of office by the Senate by simple majority, after serving for little more than a year. In public fora, her opponents complained that her response to the 2008 hurricane season had been slow and inept. But others suspected that her ousting had more to do with the threat she may have posed to her superior, although Pierre-Louis had never expressed any intention of running for president. For example, Mario Joseph, a human rights lawyer, suggested that "Préval was threatened by the growing power and connections of Pierre-Louis, particularly after the visits of Bill Clinton. She was becoming the darling of the donors, who called her capable, and I think he felt she was getting too big for her britches." See Joseph Guyler Delva. "Haiti President Designates Economist to Be Premier." Reuters (October 29, 2009). Available: http://in.reuters.com/article/2009/10/30/haiti-primeminister-idINN3039324720091030; Joseph quoted in Kim Ives. "Haitian Prime Minister Ousted by Senate." *Pacific Free Press* (November 5, 2009). Available: http://www.pacificfreepress.com/news/1/4999-haitian-prime-minister -ousted-by-senate.html (accessed April 15, 2011).

4. "Former President Clinton on Haiti." *Real Clear Politics:* January 13, 2010. Available: http://www.realclearpolitics.com/articles/2010/01/13/interview_with_ fmr_president_clinton_on_haiti_99900.html (accessed April 15, 2011).

5. Ibid.

6. Louise Ivers. "A Doctor's Story." *Irish Times:* January 18, 2010. http://www. irishtimes.com/newspaper/world/2010/0118/1224262564631.html (accessed April 15, 2011).

7. The interview was broadcast on CBS's *60 Minutes* on January 17, 2010. Available: http://www.cbsnews.com/video/watch/?id=6108550n&tag=api (accessed April 15, 2011).

8. For an extended discussion of the challenges of coordinating humanitarian aid efforts in general and after the earthquake in Haiti, see Chapter 7, "Reconstruction in the Time of Cholera" and *passim*, frankly, because that is what this book is about. For an account of these issues in the press, see Patricia Zengerle and Jackie Frank. "Haiti Needs Better Coordination." *Reuters* (January 27, 2010) Available: http://www.reuters.com/article/2010/01/27/us-quake-haiti-idUSTRE60O29A2010- 0127 (accessed April 15, 2011).

9. Dean Lorich, Soumitra Eachempati, David Helfet. "Doctors: Haiti Medical Situation Shameful." *CNN*, January 25, 2010. Available: http://articles.cnn.com/ 2010-01-25/opinion/doctors.haiti.hardships_1_haiti-trauma-surgeons-medical -supplies?_s=PM:OPINION (accessed April 15, 2011).

10. P. Farmer. "Gram-Negative Sepsis of Uncertain Etiology." *New England Journal of Medicine* 340, 11 (1999): 869–876; See also Paul Farmer. "Haiti, l'embargo et la typhoide." *Le Monde Diplomatique* (July 2003): 26–27.

11. In 2002, Haiti was ranked 147 out of 147 countries on the Water Poverty Index, and 101 out of 122 countries for water quality—dead last in the hemisphere in both studies. See P. Lawrence et al. "The Water Poverty Index: An International Comparison." *Keele Economic Research Papers* (2002); D. C. Esty and P. K. Cornelius, eds. *Environmental Performance Measurement: Global Report 2001–2002* (2002). Comparison chart available at http://www.unesco.org/bpi/wwdr/WWDR_chart2_eng.pdf (accessed April 15, 2011); see also Farmer. "Political Violence and Public Health in Haiti."

12. For more on the role of universities during the earthquake response, see Andrea Fuller. "American Universities Rush to Front Lines in Haiti." *Chronicle of Higher Education:* January 21, 2010. Available: http://chronicle.com/article/American-Universities-Rush-to/63692/ (accessed April 15, 2011).

13. Paul Farmer, Louise Ivers, and Claire Pierre. "Tales from the Front." *Miami Herald* (January 23, 2010). Available: http://www.haitispecialenvoy.org/press/op-eds/drs-farmer-ivers-pierre-tales-from-the-front/ (accessed April 15, 2011).

14. See Peter Baker and Joseph Berger. "U.S. to Resume Airlift of Injured Haitians." *New York Times:* January 31, 2010. Available: http://www.nytimes.com/2010/02/01/world/americas/01airlift.html (accessed April 15, 2011); Alex Lantier. "U.S. Halts Military Flights to Evacuate Haiti Earthquake Victims." *WSWS.org*: February 1, 2010. Available: http://www.wsws.org/articles/2010/feb2010/hait-f01.shtml (accessed April 15, 2011).

15. Farmer. *AIDS and Accusation: Haiti and the Geography of Blame.*

16. We also discussed his visit to Rwanda earlier that month, which was meant to improve Franco-Rwandan relations. The diplomatic relationship between the two countries had been strained since the genocide and was severed by Kigali in 2006, when a French judge issued arrest warrants for a number of top aides to Paul Kagame, the current Rwandan president, on the grounds that they were somehow involved in the downing of Rwandan dictator Juvenal Habyarimana's plane on April 6, 1994—the event marking the start of the hundred-day genocide. Most observers didn't find the evidence against the Kagame aides to be credible. Kouchner's trip to Kigali aimed at a return to amicable relations, including the resuscitation of cultural exchanges and development assistance. Franco-Rwandan relations would be strengthened further a month later with President Nicholas Sarkozy's visit on February 24; Sarkozy allowed that the French government had made "grave errors of judgment" during the genocide. For news coverage of Kouchner's visit to Rwanda, see "Rwanda and France Pledge to Boost Ties after Three-Year Freeze." RFI (January 7, 2010). Available: http://www.rfi.fr/actuen/articles/121/article_6426.asp (accessed April 15, 2011). For coverage of Sarkozy's trip, see Anjan Sundaram. "On Visit to Rwanda, Sarkozy Admits 'Grave Errors' in 1994 Genocide," *New York Times* (February 25, 2010). Available: http://www.nytimes.com/2010/02/26/world/europe/26france.html (accessed April 15, 2011).

17. Peter Walker. "Haiti Can Lead Earthquake Relief Effort." *Guardian* (January 25, 2010). Available: http://www.guardian.co.uk/world/2010/jan/25/haiti-earthquake-relief-effort-summit (accessed April 15, 2011).

18. Quoted in Rob Gilles. "Haiti Conference: Nations Call for Haitian Government to Lead Rebuilding," *Huffington Post:* (January 26, 2010). Available: http://www.huffingtonpost.com/2010/01/26/haiti-conference-nations_n_436495.html (accessed April 15, 2011).

19. Quoted in Marc Lacey and Ginger Thompson. "Agreement on Effort to Help Haiti Rebuild," *New York Times*: January 25, 2010. Available: http://www.nytimes.com/2010/01/26/world/americas/26haiti.html (accessed April 15, 2011).

20. Christine Welter. "Montreal Hosts Haiti Reconstruction Conference," *Suite 101*: January 26, 2010. Available: http://www.suite101.com/content/montreal-hosts-haiti-reconstruction-conference-a194024 (accessed April 15, 2011).

21. To those eager to level corruption charges against the Haitian government, I would push on two fronts. First, it's not very helpful to criticize a government such as Haiti's in a vacuum. A sound analysis situates Haitian politics and bureaucratic performance in a broader context, historical and geographical. Few years in Haiti's history are unmarked by foreign intervention or meddling of some kind. What we know about democracy in Haiti is this: whenever a popular leader (elected by significant margins) is given a chance to hold office, he will, as surely as night follows day, soon face embargoes and bad press and possibly worse. No one would deny that the current government has certain inveterate weaknesses, but perhaps it's time to let Haitian democracy run its course, to let the Haitian civil services grow and take root. Second, to avoid corruption, public institutions—from the line ministries to facilities such as the General Hospital—need an infrastructure of transparency: modern bookkeeping, electronic disbursement of payroll, performance-based financing, effective communications technology. For the last two decades, the Haitian state has been starved of resources. Long accustomed to paltry tax revenues, embargoes intended to pressure the governments in the direction of foreign business interests emptied the meager federal coffers. Instead, money flowed to NGOs, which wittingly or unwittingly weakened the public sector. By the close of the millennium, the Republic of NGOs had undermined the Republic of Haiti's capability to fulfill its government mandate. In these conditions, corruption charges sometimes seem misplaced.

22. Lacey and Thompson. "Agreement on Effort to Help Haiti Rebuild."

23. Amy Wilentz, who has written extensively about recent Haitian political history, made the point that Préval's leadership style was a welcome break from a history of "strongman" politics she connects with Duvalierism. Préval's administration, "while certainly not incandescent," she writes, "had a calming influence on the roiling tide of Haitian politics. . . . The quiet president, operating behind the scenes with the international community, instead of strutting before the foreign press and claiming he'll fix everything, is perhaps at this moment not such a bad leader for Haitian democracy, after all." See Amy Wilentz. "The Dechoukaj This Time." *New York Times,* February 7, 2010. Available: http://www.nytimes.com/2010/02/07/opinion/07wilentz.html?_r=1&adxnnl=1&pagewanted=all&adxnnlx=1292446954-gjxDURsrwoKQhLo4k/EZpw (accessed April 15, 2011). Wilentz's perspective is a helpful counterweight to the heavy doses of criticism laid on

Préval and his administration after the quake. But it is not an exaggeration to say that the government's efforts often have been anemic at best.

24. Jonathan Demme's 2003 documentary *The Agronomist* follows Jean Dominique's and Michèle Montas's struggle to make Radio Haiti-Inter a mouthpiece of the people.

25. Régine Chassagne. "I Let Out a Cry, as if I Had Just Heard that Everybody I Love Had Died." *Irish Times:* January 17, 2010.

26. For more about their organization, *Kanpe*, see http://www.kanpe.org/home .html (accessed April 15, 2011).

27. There were many such stories from the early days after the earthquake. Some aid workers were stuck en route to Haiti; others had trouble leaving. See, for example, Alan McDowell. "Aid Workers Face Logistical Problems." *National Post* (January 14, 2010). Available: http://www.nationalpost.com/news/story.html?id= 2442757.

28. The full text of President Obama's speech is available here: http://abcnews .go.com/Politics/State_of_the_Union/state-of-the-union-2010-president-obama-speech-transcript/story?id=9678572 (accessed April 15, 2011).

29. The full text of the 2003 testimonial is available here: http://foreign. senate.gov/imo/media/doc/FarmerTestimony030715.pdf (accessed April 15, 2011).

30. For evidence on this score, see Tracy Kidder's piece in the *Nation*, "The Trials of Haiti" (October 27, 2003). Available: http://www.thenation.com/archive/trials-haiti.

31. Paul Farmer, Joseph P. Kennedy, and Jeffrey Sachs. "U.S. Owes Aristide a Fair Chance to Govern." *Boston Globe* (June 30, 2001), Sect. A:15; P. Farmer, M. C. Smith Fawzi, and P. Nevil. "Unjust Embargo of Aid for Haiti." *Lancet* 361 (2003): 420–423.

32. Full coverage of the hearing is available here: http://www.cspan.org/Watch/ Media/2010/01/28/HP/A/28965/Senate+Foreign+Relations+Cmte+Hearing+on+ Haiti+Relief.aspx (accessed April 15, 2011).

33. The Foreign Assistance Act was signed into law by President John F. Kennedy in 1961. A product of Cold War politics, its stated goal was to win "hearts and minds" in developing countries declaring intentions to adopt socialist or communist tactics. Cold War mentalities still influence the U.S. foreign aid strategy. For example, Jeff Sachs notes that only one of the five operational goals outlined by the U.S. Agency for International Development (USAID) contributes to long-term development ("promoting transformational development"). The other four ("supporting strategic sites, strengthening fragile states, providing humanitarian relief, and addressing global challenges such as the HIV/AIDS epidemic and climate change") are important components of foreign policy but do too little to take on poverty and economic development. Sachs tracks the meager $2.8 billion (out of $16 billion total) that went to transformational development. "The entire sum," he writes, "went to technical cooperation: payments made primarily to U.S. entities— consultants from government agencies or nongovernmental organizations (NGOs)—for assignments in recipient nations. These missions may be useful, but the expenditures are not long-term investments in local clinics, schools, power plants, sanitation, or other infrastructure." Further, the benefits of the aid that is

disbursed are tempered by high overhead and policies promoting U.S. interests: food aid comes most often in the form of grain shipments—great for subsidized American agribusiness and perhaps less so for local farmers—and almost half the money for food aid goes to transportation costs, instead of food (see Jeffrey Sachs. "The Development Challenge." *Foreign Affairs* 84, no. 2, pp. 78–79). In addition to its Cold War legacies, U.S. foreign aid struggles under the weight of great bureaucratic inefficiencies. Aid disbursement, for example, is splintered into eighteen institutions within the State Department and the U.S. Agency for International Development alone, and an additional twenty or more government institutions also have aid programs. Stewart Patrick of the Center for Global Development has called for a new cabinet-level agency that would centralize foreign assistance for international development under one roof. See Stewart Patrick. "U.S. Aid Reform: Will It Fix What Is Broken?" (September 2006), available: http://www.cgdev.org/content/publications/detail/10497 (accessed April 15, 2011). All these problems have led a growing number of government officials, development practitioners, and academics to endorse far-reaching reform of the Foreign Assistance Act. The Bush Administration proposed reform legislation in 2006, which has since been shelved. Oxfam America and ActionAid have both proposed more substantial reforms. See also "New Day, New Way" (June 1, 2008), a proposal made by a coalition of development and foreign affairs practitioners and policymakers known as the Modernizing Foreign Assistance Network. The report is available at: http://modernizing foreignassistance.net/documents/newdaynewway.pdf (accessed April 15, 2011).

34. The history of Haitian debt runs deep: after independence, the French claimed a debt of 150 million francs for property—including slaves—lost during the Haitian Revolution (see p. 127 and n. 14). In 2008, the government of Haiti owed almost $2 billion in foreign debt, half of which was canceled after a donor conference in June 2009. G9 countries announced the cancellation of the remaining half in February 2010, as part of the earthquake relief effort. See "G7 Nations Pledge Debt Relief for Quake-Hit Haiti." *BBC* (February 7, 2010). Available: http://news.bbc.co.uk/2/hi/8502567.stm (accessed April 15, 2011).

35. Increasing evidence points toward the value of cash transfers, especially those targeted at women, at strengthening families and spurring grassroots development. See, for example, Joseph Hanlon, David Hulme, and Armando Barrientos. *Just Give Money to the Poor: The Development Revolution from the Global South* (West Hartford: Kumarian Press, 2010).

36. Transcript available: http://www.haitispecialenvoy.org/press/transcripts/testimony-of-dr-paul-farmer-to-the-us-senate-committee-on-foreign-relations/ (accessed April 15, 2011).

37. The full text of the 2003 testimonial is available here: http://foreign.senate.gov/imo/media/doc/FarmerTestimony030715.pdf (accessed April 15, 2011).

38. For more on Partners In Health's efforts to manufacture vitamin-enriched peanut butter as a ready-to-use therapeutic food, see Andrew Rice's long exposé "The Peanut Solution" in the *New York Times Magazine* (September 2, 2010). Available: http://www.nytimes.com/2010/09/05/magazine/05plumpy-t.html?page wanted=all (accessed April 15, 2011). As the article notes, producing such vitamin-

enriched peanut butter led to legal threats from a company that claimed exclusive rights to the product. But can you patent peanut butter?

39. Yesica Fisch and Martha Mendoza. "Haiti Government Gets 1 Penny of U.S. Quake Aid Dollar." Associated Press (January 27, 2010). Available: http://www. usatoday.com/news/world/2010-01-27-Haiti-aid_N.htm (accessed April 15, 2011).

40. Our colleagues at the Office of the Special Envoy have been militant about tracking these numbers. The most recent report on relief and reconstruction financing is available here: http://s3.amazonaws.com/haiti_production/assets/22/1._Overall_financing_key_facts_FINAL_6_original.pdf (accessed April 15, 2011).

41. Jonathan Katz, "Billions for Haiti, A Criticism for Every Dollar," Associated Press (March 5, 2010). Sources compiled from USAID and the United Nations. Available: http://www.informationclearinghouse.info/haitiaid.jpg (accessed April 15, 2011).

42. See Farmer. *The Uses of Haiti.*

43. Although I've probably spilled too much ink about the Peligré Dam in *AIDS and Accusation* and elsewhere, it has appeared again in headlines: the Inter-American Development Bank is considering a $40 million rehabilitation program. The dam currently operates at half capacity because of residual silt buildup; this has contributed to the country's 30 percent drop in electricity production in the past decade. The bank hopes to amend this shortage by getting the 54-megawatt dam back on its feet. See Jennifer Wells. "A Dam for the People, and a People Damned." *The Star* (August 2010). Available: http://www.thestar.com/article/894096---peligre-dam-project-brought-floods-and-darkness (accessed April 15, 2011).

44. Giuseppe Raviola, Eddy Eustache, Catherine Oswald, Gary Belkin. "Mental Health Response in Haiti in the Aftermath of the 2010 Earthquake: A Case Study for Building Long-Term Solutions." *Harvard Review of Psychiatry*, 2012 (In Press).

45. Stephen Smith and James F. Smith. "Rising to Meet an Infinite Need." *Boston Globe* (January 24, 2010). Available: http://www.boston.com/news/world/latinamerica/articles/2010/01/24/boston_based_nonprofit_has_been_thrust_into_leadership_role_in_haiti/ (accessed April 15, 2011).

46. With the help of the logistics wizards in Boston, Thierry was able to escort his cousins to their new home, and he soon returned to Cange. He is still planning a career in surgery and hopes to begin his training, in Canada or the United States, by the summer of 2011.

47. To see and hear Shelove, see the wonderful short video, "Walking the Walk," by Rebecca Rollins (translated by Caroline Hilaire). Available: http://vimeo.com/13281822 (accessed April 15, 2011).

48. The blind and otherwise handicapped had never fared much better. Graham Greene's Haiti novel, *The Comedians*, evokes the terror of the Duvalier years but also the link between disability and poverty. When a well-meaning American man visits the post office, he is swarmed by beggars with severe disabilities: "Two one-armed men and three one-legged men hemmed him round. Two were trying to sell him dirty old envelopes containing out of date Haitian postage stamps: the others were more frankly begging. A man without legs at all had installed himself be-

tween his knees and removed his shoe-laces preparatory to cleaning his shoes. Others seeing a crowd collected were fighting to join in. A young fellow, with a hole where his nose should have been, lowered his head and tried to ram his way through towards the attraction. A man with no hands raised his pink polished stumps over the heads of the crowd to exhibit his infirmity to the foreigner. It was a typical scene in the Post Office" (New York: Penguin, 1965), p. 155.

49. Rollins. "Walking the Walk."

50. David Brown. "Surgeon Seeks to Prevent 'Unnecessary Amputations' in Haiti's Earthquake Zone." *Washington Post* (January 21, 2010). Amputation has a fraught history during humanitarian aid efforts. The notorious international response to the amputated victims of Sierra Leone's civil war, for example, triggered unintended, and perhaps perverse, consequences. Some have suggested that the surge of foreign money sent to Sierra Leone after photos of amputated children and women circulated in the western media only encouraged rebels to continue chopping off limbs as a political tactic. See, for example, Linda Polman. *The Crisis Caravan: What's Wrong with Humanitarian Aid?* (New York: Macmillan Books, 2010), pp. 66–69.

51. For more on the graduation of the Global Health Delivery fellows, see "Global Health Delivery Fellows Honored for Accomplishments and Leadership." Partners in Health Online (March 30, 2010). Available: http://www.pih.org/haiti/news-entry/global-health-delivery-fellows-honored-for-accompishments-and-leadersh/ (accessed April 15, 2011). One of the graduates had the following to say about the practice of social medicine in the rural reaches of his homeland: "My first day at Zanmi Lasante, I was greeted by Dr. Maxi and Dr. Léandre, and to be honest, I thought they were nuts. They spoke to me about everything except medicine—such as transport costs, income-generating activities, construction of houses, compensation for community health workers. In fact I stayed lost. I wasn't even sure they were doctors. But I needed to learn, I needed time to live this reality . . . Later in my first year, I was annoyed, I did not think doctors should do home visits. I remember one of our faculty asked me to go find a TB patient, who had left without finishing his therapy . . . the attending insisted that any doctor taking care of a patient has a responsibility if the patient leaves the hospital. After returning to the hospital with the patient from the village of Kay Epin, I began to think differently about the doctor-patient relationship; about how my talking with and spending time with the patient changed his outcome. We decided to stay in a rural place, not to return to the city, or to do a residency—but to become "Dokte Mon"—a mountain doctor. You must understand, that we were among the best students in our classes in medical school, each of us was expected to do a residency. Generally, those who are called "mountain doctors" are surrounded by rumors of incompetence . . . but for us, choosing this path is our core engagement to join this determined team, Haitian and foreign, who in a noble mission, serve the Haitian poor. It is not easy to be devoted to this mission, there are sacrifices in these rural places, far from the lucrative and prestigious jobs in the capital that garner a private clinic or a car. But you all have accompanied us to a much greater goal, to see the medicine in a community way, medicine in service to all those who require it."

52. J. Helprin. "Bill Clinton Chides Nations over Help to Haiti." Associated Press (September 9, 2009). Available: http://www.newsvine.com/_news/2009/09/09/3243861-bill-clinton-chides-nations-over-help-for-haiti (accessed April 15, 2011).

53. "Haiti—No Leadership, No Elections." Senate Foreign Relations Committee Report. 111th Congress, 2nd Session (June 10, 2010). Available: http://www.gpoaccess.gov/congress/index.html (accessed April 15, 2011).

54. Roberts. "Responding in a Crisis."

55. A report by Merlin underscores this conclusion: "The overall emergency response could have benefited from wider participation in the effort to build capacity of the Ministry [of Health] and to support systems development and coordination, but most international agencies opted to focus on providing direct emergency care in the initial phase." Roberts. "Responding in a Crisis," p. 6.

## Chapter 4

1. This, again, resonates with the lessons drawn by Halberstam. Of the U.S. general sent to Vietnam in 1962, Halberstam writes that, "Like almost all Americans who arrived in Vietnam, Harkins was ignorant of the past, and ignorant of the special kind of war he was fighting. To him, like so many Americans, the war had begun the moment he arrived; the past had never happened and need not be taken seriously." Halberstam. *The Best and the Brightest*, p. 185.

2. Mark Danner. "To Heal Haiti, Look to History, not Nature." *New York Times* (January 21, 2010). Available: http://www.nytimes.com/2010/01/22/opinion/22danner.html?_r=2&pagewanted=all (accessed April 15, 2011).

3. See Thomas Madiou's monumental history of Haiti: *Histoire d'Haïti*. 9 vols. (Port-au-Prince: Imprimerie Henri Deschamps, 1989). The U.S. occupation is chronicled in six volumes by Roger Gaillard in *La République Exterminatrice*. 6 vols. (Port-au-Prince: Imprimerie Le Natal, 1984–1998).

4. See Noble David Cook, *Born to Die: Disease and New World Conquest, 1492–1650* (Cambridge: Cambridge University Press, 1998), p. 23, table 1.1.

5. Léon Dénius Pamphile. *Haitians and African-Americans: A Heritage of Tragedy and Hope* (Gainesville: University of Florida Press, 2003), p. 2.

6. M.-L.-E. Moreau de Saint-Méry. *Description Topographique, Physique, Civile, Politique et Historique de la Partie Française de l'Isle Saint-Domingue (1797–1798)*. 3 vols. New ed., B. Maurel and E. Taillemite, eds. (Paris: Société de l'Histoire des Colonies Françaises and Librairie Larose).

7. Cited in Robert Heinl and Nancy Heinl. *Written in Blood* (Boston: Houghton Mifflin Co., 1978), pp. 26–27.

8. Eric Williams. *From Columbus to Castro: The History of the Caribbean, 1492–1969* (London: Andre Deutsch), p. 246.

9. Cited in Claude Auguste and Marecel Auguste. *L'Expédition Leclerc 1801–1803* (Port-au-Prince: Imprimerie Henri Deschamps), p. 236; Farmer. *The Uses of Haiti*, p. 70.

10. Quoted in Laurent Dubois. *Avengers of the New World* (Cambridge: Harvard University Press, 2004), p. 301.

11. For one of the best accounts of the abolition of the slave trade in England, see Adam Hochschild. *Bury the Chains: Prophets and Rebels in the Fight to Free an Empire's Slaves* (New York: Houghton Mifflin, 2005).

12. After fifty years of searching for the eight-page document, the second independence declaration in history (after the U.S. Declaration in 1776) was found by Julia Gaffield, an American graduate student, in the British National Archives in Kew. For more information, see "Haiti's Declaration of Independence discovered at The National Archives," April 1, 2010. Available: http://www.nationalarchives.gov.uk/news/453.htm (accessed April 15, 2011). Full text of the Declaration of Independence available here: http://www.nathanielturner.com/haitiandeclarationof independence1804.htm (accessed April 15, 2011).

13. Cited in Hans Schmidt. *The United States Occupation of Haiti, 1915–1934* (New Brunswick, NJ: Rutgers University Press, 1971), p. 312.

14. Haun Saussy recently published a short piece revealing the Kingdom of France's logic behind indemnification. The order, issued by King Charles X on April 17, 1785, reads: "The present inhabitants of the French part of the island of Santo Domingo shall pay to the Caisse des Dépôts et Consignations de France in five equal yearly installments, from year to year . . . the sum of 150,000,000 francs, intended to make whole those former colonists who require reimbursement. We concede, on these conditions, by the present Order, to the *inhabitants of the French part of Santo Domingo* the full and complete independence of their government" (italics added). In the eyes of Charles X, the Haitian Revolution hadn't happened; Haiti still belonged to France. See "That Is One Odious Debt." *Printculture* (December 27, 2010). Available: http://printculture.com/item-2781.html (accessed April 15, 2011).

15. Danner. "To Heal Haiti Look to History, not Nature."

16. I've written about this and earned some scorn from French officialdom for my troubles. See, for example, P. Farmer. "Douze Points en Faveur de la Restitution à Haïti de la Dette Française." *L'Union* (November 11, 2003): 1, 3, 4. More recently, after the quake, more than ninety academics, journalists, and activists signed an open letter to President Sarkozy urging restitution of the French debt. See "M. Sarkozy, Rendez à Haïti Son Argent Extorqué." *Libération.* August 16, 2010. Available: http://www.liberation.fr/monde/0101652216-m-sarkozy-rendez-a-haiti-son-argent-extorque (accessed April 15, 2011).

17. Jean Price-Mars. *La République d'Haïti et la République Dominicaine: Les Aspects Divers d'un Problème d'Histoire, de Géographie et d'Ethnologie* (Lausanne: Imprimerie Held, 1953), pp. 169–170.

18. Quoted in Rayford Logan. *Haiti and the Dominican Republic* (London: Oxford University Press, 1968), p. 119.

19. Roger Gaillard. *Le Guerilla de Batraville* (Port-au-Prince: Imprimerie Le Natal, 1983), pp. 261–262. The authoritative North American version of the history finds 3,250 peasant deaths in the twenty months of active resistance. See Hans Schmidt. *The United States Occupation of Haiti, 1915–1934* (New Brunswick, NJ: Rutgers University Press, 1971), p. 103.

20. Balch won the prize in 1946 for her efforts to promote peace between the World Wars. (John Mott also won the Peace Prize in 1946.) While serving on the Women's International League for Peace and Freedom's committee investigating the occupation of Haiti, Balch wrote "Occupied Haiti," a report calling for the immediate withdrawal of U.S. marines from Haiti. For more on Balch, see Kristen Gwinn's biography, *Emily Greene Balch: The Long Road to Internationalism* (Chicago: University of Illinois Press, 2011).

21. Military historians Heinl and Heinl estimated that 2,250 had been killed from 1915 to 1920 during the Cacos uprisings. See Heinl and Heinl. *Written in Blood*, p. 441, n. 24., pp. 463, 470.

22. Cited in Rod Prince. *Haiti: Family Business* (London: Latin American Bureau, 1985), p. 21.

23. See e.g. Heinl and Heinl. *Written in Blood*, p. 441, n. 24.

24. In one scene, the narrator watches a photograph of Papa Doc Duvalier—required by law to be posted in every building—burn in the fire of a Voodoo ceremony: "The flames lit the photograph nailed on the pillar, the heavy spectacles, the eyes staring at the ground as though at a body ready for dissection. Once he had been a country doctor struggling successfully against typhoid; he had been a founder of the Ethnological Society . . . *Corruptio optimi.*" Greene. *The Comedians*, p. 180.

25. For more on this violent interregnum, see Erica James' book *Democratic Insecurities: Violence, Trauma, and Intervention in Haiti* (Berkeley: University of California Press, 2010), which examines the terror apparatus of the Duvalier dictatorships. Violation of sex, gender, and kinship norms through rape, torture, and shame was a strategy of state and, indeed, a locus of Duvalierist power. James analyzes the practice of documenting trauma narratives as a means of marshalling resources in the subsequent aid economy, and the varied implications of this practice for both the donors and recipients of aid dollars. She describes the "bureaucraft" culture that arose in Haiti amidst failures of aid transparency: a public trade in accusations about hidden or occult activity amongst government and non-government organizations that have led to violence and civil unrest.

26. Amy Wilentz. *The Rainy Season: Haiti After Duvalier* (New York: Simon and Schuster, 1989), p. 335. Leslie Francois Saint Roc Manigat, born August 16, 1930 in Port-au-Prince, was elected president of Haiti in an election tightly controlled by the military in January 1988.

27. Aristide wrote about the massacre: "Everyone was running, trying to find a place to hide. One man was shot in the outside courtyard, with his Bible in his hand. Bullets were zinging left and right. I saw a pregnant woman screaming for help in the pews, and holding onto her stomach. A man had just speared her there, and she was bathed in red blood . . . this was a prophetic, historic resistance that we will never forget." Jean Bertrand Aristide. *In the Parish of the Poor: Writings from Haiti* (MaryKnoll, New York: Orbis, 1990), p. 55.

28. I wrote an account of the elections for a Jesuit magazine shortly after Aristide's inauguration. I cribbed the title from the liberation theologian, Gustavo Gut-

tiérrez. See Paul Farmer. "The Power of the Poor in Haiti." *America* 164, 9 (1992): 260–267.

29. Bob Shacochis. *The Immaculate Invasion* (New York: Penguin, 1999).

30. Oscar Arias. "Only the marching band." *The Washington Post* (March 12, 2004).

31. Some of the most thorough accounts of the period include: Randal Robinson. *An Unbroken Agony: Haiti, From Revolution to the Kidnapping of a President* (New York: Basic Civitas Books, 2007); Peter Hallward. *Damming the Flood: Haiti, Aristide, and the Politics of Containment* (London: Verso, 2008); and Isabel Macdonald. "'Parachute Journalism' in Haiti: Media Sourcing in the 2003–2004 Political Crisis." *Canadian Journal of Communication* 33: 213–232. Also be sure to see Jeb Sprague's forthcoming book *Haiti and the Roots of Paramilitarism* (New York: Monthy Review Press, 2012).

32. Madison Smartt Bell. "Mine of Stones: With and Without the Spirits Along the Cordon de l'Ouest." *Harper's* (January 2004), p. 65.

33. Peter Hallward's book, *Damming the Flood*, is a grueling and instructive exploration of this slow-motion coup.

34. See Paul Farmer. "Who Removed Aristide?" *London Review of Books* 26, 8 (2004): 28–31. See also Randall Robinson's book, *An Unbroken Agony: Haiti, from Revolution to the Kidnapping of a President* (New York: Perseus Books, 2007).

35. Amy Wilentz. "Coup in Haiti." *Nation* (March 22, 2004). Available: http://amywilentz.com/blog/coup-in-haiti/ (accessed April 15, 2011). Wilentz continues: "One thing about coups: They don't just happen. In a country like Haiti, where the military has been disbanded for nearly a decade, soldiers don't simply emerge from the underbrush; they have to be reorganized, retrained and resupplied . . . In the current coup, there are several players. There is the disgruntled former Haitian army (an institution with a violent and unpalatable recent history), which has been wielded many times in the service of coups d'état, often subsidized by its masters, the elite of Haiti. The elite, too, had their hand in this coup–it's hard to believe in this day and age, but they must be called the entrenched class enemies of the Haitian people. There is 'a growing enthusiasm among businessmen to use the rebels as a security force,' said a news report from the *Los Angeles Times* after the remnants of the Haitian army that helped engineer the coup descended on the capital. '[The businessmen] welcomed the rebels.'"

34. Peter Heinlein. "UN Peacekeeping Chief: Haiti Worse than Darfur." *Voice of America* (June 28, 2005). Available: http://www.voanews.com/english/2005-06-28-voa63.cfm (accessed April 15, 2011).

## Chapter 5

1. For more on internally displaced persons in Africa and around the world see Internal Displacement Monitoring Centre, "Internal Displacement: Global Overview of Trends and Developments in 2010," March 2011 Report. Available:

http://www.internal-displacement.org/publications/global-overview-2010.pdf (accessed April 14, 2011).

2. The memo was leaked to Turtle Bay on February 17, 2010. Available: http://turtlebay.foreignpolicy.com/posts/2010/02/17/top_un_aid_official_critiques_haiti_aid_efforts_in_confidential_email (accessed April 15, 2011).

3. Kimberly A. Cullen and Louise C. Ivers. "Human Rights Assessment in Parc Jean-Marie Vincent, Port-au-Prince, Haiti." *Health and Human Rights in Practice* 12, no. 2: 1–12.

4. See Didi Bertrand Farmer. "Bearing Witness: Girls and Women in Haiti's Camps." *World Pulse* (November 4, 2010). Available: http://www.worldpulse.com/node/30500/ (accessed April 15, 2011); see also her essay in this book, "Mothers and Daughters of Haïti," where this topic is explored at greater length.

## Chapter 6

1. A recording of the hearing is available here: http://foreign.senate.gov/hearings/hearing/?id=3f546a93-d363-da0b-b25f-f1c5d096ddb1 (accessed April 15, 2011). For more on food assistance in Haiti, see the recent report by the Center for Human Rights and Global Justice and the Global Justice Clinic at New York University's School of Law, Partners In Health, Zanmi Lasante, and the Robert F. Kennedy Center for Justice and Human Rights. *Sak Vid Pa Kanpe: The Impact of U.S. Food Aid on Human Rights in Haiti* (2010). Available: http://parthealth.3cdn.net/3f82f61a3316d7f1a0_pvm6b8of3.pdf.

2. Anna Zingg et al. "Haiti-Hurricane Season 2008." International Committee of the Red Cross Report (September 23, 2008).

3. Jean-Claude Duvalier, for example, often spoke of making Haiti the "Taiwan of the Caribbean" to attract foreign businesses and investment. More often than not, what he attracted were offshore assembly plants which had mixed effects on Haitian employment (many offered impossibly low wages, less than $5 per day in most cases) and long-term growth. See Maguire. *Haiti After the Donor Conference.*

4. This estimate of 2009 disbursements was prepared in January 2010 in an internal memorandum of the UN Office of the Special Envoy for Haiti. President Clinton, in his capacity as UN Envoy, frequently appealed to donors to fulfill their commitments. See Helprin, "Bill Clinton Chides Nations over Help to Haiti."

5. Madeline Kristoff and Liz Panarelli. *Haiti: A Republic of NGOs?* U.S. Institute for Peace, Peace Brief (April 26, 2010). Available: http://www.usip.org/publications/haiti-republic-ngos (accessed April 15, 2011).

6. In 2004, the de facto government published a set of ground rules following the forced departure of President Aristide. The Haitian government put out two reports in 2007, one on political decentralization (the government had little presence outside Port-au-Prince) and another on poverty reduction, and then another report in 2009 that spelled out a rebuilding strategy after the previous year's hurricanes. The RAND Corporation summarized the Haitian Government's strategic plans in a report in 2010, which can be found online at www.rand.org/pubs/monographs/2010/RAND_MG1039.pdf (accessed April 15, 2011).

7. Neil MacFarquhar. "Haiti Frets over Aid and Control of Rebuilding." *New York Times* (March 30, 2010). Available: http://www.nytimes.com/2010/03/31/world/americas/31haiti.html?ref=haiti (accessed April 15, 2011).

8. These pledges for reconstruction aid were separate from the $2 billion or so already promised or disbursed in Haiti for immediate disaster relief.

9. Jonathan Katz. "US and EU Pledge $9.8 Billion to Rebuild Haiti After Earthquake." Associated Press (April 1, 2010). Available: http://www.huffingtonpost.com/2010/03/31/us-and-eu-pledge-billions_n_520560.html (accessed April 15, 2011). The story notes that Venezuela's $2 billion contribution may have included money already sent to Haiti as relief funds.

10. Quoted in "Over US $5 Billion Pledged for Haiti's Recovery." http://www.haiticonference.org/story.html (accessed April 15, 2011).

11. Pamela Falk. "Haiti Donor Meeting Far Exceeds $4B Goal." *CBC News* (March 31, 2010). Available: http://www.cbsnews.com/stories/2010/03/31/world/main6350269.shtml.

12. One report found that the quake left 40 percent of the civil service injured or dead, along with twenty-eight out of twenty-nine federal buildings down. *Haiti—no leadership, no elections.* Senate Foreign Relations Committee Report. 111th Congress, 2nd Session (June 10, 2010). Available: http://www.gpoaccess.gov/congress/index.html (accessed April 15, 2011).

13. This is not meant as an ideological claim; telecommunications is a case in point. The public sector was unable to meet demand for telephones in Haiti—only a few thousand firms and families had landlines. It was not until the cell phone revolution, over the past decade, that privatized phones became valuable, even to the very poor, who use them as banking tools as well as a means of communicating with family and friends. More people had access to cell phones now than had they waited for a publicly controlled company to deliver. Similarly, independent service providers and NGOs might do a better job getting social services to the poor now. But should we compare providing cell phones to providing health care or safe water or education?

14. Jonathan Katz. "Clinton-Led Commission Starts Up in Haiti." *ABC News* (June 17, 2010). Available: http://abcnews.go.com/Business/wireStory?id=10943320&page=1 (accessed April 15, 2011).

15. See Charity Navigator's special report on the anniversary of the quake. Available: http://www.charitynavigator.org/index.cfm?bay=content.view&cpid=1186 (accessed April 15, 2011).

16. At the Skoll Foundation Conference on April 30, 2010, we brainstormed this question as a problem of catalysis, hoping that the entrepreneurs gathered there would seek new technologies and delivery strategies that might fill the gap between goodwill and implementation in Haiti. *Catalyzing Collaboration: Our Humanity at Stake.* http://www.skollworldforum.com/forum-2010 (accessed April 15, 2011).

17. See Walter Rodney's forceful argument that colonialism led to the underdevelopment of Africa. Walter Rodney. *How Europe Underdeveloped Africa* (Dar-Es-Salaam, Tanzania: London and Tanzanian Publishing House, 1973). Available:

http://www.blackherbals.com/walter_rodney.pdf (accessed April 15, 2011). On so-called dependency theory see the work of Hans Singer ("The Distribution of Gains between Investing and Borrowing Countries," *American Economic Review* 40, no. 2, 1950) and Raúl Prebisch. (*The Economic Development of Latin America and Its Principal Problems*. [New York: United Nations, 1950].) Dependency theory emerged in the post-War era to counter reigning modernization theory, which held that all countries progressed along a series of stages of economic development. In contrast to this progressivist vision of development, dependency theorists posited that the poverty of countries at the periphery was intimately linked to the wealth of countries at the core. According to this narrative, the rich get richer because the poor get poorer.

18. Paul Collier has argued the combination of high population growth and un-employment in Haiti has created a large and volatile group of unemployed young people—a "youth tsunami," in his words. "Haiti has exceptionally rapid popula-tion growth," he writes, "which adds to an already acute pressure on land. This youth tsunami is accelerating the process of environmental degradation and adding to the potentially explosive pool of underemployed youth." See Paul Col-lier. "Haiti: From Natural Catastrophe to Economic Recovery." *United Nations* (Jan-uary 2009). Available: http://www.scribd.com/doc/26835870/Paul-Collier-on-Haiti (accessed April 15, 2011). Secretary Clinton referred to this concept in her speech at the 2009 donors' conference: "Haiti has the highest unemployment rate in our hemisphere. Seventy percent of its people do not have jobs. It also has one of the region's highest growth rates. Together, these trends have created what Paul Collier has called a youth tsunami. Nearly one million young people are expected to come into the job market in the next five years." Available: http://www.haiti innovation.org/en/2009/04/14/secretary-clintons-remarks-haiti-donors-conference (accessed April 15, 2011).

19. Jonathan Katz. "Does Camp Corail Explain How Haiti Relief Can Be Done Right?" *Center for Economic and Policy Research* (April 26, 2010). Available: http://www.cepr.net/index.php/relief-and-reconstruction-watch/does-camp-corail-demonstrate-how-haiti-relief-can-be-done-right/ (accessed April 15, 2011).

20. Jonathan Katz. "Haiti Recovery Paralyzed 6 Months after Deadly Quake." Associated Press (July 11, 2010). Available: http://www.msnbc.msn.com/id/38184951/ns/world_news-americas/ (accessed April 15, 2011).

21. Jonathan Katz and Marko Alvarez. "Haiti: Summer Storm Floods 'Safe' Refugee Camp." Associated Press (July 13, 2010). Available: http://seattletimes .nwsource.com/html/nationworld/2012347420_apcbhaitihomelesscamp.html (ac-cessed April 15, 2011).

22. For more information on *Zanmi Beni*, see "Update: A New Home at Zanmi Beni." Available: http://www.pih.org/news/entry/update-a-new-home-at-zanmi-beni/ (accessed April 15, 2011).

23. Remarks by Paul Weisenfeld, USAID Haiti Task Team coordinator, at a me-dia roundtable on July 19, 2010. Available: http://www.usaid.gov/press/speeches/2010/sp100719_1.html (accessed April 15, 2011).

24. Ibid.

25. Franklin D. Roosevelt, First Inaugural Address. March 4, 1933.

26. See Martin Luther King, Jr. *All Labor Has Dignity* (Boston: Beacon Press, 1963).

27. Conrad Black. *Franklin Delano Roosevelt: Champion of Freedom* (New York: PublicAffairs, 2003), p. 194.

28. The crisis had finally imposed some discipline of responsibility even on the Republican legislators, who with uncharacteristic docility did what the governor asked. (The New York voters would overwhelmingly approve the bond issue in November 1932.) Faithful to his own romantic notions of rural life, Roosevelt had TERA subsidize the resettlement of as many unemployed as possible on marginal farmland, with tools and instruction on how to cultivate it. In six years TERA assisted five million people, 40 percent of the population of New York State, at a cost of $1,555,000. At the end of the period, 70 percent of these were no longer reliant on government assistance. See Black. *Franklin Delano Roosevelt,* pp. 216–217.

29. Robert Maguire has written eloquently of the need for similar programs in Haiti. See, for example, *Haiti Held Hostage: International Responses to the Quest for Nationhood, 1986–1996.* Occasional Paper #23. (Providence, RI: Thomas J. Watson Jr. Institute for International Studies, Brown University: 1996). See also his more recent *Haiti after the Donors' Conference: A Way Forward.* This article calls for a national civic service corps that would generate shovel-ready projects, akin to President Roosevelt's Works Progress Administration and its subsidiary Civilian Conservation Corps. Not only would such an initiative grease the wheels of economic growth, he contends, but it could also combat the cycles of deforestation and erosion that—along with dumping subsidized American produce in Haitian markets—fuel rural poverty and urban crowding.

30. Jonathan Katz. "Associated Press Impact: Haiti Still Waiting for Pledged U.S. Aid," Associated Press (September 28, 2010). Available: http://www.newsvine.com/_news/2010/09/28/5195300-ap-impact-haiti-still-waiting-for-pledged-us-aid (accessed April 15, 2011).

31. See Nicolai Ouroesoff, "A Plan to Spur Growth Away from Haiti's Capital." *New York Times* (March 30, 2010). Available: http://www.nytimes.com/2010/03/31/arts/design/31planning.html?pagewanted=2&ref=haiti (accessed April 15, 2011).

32. Those interested in this topic should read Sidney Mintz's *Sweetness and Power: The Place of Sugar in Modern History* (New York: Viking Penguin, 1985). The book provides an excellent account, although completed before the era of biofuels. Mintz's ethnographic work on Haiti, which spans three decades, is also always instructive to read, as are his books on the rest of the Caribbean.

33. For more on the Butaro hospital, see: http://act.pih.org/page/s/watch-butaro (accessed April 15, 2011).

34. Denis Lai Hang Hui. "Politics of Sichuan Earthquake," *Journal of Contingencies and Crisis Management* 17, No. 2 (June 2009).

35. Jonathan Watts. "Sichuan Earthquake: Tragedy Brings New Mood of Unity." *The Guardian* (June 20, 2008): http://www.guardian.co.uk/world/2008/jun/10/chinaearthquake.china (accessed April 15, 2011).

36. "Katrina, Five Years Later," *New York Times* (September 1, 2010): http://www.nytimes.com/2010/09/02/opinion/02thu1.html (accessed April 15, 2011).

37. The best example is Amy Wilentz' *The Rainy Season,* which spoofs her journalist colleagues' prejudices about Haiti. Most journalists with deep knowledge of the place have also mocked the Haiti set piece. A case in point set of platitudes comes from an American journalist in 1991: "It's hard to sell Haiti as a tourist paradise when popular perceptions of the place make a visit fall into the category of 'Holidays from Hell.' Dire poverty, AIDS, child slavery, zombies, voodoo animal sacrifices and political violence are just some of the negative images facing tour operators. A U.S. government travel warning 'strongly advises' Americans to avoid Haiti." (San Francisco *Sunday Punch,* March 31, 1991). Also see Robert Lawless. *Haiti's Bad Press* (Rochester, VT: Schenkman Books, 1992). The same sort of template-driven reporting has been critiqued after the quake. Dr. Evan Lyon sent us a wry (and perhaps rueful) article titled "How to Write About Haiti" by an irritated, Haiti-based journalist that captures some of the tropes found in popular press articles after the earthquake. The following passage is representative: "You are struck by the 'resilience' of the Haitian people. They will survive no matter how poor they are. They are stoic, they rarely complain, and so they are admirable. The best poor person is one who suffers quietly. A two-sentence quote about their misery fitting neatly into your story is all that's needed. On your last visit you became enchanted with Haiti. You are in love with its colorful culture and feel compelled to return. You care so much about these hard-working people. You are here to help them. You are their voice. They cannot speak for themselves." See Ansel Hertz. "How to Write about Haiti." *Huffington Post* (July 23, 2010). Available: http://www.huffingtonpost.com/crossover-dreams/a-guide-for-american-jour_b_656689.html (accessed April 15, 2011). As noted throughout this book, the Haitians, however resilient, did not in fact suffer in silence.

38. "Plans and Benchmarks for Haiti," *New York Times* (August 29, 2010). Available: http://www.nytimes.com/2010/08/30/opinion/30mon2.html (accessed April 15, 2011).

39. Estimates of the amount of debris have ranged between 10 and 20 million cubic meters. Katz. "AP Impact: Haiti Still Waiting for Pledged U.S. Aid."

40. The Associated Press reported that of 1,583 U.S. contracts for Haiti relief efforts made by December, only 20 went to Haitian companies (worth $4.3 million out of $267 million). Most went to beltway contractors, including one quarter disbursed through a no-bid process that didn't include Haitian participants. See Martha Mendoza. "Would-Be Haitian Contractors Miss Out on Aid." Associated Press (December 12, 2010). Available: http://news.yahoo.com/s/ap/20101212/ap_on_re_us/cb_haiti_outsourcing_aid_1.

41. When we gathered to lay the cornerstone of the new hospital, Ann read a letter I'd sent her in March of 1989: "When we last spoke, you were teetering between business and art. If business won out, would you please help me to build a hospital for the poor in Haiti? If you stayed with art, would you please send us a painting to cheer up our patients?" We are grateful she became an architect.

42. For information on the Mirebalais hospital, including recent updates about

construction and videos onsite, see http://www.pih.org/six-months/subject/mirebalais-teaching-hospital (accessed April 15, 2011).

### Chapter 7

1. P. Lawrence et al. "The Water Poverty Index."

2. Cholera thrives in the poor sanitation and water conditions of refugee camps. After the genocide in Rwanda, millions of refugees, including most surviving *génocidaires*, streamed across the Congolese border and took shelter in the region around Goma. Before long, they were housed and fed by the humanitarian machine that now follows conflict as surely as day follows night. Cholera exploded in those camps, drawing ever greater numbers of humanitarian groups to the region. For more on this episode, see Linda Polman. *The Crisis Caravan*, chapter 1.

3. *Acute Watery Diarrhea and Cholera: Haiti Pre-decision Brief for Public Health Action.* CDC (2010). Available: http://www.bt.cdc.gov/disasters/earthquakes/haiti/waterydiarrhea_pre-decision_brief.asp (accessed April 15, 2011).

4. Farmer et al. "Unjust Embargo of Aid for Haiti."

5. For an extended discussion of the effect of the aid embargo on Haiti, see the 2008 report by the Center for Human Rights and Global Justice and the Global Justice Clinic at New York University's School of Law, Partners In Health, Zanmi Lasante, and the Robert F. Kennedy Center for Justice and Human Rights. *Wòch nan Soley: The Denial of the Right to Water in Haiti*. Available: www.pih.org/page/-/reports/Haiti_Report_FINAL.pdf (accessed April 15, 2011).

6. Farmer. *AIDS and Accusation.*

7. Karen McCarthy Brown. "Systematic Remembering, Systematic Forgetting: Ogou in Haiti." In *Africa's Ogun: Old World and New*. Sandra Barnes, ed. (Bloomington: Indiana University Press, 1989), p. 67. This topic is more fully explored in Alfred Métraux's classic study, *Haitian Voodoo*. Métraux traces the lineage of modern Haitian sorcery accusations to the same source: "Man is never cruel and unjust with impunity: the anxiety which grows in the minds of those who abuse power often takes the form of imaginary terrors and demented obsessions. The master maltreated his slave, but feared his hatred. He treated him like a beast of burden but dreaded the occult powers which he imputed to him. And the greater the subjugation of the Black, the more he inspired fear; that ubiquitous fear which shows in the records of the period and which solidified in that obsession with poison, which throughout the eighteenth century, was the cause of so many atrocities. Perhaps certain slaves did revenge themselves on their tyrants in this way—such a thing is possible and even probable—but the fear which reigned in the plantations had its source in deeper recesses of the soul: it was the witchcraft of remote and mysterious Africa which troubled the sleep of people in 'the big house.'" Alfred Métraux. *Haitian Voodoo*. Hugo Charteris, trans. (New York: Schocken, 1972), p. 15.

8. E. Mintz and R. Guerrant. "A Lion in Our Village—the Unconscionable Tragedy of Cholera in Africa." *New England Journal of Medicine* 360 (2009): 1060–1063.

9. Randal Archibold. "Cholera Moves into Beleaguered Haitian Capital." *New York Times* (November 9, 2010). Available: http://www.nytimes.com/2010/11/10/world/americas/10haiti.html (accessed April 15, 2011).

10. Pan American Health Organization. "Health Cluster Bulletin: Cholera Outbreak in Haiti—#15." (January 21, 2011). Available: http://new.paho.org/blogs/haiti/?p=1739 (accessed April 15, 2011).

11. Jonathan Katz. "Cholera Confirmed for Resident of Haiti's Capital." Associated Press (November 9, 2010). Available: http://www.physorg.com/news/2010-11-cholera-resident-haiti-capital.html (accessed April 15, 2011).

12. Ibid.

13. My visit there eleven months earlier, with Luis-Alberto Moreno, the president of the Inter-American Development Bank, and our families, was designed to showcase our efforts with the Haitian public health sector in Lascahobas and, thus, to signal the potential for a similar partnership in Mirebalais, the closest town. None of us would ever have imagined that the two words, Nepal and Mirebalais, would come to have such significance less than a year later—although we should have. As noted twenty years ago, there is, in a global economy, no reason to believe that our pathogens will not be shared as freely as our products, our profits, and our losses. See P. Farmer. "The Exotic and the Mundane: Human Immunodeficiency Virus in Haiti." *Human Nature* 1, 4 (1990): 415–446.

14. Jonathan Katz. "UN Worries Its Troops Caused Cholera in Haiti." Associated Press (November 20, 2010). Available: http://www.msnbc.msn.com/id/40280944/ns/health/ (accessed April 15, 2011).

15. Ibid.

16. Some took this to mean that the peacekeepers could not be cholera's source. But this view does not take into account the frequency of asymptomatic cholera cases as well as false negatives. Katz goes on to explain: "The tests were taken from leaking water and an underground waste container at the base a week after the epidemic was first noted and processed at a lab in the neighboring Dominican Republic, UN spokesman Vincenzo Pugliese said. Mekalanos said that it is extremely difficult to accurately isolate cholera in environmental samples and that false negatives are common. The Nepalese troops were not tested for cholera before their deployment if they did not present symptoms. But health officials say 75 percent of people infected with cholera bacteria do not show symptoms and can still pass on the disease for weeks." Katz. "UN Worries Its Troops Caused Cholera in Haiti."

17. World Health Organization. "Cholera Vaccines: WHO Position Paper." *Wkly Epidemiol Rec* 85 (2010): 118.

18. Ivan Watson. "Medical Group Blasts 'Inadequate' Response to Haiti Cholera Outbreak." *CNN* (November 19, 2010). Available: http://articles.cnn.com/2010-11-19/world/haiti.cholera_1_haiti-cholera-outbreak-peacekeepers-nepal?_s=PM:WORLD (accessed April 15, 2011).

19. Ibid.

20. Katz. "UN Worries Its Troops Caused Cholera in Haiti."

21. Watson. "Medical Group Blasts 'Inadequate' Response to Haiti Cholera Outbreak."

22. C. S. Chin et al. "The Origin of the Haitian Cholera Outbreak Strain." *New England Journal of Medicine* 164 (2011): 1.

23. See, for example, Richard Knox. "Cholera Vaccine Isn't the Answer for Haiti." *NPR* (October 28, 2010). Available: http://www.npr.org/blogs/health/2010/10/28/130884642/why-the-cholera-vaccine-isn-t-the-answer-for-haiti (accessed April 15, 2011).

24. U.S. Centers for Disease Control and Prevention. *Update: cholera outbreak—Haiti 2010*. (December 8, 2010). Available at http://www.cdc.gov/mmwr/preview/mmwrhtml/mm5948a4.htm (accessed April 15, 2011).

25. See Partners In Health. "Curbing Cervical Cancer in Haiti." *Partners In Health Bulletin* (August 27, 2010). Available: http://www.pih.org/news/entry/curbing-cervical-cancer-in-haiti/ (accessed April 15, 2011).

26. A project at the National Penitentiary of Port-au-Prince found that providing antibiotics (along with potable water, soap, and sanitation services) to prisoners sharing living quarters with others with confirmed cholera helped to reduce incidence within the institution. See May J., Joseph P., Pape J., Binswanger I. "Healthcare for Prisoners in Haiti," *Ann Intern Med.* 153 (2010): 407–410.

27. Jeff Sachs. "The Fire This Time Was US-Fueled." *Taipei Times* (March 1, 2009). Available: http://www.taipeitimes.com/News/editorials/archives/2004/03/01/2003100742/3 (accessed April 15, 2011).

28. Ingrid Arnesen and Betsey Mckay. "Cholera Spreading in Haiti Faster than Thought." *Wall Street Journal* (November 25, 2010). Available: http://online.wsj.com/article/SB10001424052748703572404575635533532154818.html (accessed April 15, 2011).

29. Some studies also indicate that the proportion of severe cases may be underestimated in El Tor epidemics. See, for example, K. Bart et al. "Seroepidemiologic Studies During a Simultaneous Epidemic of Infection with El Tor Ogawa and Classical Inaba *Vibrio cholerae*." *Journal of Infectious Diseases* 121 (1970): 17–24. This paper compares the spectrum of illness for El Tor and classic biotype strains of *Vibrio cholerae*. The classic biotype produced a lower proportion of asymptomatic infections (59% vs. 75%) and a higher proportion of severe infections (11% vs. 2%) than the El Tor biotype. Some have hypothesized that the spectrum of variant El Tor biotype strains with classic toxin type would more closely resemble that of the classic biotype, though evidence is anecdotal to date.

30. See L. Ivers et al. "Five Complementary Interventions to Slow Cholera: Haiti." *Lancet* 376 (2010): 2048–2051; D. Walton and L. Ivers. "Responding to Cholera in Post-Earthquake Haiti." *New England Journal of Medicine* 364 (2011): 3–5, published online on December 9, 2010.

31. Don McNeil. "Use of Cholera Vaccine in Haiti Is Now Viewed as Viable." *New York Times* (December 10, 2010).

32. Ibid.

33. Paul Farmer and Jean-Renold Réjouit. "How We Can Stop Cholera in Haiti." *Newsweek* (November 20, 2010).

34. In Press: *PLoS Neglected Tropical Diseases:* e1145. (2011) doi: 10.1371/journal.pntd.0001145

35. OCHA Cholera Situation Report # 33 (January 21, 2011). Available: http://www.reliefweb.int/rw/rwb.nsf/db900SID/MCOI-8DDCXY?OpenDocument (accessed April 15, 2011).

36. R. Tuite et al. "Cholera Epidemic in Haiti, 2010: Using a Transmission Model to Explain Spatial Spread of Disease and Identify Optimal Control Interventions." *Annals of Internal Medicine* (March 7, 2011).

37. J. Andrews et al. "Transmission Dynamics and Control of Cholera in Haiti: An Epidemic Model." *Lancet* (March 16, 2011), DOI: 10.1016/S0140-6736(11)60273-0.

38. Unni Karunakara. "Haiti: Where Aid Failed." *Guardian* (December 28, 2010). Available: http://www.guardian.co.uk/commentisfree/2010/dec/28/haiti-cholera-earthquake-aid-agencies-failure (accessed April 15, 2011).

39. Jonathan Katz. "Six Killed in Sept. 24 Rainstorm in Port-au-Prince." Associated Press (September 24, 2010). Available: http://canadahaitiaction.ca/content/six-killed-sept-24-rainstorm-port-au-prince (accessed April 15, 2011).

40. For a summary of Kouchner's trip to Haiti, see "Visit of Bernard Kouchner to Haïti (September 25 and 26, 2010)." *Diplomatie* (September 26, 2010). Available: http://www.diplomatie.gouv.fr/en/country-files_156/haiti_473/france-and-haiti_2641/political-relations_6180/visit-of-bernard-kouchner-to-haiti-25-26.09.10_14309.html (accessed April 15, 2011).

41. Deborah Sontag. "In Haiti, Rising Call for Displaced to Go Away." *New York Times* (October 4, 2010). Available: http://www.nytimes.com/2010/10/05/world/americas/05haiti.html (accessed April 15, 2011).

42. There are other reminders, too. In an article titled "Haiti: Humanitarian Crisis or Crisis of Humanitarianism?" Jane Regan points out that a few days before Hurricane Tomas hit the island on November 5, Port-au-Prince's canals—critical drainage arteries—had not yet been cleared. *Huffington Post* (November 5, 2010). Available: http://www.huffingtonpost.com/jane-regan/haiti---humanitarian-cris_b_779503.html.

43. Jonathan Katz and Martha Mendoza. "Haiti Still Waiting for Pledged U.S. Aid." Associated Press (September 29, 2010). Available: http://www.huffington post.com/2010/09/29/haiti-still-waiting-for-p_n_743002.html (accessed April 15, 2011).

44. See Ma. Rizza Leonzon. "Bureaucracy Delays US Aid for Haiti Reconstruction." *Devex* (September 29, 2010). Available: http://www.devex.com/en/blogs/the-development-newswire/us-aid-pledge-for-haiti-stalled-by-bureaucray-ap-says (accessed April 15, 2011). See also Jonathan Katz and Martha Mendoza. "Another Obstacle Stalls $1.15 Billion in U.S. Aid to Haiti." Associated Press (November 6, 2010). Available: http://finance.yahoo.com/news/Another-obstacle-stalls-115B-apf-3649074743.html?x=0 (accessed April 15, 2011). A number of Republican senators, led by Tom Coburn of Oklahoma, raised concerns about corruption, stalling the money for months. The authors report, "President Barack Obama wasn't able to sign the appropriations bill containing the money until July 29. A subsequent bill to authorize release of the funds stalled, and it took until September 20 for the Obama administration to submit a spending plan in an attempt to free up the money."

45. Katz and Mendoza. "Haiti Still Waiting for Pledged U.S. Aid."

46. Martha Brannigan and Jacqueline Charles. "US Firms Want Part in Haiti Cleanup." Associated Press (February 9, 2010). Available: http://www.truthout.org/us-firms-want-part-haiti-cleanup56775 (accessed April 15, 2011). Competing for roles like these was, of course, unseemly for universities. Whether speaking of a Harvard doctor helping a colleague from Dartmouth perform, with Haitian colleagues, the first dialysis in a town in central Haiti or an American plastic surgeon addressing complex surgical problems in a quake-affected hospital, there was purity of purpose for the American research university. Whether it was a group of students and faculty coordinating volunteers and planes and helping to transfer patients, or students and other university-affiliated groups willing to raise money for relief and reconstruction, it was evident that universities had much to offer even before we got to the in-kind donations of research and teaching that we are uniquely qualified to offer. The alternative was to curry favor with power qua power, with the sort of results laid out so clearly in *The Best and the Brightest*. Halberstam mentioned the story of how, in 1967, a leader of the Urban League "defended the war and ended up in a bitter confrontation with Dr. King; [Whitney] Young told King his criticism of the war was unwise, it would antagonize the President and they wouldn't get anything from him. King, genuinely angry, told him, 'Whitney, what you're saying may get you a foundation grant, but it won't get you into the kingdom of truth.'" (David Halberstam. *The Best and the Brightest*, p. 185.) It wasn't as if we didn't need foundation grants to respond effectively to the sorts of problems we encountered in Haiti. But we didn't need to sell our souls to get them.

47. Trenton Daniel. "Bill Clinton Tells Diaspora: 'Haiti Needs You Now.'" *Miami Herald* (August 9, 2009). Available: http://www.miamiherald.com/news/americas/haiti/story/1179067.html.

48. Even the U.S. Government Accounting Office, an independent evaluative body, long ago reached dim conclusions about the effectiveness of our government's programs. It concluded: "The aid program to date has had limited impact on Haiti's dire poverty, and many projects have had less than satisfactory results." See U.S. General Accounting Office. *GAO Report-Assistance to Haiti: Barriers, Recent Program Changes and Future Options* (1982). Available: http://archive.gao.gov/d41t14/117663.pdf (accessed April 15, 2011).

49. The "late Victorian holocausts" resulted in fifty million deaths, leading Davis to the conclusion that "we are not dealing, in other words, with 'lands of famine' becalmed in stagnant backwaters of world history, but with the fate of tropical humanity at the precise moment (1870–1914) when its labor and products were being dynamically conscripted into a London-centered world economy. Millions died, not outside the 'modern world system,' but in the very process of being forcibly incorporated into its economic and political structures." Mike Davis. *Late Victorian Holocausts: El Nino Famines and the Making of the Third World* (London: Verso, 2001), p. 9. See also Amartya Sen's analysis of why no famine has occurred in a functioning democracy. "Any government that is accountable to its citizens," he writes, "can without great difficulty ration food provisions and prevent death

by starvation; famines occur, instead, in states without the will to provide services for their citizens." Amartya Sen. *Poverty and Famines: An Essay on Entitlement and Deprivation* (London: Oxford University Press, 1981).

50. Nor could other poor countries. The rich world pays out an estimated $300 billion in annual agribusiness subsidies, while preventing poor countries from doing the same under the banner of free trade. (See "The White Man's Shame." *The Economist*, September 25, 1999: p. 89.) Tariffs, which are on average four times higher in rich countries, are disbanded in poor countries, and subsidized crops are sold at artificially low prices, making agriculture unprofitable across much of the developing world. This also fuels erosion, deforestation, and urbanization, along with poverty and inequality. See Thomas Pogge. *World Poverty and Human Rights* (Cambridge, UK: Polity Press, 2008), pp. 15–22.

51. Polman. *The Crisis Caravan: What's Wrong with Humanitarian Aid?*, p. 39.

52. Mark Danner. "To heal Haiti look to history, not nature." *New York Times* (January 21, 2010). Available: http://www.nytimes.com/2010/01/22/opinion/22danner.html?_r=2&pagewanted=all (accessed April 15, 2011).

53. Philip Gourevitch. "Alms Dealers: Can You Provide Humanitarian Aid without Facilitating Conflicts?" *The New Yorker* (October 11, 2010). Available: http://www.newyorker.com/arts/critics/atlarge/2010/10/11/101011crat_atlarge_gourevitch (accessed April 15, 2011), p. 105.

54. Two other accounts Gourevitch mentions of the unintended consequences of humanitarian aid are Michael Maren's *The Road to Hell: The Ravaging Effects of Foreign Aid and International Charity* (New York: Simon & Schuster, 1997), and Alex de Waal's *Famine Crimes: Politics and the Disaster Relief Industry in Africa* (Bloomington, IN: Indiana University Press, 1997).

55. On restavèks, Mildred Aristide's 2003 book *Child Domestic Service in Haiti and Its Historical Underpinnings* underlines this link. Border conflicts occupy a large place in the Gourevitch-Polman litany, from Haiti-D.R. to Rwanda-Zaire to Cambodia-Thailand. "Consider how, in the early eighties, aid fortified fugitive Khmer Rouge killers in camps on the Thai-Cambodian border," Gourevitch writes, "enabling them to visit another ten years of war, terror, and misery upon Cambodians." Gourevitch. "Alms Dealers," p. 105.

56. Gourevitch. "Alms Dealers," p. 105.

57. See the long exposé in the *New York Times* by Walt Bogdanich and Jenny Nordberg (2006), "Mixed U.S. Signals Help Tilt Haiti Toward Chaos." One passage reads, "Haiti has had a long, tense relationship with the Dominican Republic, its more affluent neighbor on the island of Hispaniola. Haitians who work there are often mistreated, human rights groups say, and the country has been a haven for those accused of trying to overthrow Haitian governments. In December 2002, the I.R.I. began training Haitian political parties there, at the Hotel Santo Domingo, owned by the Fanjul family, which fled Cuba under Mr. Castro and now runs a giant sugar-cane business. The training was unusual for more than its location: only Mr. Aristide's opponents, not members of his party, were invited." Available: http://www.nytimes.com/2006/01/29/international/americas/29haiti.html?pagewanted=all (accessed April 15, 2011).

## Chapter 8

1. Modern Haitian history surely also bears the imprint of the conquests and genocides visited upon the island between the close of the fifteenth century, when the Columbian exchange began to extinguish Haiti's natives, and the late eighteenth century, when slavery made Haiti the largest source of prerevolutionary France's foreign exchange and its most unstable colony. When Jared Diamond writes that "guns, germs, and steel" play, along with geography, the chief roles in determining why some regions are rich and others poor, he could find few examples more illustrative than the island of Hispaniola, especially its crowded and mountainous western portion; see Jared Diamond. *Guns, Germs, and Steel: The Fates of Human Societies* (New York: Norton, 1997), p. 213. "There is no doubt," Diamond writes, "that Europeans developed a big advantage in weaponry, technology, and political organization over most of the non-European peoples that they conquered. But that advantage alone doesn't fully explain how initially so few European immigrants came to supplant so much of the native population of the Americas and some other parts of the world. That might not have happened without Europe's sinister gift to other continents—the germs evolving from Eurasians' long intimacy with domestic animals." Cholera may be the next chapter of this dark saga.

2. Reflecting on her experiences working for Médecins Sans Frontières in the Goma (Zaïre) refugee camps, Terry describes "the paradox of humanitarian action: it can contradict its fundamental purpose by prolonging the suffering it intends to alleviate." See Fiona Terry. *Condemned to Repeat?* (Ithaca: Cornell University Press, 2002), p. 89.

3. Gourevitch. "Alms Dealers," p. 105.

4. This book, written in the aftermath of an earthquake in Haiti does not seek to explore competing claims of causality regarding the violence in the Congo. For more on this topic, see the sometimes conflicting accounts by John Pottier (*Reimagining Rwanda: Conflict, Survival and Disinformation in the Late Twentieth Century* [New York: Cambridge University Press, 2002]); Gérard Prunier (*Africa's World War: Congo, the Rwandan Genocide, and the Making of a Continental Catastrophe* [Oxford: Oxford University Press, 2009]); and Jason Stearns (*Dancing in the Glory of Monsters: The Collapse of the Congo and the Great War of Africa* [New York: PublicAffairs, 2011]), as well as the broader review of postcolonial African history by Martin Meredith (*The Fate of Africa* [New York: PublicAffairs, 2005]).

5. In 1996, Rwanda had a gross national income per capita of 730 (PPP international dollars). See the World Bank's *World Development Report 1996: From Plan to Market* (New York: Oxford University Press, 1996).

6. Jared Diamond. *Collapse: How Societies Choose to Fail or Succeed* (New York: Viking, 2005). In *Collapse*, Diamond interprets the Rwandan genocide as, in part, a Malthusian crisis in which population growth outpaces food production. In the 1990s (and today), it was the most densely populated country in Africa and one of the most densely populated in the world. As trees were chopped down and land overused, disputes—often violent—over land became frequent in the years before

the genocide. "Even before 1994," Diamond writes, "Rwanda was experiencing rising levels of violence and theft, perpetrated especially by hungry landless young people without off-farm income. When one compares crime rates for people of age 21–25 among different parts of Rwanda, most of the regional differences prove to be correlated statistically with population density and per-capita availability of calories: high population densities and worse starvation were associated with more crime." (*Collapse*, p. 324–325.) Competition over land and food were important factors, among others, in the lead up to the Rwandan civil war and genocide.

Diamond brings a similar lens to a question this book considers as well: why have the fates of Haiti and the Dominican Republic—sharing a single island and once home to a single people—diverged dramatically in the last two centuries? (Diamond also notes the visible differences in forest cover across the border: the Dominican side is 28% forested; the Haitian side, 1%. See *Collapse*, p. 329.) His answer is complex and multifaceted, but he again calls the reader's attention to the twin problems of population density and environmental strain: "France imported far more slaves into its colony than did Spain. As a result, Haiti had a population seven times higher than its neighbor during the colonial times, and it still has a somewhat larger population today, about 10,000,000 versus 8,800,000. But Haiti's area is only slightly more than half of that of the Dominican Republic, so that Haiti with a large population and smaller area has double the Republic's population density. The combination of that higher population density and lower rainfall was the main factor behind the more rapid deforestation and loss of soil fertility on the Haitian side." (*Collapse*, p. 340.)

7. See "Rwanda Vision 2020." (Updated July 2000.) Available: http://www.gesci .org/assets/files/Rwanda_Vision_2020.pdf (accessed April 15, 2011).

8. For more on the interim government's anti-corruption campaign see Frederick Golooba-Mutebi, "Collapse, War, and Reconstruction in Rwanda: An Analytical Narrative on State-making." *Crisis States Working Paper No. 28* (2008), p. 31. Available: http://www.dfid.gov.uk/r4d/PDF/Outputs/CrisisStates/wp28.2.pdf (accessed April 15, 2011).

9. For more on the immediate responses of the international community to the genocide and the interim governments, see Gérard Prunier, *The Rwanda Crisis: History of a Genocide* (New York: Columbia University Press, 1994), pp. 336–345.

10. As noted, see the Internal Displacement Monitoring Centre's 2011 report "Internal Displacement: Global Overview of Trends and Developments in 2010."

11. See, for example, D. Hilhorst and M. van Leeuwen, "Emergency and Development: The Case of *Imidugudu*, Villagization in Rwanda," *Journal of Refugee Studies* 13 (2000): 264–280; E. Brusset, "Imidugudu and Humanitarian Aid: The Influence of NGOs on Post-war Conditions in Rwanda." *Autrepart* 26 (2003): 107–121.

12. Stephen Kinzer. *A Thousand Hills: Rwanda's Rebirth and the Man Who Dreamed It* (New Jersey: John Wiley and Sons Inc., 2008), p. 199.

13. This topic is explored in greater detail by Jason K. Stearns in *Dancing in the Glory of Monsters: The Collapse of the Congo and the Great War of Africa* (New York: PublicAffairs, 2011), which details Mobutu's assistance to Juvénal Habyari-

mana's government, including its armed forces, before and after the genocide: "The army's flight across the border did not end the civil war in Rwanda but constituted a hiatus in the hostilities. The Rwandan Armed Forces (FAR), as the Hutu-dominated army was called, used the protection provided by the border to regroup, rearm, and prepare to retake power in Kigali. One of their leaders, Colonel Théoneste Bagosura, said in an interview that they would 'wage a war that will be long and full of dead people until the minority Tutsi are finished and completely out of the country.' Crucially, they enjoyed the support of Zaïre's ailing president, Mobutu Sese Seko, who had sent troops to support the FAR against the RPF [Rwandan Patriotic Front], and who had been close friends with President Juvénal Habyarimana. In part, what was to play out over the next decade in the Congo was a continuation of the Rwandan civil war, as the new government attempted to extirpate the *génocidaires* and the remnants of Habyarimana's army on a much broader canvas" (Stearns, 2011, p. 15).

14. Kinzer. *A Thousand Hills*, pp. 203–204.

15. Dorothea Hilhorst and Mathijs van Leeuwen. "Villagisation in Rwanda: A Case of Emergency Development?" *Wageningen Disaster Studies* Disaster Sites No. 2 (1999).

16. Saskia van Hoyweghan. "The Urgency of Land and Agrarian Reform in Rwanda." *African Affairs* 98 (1999): 353–372.

17. Minh Day. "Alternative Dispute Resolution and Customary Law: Resolving Property Disputes in Post-conflict Nations, a Case Study of Rwanda." *Georgetown Immigration Law Journal* 16 (2001): 235–256.

18. See, for example, Chris Higgins and Herman Musahara. "Land reform, land scarcity and post-conflict reconstruction: A case study of Rwanda." In: Chris Huggins and Jenny Clover, eds. *From the Ground Up: Land Rights, Conflict and Peace in Sub-Saharan Africa.* (Nairobi and Pretoria: African Centre for Technology Studies and Institute for Security Studies, 2005), pp. 269–346. Available at: http://www.iss.co.za/pubs/Books/GroundUp/6Land.pdf. (See pp. 287, 313–314 for the actual citations.)

19. The extent to which the government directed such efforts is debated. For example, Pottier's *Re-imagining Rwanda*, pp. 186–190, describes land allocation as an organic process that was determined principally by local actors.

20. Here the Rwandan and Haitian national experiences diverge. Although Haitian prisons are overcrowded, leading to outbreaks of disease (including cholera, which immediately hit the prisons in Saint-Marc and Mirebalais), and most detainees had not enjoyed anything approaching due process, the Haitian prison population is small compared to that in Rwanda. For a comparison of various truth and reconciliation commissions, see Patricia Hayner's *Unspeakable Truths: Facing the Challenge of Truth Commissions* (New York: Routledge, 2002).

21. Quoted in Kinzer. *A Thousand Hills*, p. 257.

22. The *gacaca* process, based in part on traditional law and in part on the exigencies of the moment, has been the subject of a great deal of commentary, much of it negative. Some have pointed out, for example, that RPF crimes went largely unjudged (Kinzer, p. 259). Peter Uvin sums up the freighted debate: the *gacaca*

system "profoundly compromises on principles of justice as defined in internationally agreed-upon human rights or criminal law standards," but respects the "spirit of international criminal and human rights law, if not the letter." He ultimately concludes that it is the "locally appropriate form." Quoted in Kinzer, p. 258. Also see E. Daly. "Between Punitive and Reconstructive Justice: The Gacaca Courts in Rwanda." *New York University Journal of International Law & Politics* 34 (2002): 355; J. Sarkin. "The Tension between Justice and Reconciliation in Rwanda: Politics, Human Rights, Due Process and the Role of the Gacaca Courts in Dealing with the Genocide." *Journal of African Law* 45 (2001): 143–172.

23. Jean Hatzfeld. *The Antelope's Strategy: Living in Rwanda After the Genocide* (New York: Farrar, Straus and Giroux, 2007), p. 204.

24. Gender equity is another topic that is much discussed and little implemented. More money is spent on empty "empowerment workshops" than in making sure that women have fair pay, equal representation in government, and ready access to health care and education. Here again, Rwanda is ahead of the pack: by mandating equal representation in government, it soon boasted significant gender equity at the top levels of government (in the legislative branch and in cabinet-level positions). Today, more than half of its parliamentarians are women, as are many of the mayors of its larger cities. For more on this, see C. Devlin and R. Elgie "The effect of increased women's representation in parliament: The case of Rwanda." *Parliamentary Affairs* 61, no. 2 (2008): 237–254.

25. Peter Uvin. *Aiding Violence* (West Hartford: Kumarian Press, 1998).

26. The Rwandan campaign provoked a firestorm of criticism, of course, and was even labeled "double genocide" by some. A UN draft report released in September 2010 fanned these flames by underscoring crimes alleged to have been committed by Kagame's armies (mostly Tutsi) in the Congo campaign. The report was leaked by *Le Monde*. See http://www.lemonde.fr/afrique/article/2010/08/26/l-acte-d-accusation-de-dix-ans-de-crimes-au-congo-rdc_1402933_3212.html (accessed April 15, 2011). See also the Rwandan government's response: *Official Government of Rwanda Comments on the Draft UN Mapping Report on the DRC*. Geneva          (October          1,          2010).          Available: http://www.gov.rw/sub.php?page=print&id_article=112 (accessed April 15, 2011). See also Aldo Ajello's interview with Colette Braekman on the topic. Available: http://www.newtimes.co.rw/index.php?issue=14415&article=34668 (accessed April 15, 2011).

27. Uvin. *Aiding Violence*, p. 127. Uvin writes, "The social and political are outside the game of development. Development is done through projects, that is, well-defined technical/financial packages with limited time frames as well as functional and regional scopes. Scant attention is paid to the national or international context or to the political background against which these projects occur" (pp. 154–155). Uvin's argument builds on James Ferguson's long-standing critique of the depoliticizing nature of the development enterprise. See J. Ferguson. *The Anti-Politics Machine: "Development," Depoliticization, and Bureaucratic Power in Lesotho* (Cambridge: Cambridge University Press, 1990), for example, pp. 16–21.

28. "Our peculiar institution" was a common euphemism for slavery used in the American South before the Civil War. It was popularized by John C. Calhoun of South Carolina in his *Speech on the Reception of Abolition Petitions* (February 6, 1837). Available: http://www.wfu.edu/~zulick/340/calhoun2.html (accessed April 15, 2011).

29. Trouillot describes the process by which the poor rural population became subject to a tiny urban élite: "The chronic instability of Haitian political life," he writes, "as manifested in the rhythm of political succession, numerous constitutional crises, and recurring armed feuds is so obvious that Haitian and foreign observers alike have tended to inflate the role of politics in shaping the course of the country's history. They often see the stages of historical evolution in terms of changes to the regime, to a degree that masks underlying continuities. The point is that the state's importance came not from the power vested in individual regimes but from its role in the extraction and distribution of peasant surplus... At the bottom of the social scale, but vitally important for the entire nation, was a peasantry divided into several strata: landless people, sharecroppers, small proprietors, and rich peasants. Together, these men and women did the work and furnished almost all the country's wealth. But their techniques of production stagnated.... Statistically, peasant productivity today is only equal to that of 1843, if not lower. The touchstone of Haiti's socioeconomic system has thus been a peasantry that worked more and more but produced less and less, as population increased and the availability of fertile land decreased...most of the fruits of the peasantry's toil were seized by the alliance of rulers and merchants and transferred abroad... [T]he socioeconomic structures, and the historical and cultural context in which their effects were felt, implied a separation between the peasantry and the urban world. This separation produced two contradictory tendencies: the political marginalization of the peasantry and the concentration of urban demands in the narrow sphere of governmental decisions." Michel-Rolph Trouillot. *Haiti, State Against Nation: The Origins and Legacy of Duvalierism* (New York: Monthly Review Press, 1990), pp. 83–85.

30. Haitian farmers may also benefit from a rise in global food prices. A report published by the UN's International Fund for Agricultural Development on December 6, 2010, suggests that poor farmers around the world may receive an income boost from the surge in food prices, giving them greater income to reinvest in irrigation, better fertilizers, new farming equipment, and other means to increase yield in future seasons. See Rural Poverty Report 2011. Available: http://www.ifad.org/rpr2011/report/ (accessed April 15, 2011).

31. A December 2010 news story estimates that Haitian rice production may be compromised due to consumer fears about crops grown in cholera-affected areas. See "Cholera Outbreak Could Hurt Haiti's Rice Production." *CNN* (December 30, 2010). Available: edition.cnn.com/2010/WORLD/Americas/12/29/Haiti.cholera/ (accessed April 15, 2011).

32. The connections between economic growth and social safety nets, including those that would protect the most vulnerable from want, are not linear. Amartya Sen has often underlined the links between freedom, on the one hand, and socio-

economic conditions (what has been termed here "human security"), on the other. See, for example, *Development as Freedom* (New York: Anchor Books, 1999). "Growth of GNP or of industrial incomes," Sen writes, "can, of course, be very important as means to expanding the freedoms enjoyed by the members of the society. But freedoms depend also on other determinants, such as social and economic arrangements (for example, facilities for education and health care) as well as political and civil rights (for example, the liberty to participate in public discussion and scrutiny)." (Sen. *Development as Freedom*, p. 3)

### Epilogue

1. Aristide remained in South Africa when the narrative of this book concluded. But on March 18, 2011, Aristide returned home. For an account of his reception and the implications of his return, see Jeb Sprague. "Haiti's Movement from Below Endures." Al Jazeera (March 27, 2011). Available: http://english. aljazeera.net/indepth/features/2011/03/2011322143841972574.html (accessed April 15, 2011).

2. Stephen Smith. "Year after Haiti Quake, Agency Asks How Far It Can Go." *Boston Globe:* January 11, 2011. Available: http://www.boston.com/lifestyle/health/articles/2011/01/11/soaring_need_fuels_agencys_growth_in_haiti/ (accessed April 15, 2011).

3. See "Haiti One Year Later: The Progress to Date and the Path Forward." *Interim Haiti Recovery Commission Report* (January 12, 2011). Available: http://www.cirh.ht/sites/ihrc/en/News%20and%20Events/News/Pages/12janv11.aspx.

4. See, for example, the article about my former student, Dr. Megan Coffee, who has worked with few resources and a handful of public employees to improve care for patients with HIV and tuberculosis at the General Hospital. Bob Braun. "Maplewood Doctor Volunteers at Haiti's Largest Hospital after Devastating Earthquake." *Star-Ledger* (July 20, 2010). Available: http://blog.nj.com/njv_bob_braun/2010/07/doctor_from_maplewood_voluntee.html (accessed April 15, 2011). Nick Lobel-Weiss from Global Emergency Relief also did yeoman's work at the General Hospital. One of the more significant developments was, as noted, the American Red Cross grant to provide "performance-based" salary support for the hospital's underpaid (and overworked) staff. It is our hope that the Red Cross's commitment to accompanying the General Hospital may become a model for how nongovernmental organizations and private groups can partner with the public sector to strengthen the Haitian health system.

5. One of the reasons that Claire's job is hard is that too little of the reconstruction funds end up in Haitian hands. The December Associated Press investigation cited in Chapter 5, note 40, page 382, found that only 20 of 1,583 U.S. contracts for recovery aid went to Haitian-run enterprises. That's $1.60 out of every $100. See Martha Mendoza "Would-be Haitian Contractors Miss Out on Aid." Associated Press (December 12, 2010). Available: http://news.yahoo.com/s/ap/20101212/ap_on_re_us/cb_haiti_outsourcing_aid_1 (accessed April 15, 2011).

### Afterword

1. United Nations Office of the Special Envoy for Haiti, "Assistance Tracker." Available: http://www.haitispecialenvoy.org/assistance-tracker/ (accessed March 8, 2012).

2. See, for example, Andrew Rosenthal, "Bob the builder goes to Haiti," *New York Times* (December 1, 2011). Available: http://loyalopposition.blogs.nytimes.com/2011/12/01/bob-the-builder-goes-to-haiti/ (accessed April 6, 2012).

3. L. Ivers et al., "Five Complementary Interventions to Slow Cholera: Haiti." *Lancet* 376 (2010): 2048–2051; PAHO, "Call to Action: A Cholera-Free Hispaniola," December 29, 2011. Available: http://new.paho.org/colera/.

4. Deborah Sontag, "In Haiti, Global Failures on a Cholera Epidemic," *New York Times* (March 31, 2012). Available: http://www.nytimes.com/2012/04/01/world/americas/haitis-cholera-outraced-the-experts-and-tainted-the-un.html?_r=1&ref=deborahsontag

5. Robert Richardson, *William James: In the Maelstrom of American Modernism* (New York: Houghton Mifflin, 2006), pp. 6–7.

6. Evan Osnos, "Japan's 3/11," *The New Yorker* (March 11, 2012). Available: http://www.newyorker.com/online/blogs/evanosnos/2012/03/japans-311.html (accessed March 18, 2012).

# ACRONYMS AND INITIALISMS

CHAI: Clinton Health Access Initiative

CHOP: Children's Hospital of Philadelphia

DART: Disaster Assistance Response Team

GHESKIO: Le Groupe Haïtien d'Etude du Sarcome de Kaposi et des Infections Opportunistes (The Haitian Group for the Study of Kaposi's Sarcoma and Opportunistic Infections)

GSD: get stuff done

HELP: Haitian Education Leadership Project

HUEH: l'Hôpital Université d'Etat d'Haïti (Haitian State University Hospital)

HUP: Hospital of the University of Pennsylvania

IDP: internally displaced person

IHRC: Interim Haiti Recovery Commission

IMC: International Medical Corps

MASH: Mobile Army Surgical Hospital

MINUSTAH: UN Stabilization Mission in Haiti

MSF: Medécins Sans Frontières

NGO: nongovernmental organization

OCHA: Office for the Coordination of Humanitarian Affairs

OSE: Office of the Special Envoy

PDNA: Post-Disaster Needs Assessment

PIH/ZL: Partners In Health/Zanmi Lasante

PIH: Partners In Health

RTHC: Right to Health Care

UNICEF: United Nations Children's Fund
USAID: United States Agency for International Development
WFP: World Food Program
WHO: World Health Organization

# CONTRIBUTORS

**Jennie W. Block, O.P.,** currently serves as Paul Farmer's Chief of Staff and was his Chief Advisor at the UN Office of the Special Envoy (OSE) for Haiti overseeing the start-up and management of the OSE. She is a theologian and a disability rights activist and was a management consultant to non-profit organizations for more than twenty years. She spent six months in New Orleans leading a disaster relief team after Hurricane Katrina. She is the author of *Copious Hosting: A Theology of Access for People with Disabilities* and *Are You Ready? A Guide to Preparing for Disasters.*

**Edwidge Danticat** was born in Haiti in 1969 and came to the United States when she was twelve years old. She graduated from Barnard College and received an M.F.A. from Brown University. She is the author of many books, including the novels *Breath, Eyes, Memory, The Farming of Bones* and *The Dew Breaker*, the short story collection *Krik? Krak!,* whose National Book Award nomination made Danticat the youngest nominee ever, and the memoir *Brother, I'm Dying,* which won the National Book Critics Circle Award and the Dayton Literary Peace Prize. She recently published a collection of essays, *Create Dangerously: The Immigrant Artist at Work,* and *Eight Days,* a children's book about a young earthquake survivor illustrated by Alix Delinois. A recipient of a MacArthur Genius grant, Danticat lives in Miami with her husband and daughters.

**Nancy Dorsinville** is currently the Advisor for NGOs and Civil Society at the UN Office of the Special Envoy for Haiti, where she focuses on policy issues for vulnerable populations, namely internally displaced populations and in particular gender mainstreaming, orphans and vulnerable children and the handicapped. She is the liaison for the OSE and the government of Haiti ministries responsible for these transversal issues. Originally from

Haiti, she is an anthropologist and prior to joining the OSE was a research associate at the Harvard School of Public Health. She served as director of HIV prevention education for the city of New York and has a long standing affiliation with the Clinton Health Access Initiative, under whose umbrella she conducted a country-wide diagnostic of the health system in Haiti in conjunction with the Haitian Ministry of Health and Partners in Health. She has done extensive field work with Paul Farmer and continues to be part of his Global Health teaching team at Harvard University.

**Didi Bertrand Farmer** has worked for the last ten years as a community organizer, an activist for the rights of women and girls, and a researcher in Paris, Haiti, and Rwanda. She currently serves as the Director of the Community Health Program for Partners In Health in Rwanda and leads the Haiti-Rwanda Commission, created after the 2010 earthquake to promote cultural exchanges between the two countries.

**Louise Ivers,** M.D., is Chief of Mission for Partners In Health in Haiti. She is an Assistant Professor of Medicine at Harvard Medical School and an Associate Physician in the Division of Global Health Equity at Brigham and Women's Hospital. Dr. Ivers implements health programs and is interested in improving the delivery of health care in resource poor settings, the provision of care to the rural and urban poor, as well as patient-oriented investigation that offers solutions to barriers to healthcare. She balances her time between management of PIH Haiti, direct clinical service, and operational research.

**Dubique Kobel,** M.D., is a clinician working with Zanmi Lasante in Port-au-Prince. He attended medical school in Cuba. He and his wife, Dr. Nadège Kobel, have been providing health care to the residents of Parc Jean-Marie Vincent since the earthquake.

**Evan Lyon,** M.D., has worked in Haiti since 1996, when he first lived in Port-au-Prince as a volunteer teacher. He has worked against health inequities as a clinician, teacher, activist, and scholar for more than a decade. Dr. Lyon completed his medical degree at Harvard Medical School in 2003 and internal medicine residency at Brigham and Women's Hospital in 2007. He has been involved in many aspects of Partners in Health/Zanmi Lasante's expansion in rural Haiti, including TB and HIV care, community health work, prisoner care, health education, and human rights documentation and advocacy. After the earthquake in January 2010, Dr. Lyon helped coordinate Partners In Health's immediate relief efforts in support of the public General Hospital in downtown Port-au-Prince.

**Michèle Montas-Dominique** is an award-winning journalist and the former news director of Radio Haiti Inter, a private radio station in Port-au-Prince where she began reporting in the early 1970s. She took the direction of the radio station in 2000 when her husband, well-known Haitian broadcast journalist Jean Dominique, was gunned down in front of it. In December 2002, Michele Montas's bodyguard was killed with a bullet intended for her, and Radio Haiti Inter was closed two months later. During her third exile in New York, Montas worked as Spokesperson of the United Nations Secretary General, before returning to Haiti last January, one week before the earthquake. She is a Senior Adviser to the UN Secretary General's Special Representative in Haiti.

**Joia S. Mukherjee,** M.D., trained in Infectious Disease, Internal Medicine, and Pediatrics at the Massachusetts General Hospital and has an MPH from the Harvard School of Public Health. Since 2000, Dr. Mukherjee has served as the Medical Director of Partners In Health, an international medical charity with programs in the United States, Haiti, the Dominican Republic, Rwanda, Lesotho, Malawi, Burundi, Peru, Mexico, Guatemala, Russia, and Kazakhstan. As Medical Director, Joia coordinates and supports Partners In Health's clinical team in their efforts to provide high-quality care to the poorest and most vulnerable. She is also an Associate Professor in the Department of Global Health and Social Medicine at Harvard Medical School and in the Division of Global Health Equity at the Brigham and Women's Hospital. She teaches infectious disease, global health, and human rights to health professionals and students from around the world. Dr. Mukherjee's research and scholarship are focused on generating a body of evidence to inform the development of health care delivery systems to address the enormous burden of disease in resource-poor settings. Dr. Mukherjee consults for the World Health Organization on health systems strengthening, human resources for health, and the treatment for HIV and drug resistant tuberculosis in developing countries.

**Naomi Rosenberg** has been working for Partners In Health (PIH) since 2005 and is a second-year medical student at University of Pennsylvania School of Medicine. At PIH, she directed the Right to Health Care Program—a program that brings patients from Haiti and Rwanda to the United States and elsewhere for treatment not available in their home country. In January 2010, Naomi took a leave of absence from medical school to assist with work in Haiti and has been responsible for the transfer and care of fourteen critically ill people, who are currently living in the Philadelphia area. She also works to connect patients in Port-au-Prince to specialty care whether in Haiti or abroad.

**Timothy T. Schwartz,** Ph.D., has lived and worked on Hispaniola, the Caribbean island that Haiti shares with the Spanish speaking Dominican Republic, since 1990. Schwartz spent two years living in a Haitian fishing village, part of a dissertation project funded by the National Science Foundation, and three years living and working among peasant farmers. He has directed five major studies in rural Haiti for the German government, US-AID, and multinational NGOs. Dr. Schwartz is the author of a book about the failing of charity and aid in Haiti called *Travesty in Haiti* and an academic treatise called *Fewer Men, More Babies: Sex, Family and Fertility in Haiti.*

**Jéhane Sedky** joined the Office of the Special Envoy for Haiti in June 2009 as the Senior Advisor on Strategic Communications. Prior to her appointment, she served for two years as Senior Advisor to United Nations Assistant Secretary-General Kathleen Cravero. Previously, Ms. Sedky was Chief of Media Relations at UNICEF. When President Clinton's UN Tsunami Office was created (in 2005), Ms. Sedky was appointed Strategic Communications Advisor. Ms. Sedky began her UN career as a Press Officer at UNICEF, where for five years she worked closely with Executive Director Carol Bellamy on media issues related to the protection of children and women. She has an undergraduate degree in International Relations from Tufts University and a graduate degree in International Human Rights Law and Political Science from the Graduate Institute of International Studies in Geneva. She has authored a book on children in armed conflict.

# ACKNOWLEDGMENTS

I make two types of acknowledgments in closing this book. The first, to thank those who helped us to write or illustrate or edit the book, can be done in fairly short order. The second would necessarily include listing the thousands of friends, family, volunteers, and donors who gave us something more to describe than collapsed buildings and broken bodies. The long list (a modest way to thank those who helped us save lives) is still very incomplete, but can be found at http://www.pih.org/eqgratitude.

These short thanks do not include those credited as writers or authors or editors, even though each contributed greatly to the book, while working behind the scenes: Peter Osnos, who encouraged me to write for him long before the earthquake; Lindsay Jones, our first editor at PublicAffairs; Lisa Kaufman and Christine Marra, senior editor and editorial production manager, respectively; and Susan Weinberg who, along with Peter, is seeking to make sure this book is widely read. Whether we're writers, editors, or photographers (or the lone artist in the group), we share this gratitude to the A Team at PublicAffairs.

In Haiti, the quake has left me more thankful than ever for the valiant health care professionals (doctors, nurses, social workers, and community health workers) of Partners In Health and Zanmi Lasante, and also for all those who work in communications, procurement, logistics, and finance. A few of them appear as characters in these pages, but hundreds more have worked long hours providing care in the quake's aftermath, including a stubborn cholera epidemic and a dearth of services in the regions most affected by the quake. I hope I may be forgiven for singling out Ophelia Dahl, Ted Constan, Loune Viaud, Pa Frico, his daughter Marie-Flore Chipps (who, like most of our Haitian coworkers, faced heavy losses), Evan Lyon, Keith Joseph, Bepi Ravida, Serena Koenig, Koji Nakashima, Kate Greene, Kim Cullen, Ali Lutz, Kathryn Kempton, Jon Lascher, Andrew Marx, Maxi

Raymonville, Wesler Lambert, Fernet Léandre, Anany Gretchko Prosper, Patrick Ulysse, Leslie Tuttle, Sarah Marsh, Cate Oswald, Father Eddy Eustache, and Paul Zintl.

In the Haitian Ministry of Health, in addition to those thanked in the text, I am grateful to Alex Larsen, Gabriel Thimothe, Ariel Henry, Claude Surena, and many others struggling in Haiti's underfunded public health system, which includes the General Hospital and partners from Belladères to Saint-Marc.

Harvard Medical School and its affiliated hospitals have allowed me, Louise Ivers, Joia Mukherjee, Claire Pierre, David Walton, and many others to serve as volunteers in Haiti before and after the quake, and my gratitude to these institutions—for helping universities and academic medical centers to build a "there there" in global health—knows no bounds. President Drew Faust and Dean Jeffrey Flier share our vision of global health, as do Ophelia Dahl and Jim Yong Kim and partners, including Wes Edens, Mala Gaonkar, Bill and Daisy Helman, Dan and Annette Nova, and Stephen and Liz Kahn. At the Department of Global Health and Social Medicine, my thanks go to Emily Bahnsen, Zoe Agoos, Matt Basilico, Luke Messac, and Jen Puccetti, and also to academic colleagues, including Anne Becker and David Jones and Arthur Kleinman, who covered for me and others in teaching, clinical, and administrative duties in the weeks after the quake. Thanks, too, to Deans Rick Mills and David Golan, and to several of my medical students, who are listed below. At Brigham and Women's Hospital, thanks go to Howard Hiatt, Joe Rhatigan, Jenni Watson, Susan Radlinski, to the Global Health Equity residents, and to all the doctors and nurses, named and unnamed, who traveled to Haiti after the quake; we are all indebted to the hospital's leadership, especially Joe Loscalzo and Betsy Nabel, for making such pragmatic solidarity possible. At Partners Healthcare, my deepest debt is to Gary Gottlieb, also of Partners In Health, but many others came up with cash, supplies, transportation, and, especially, skilled medical personnel. I am thankful to many at Children's Hospital, but especially to John Meara and so many other surgeons (and anesthesiologists and surgical nurses) from all Harvard teaching hospitals. You did us proud.

Most of the UN leadership with whom President Clinton and I worked the most closely perished in the quake, but members of our OSE team were spared and continued working: Nancy Dorsinville, John Harding, Ricardo Sanchez-Sosa. Other UN officials rotated in and out of Haiti, but brevity of service was not always a marker of impact. I'm grateful to Dr. Garry Conille for his hard work and leadership, and to Katherine Gilbert for her innovations in tracking aid and also aid effectiveness. Our collective thanks go to Gabrielle Apollon, Lee Bailey, Carolina de Borbon Parma, Jennie Weiss Block, Anne Frotscher, Abbey Gardner, Kirsten Gelsdorf, Treena Huang, Hardin Lang, Francesca Lubrano di Giunno, Habila Maiga, Joel Malebranche, Violeta Maximova, Gregory Milne, Paula Montes, Lenore Price, Maria Concepcion del Rosario, Jéhane Sedky, and Anke Strauss. In addition, I'd like to offer a special thanks to Aaron Charlop-Powers, whose mother, a friend to our work, died in an accident shortly after the quake; Aaron continued his efforts in and behalf of Haiti.

Some of our friends and colleagues at the Clinton Foundation and in President Clinton's office are named in the previous pages, but I'd like to thank in particular the tireless Laura Graham and also Hannah Richert, Doug Band, Ami Desai, and Jon Davidson. Many have spent long hours responding to the cholera outbreak, but I can't help but thank Mark Rosenberg in particular for his vision in drafting the consensus statement.

In Rwanda, where we have worked (and been sheltered) for some years, we are grateful to leaders at the national, provincial, and district levels for their support of our efforts and for their warm welcome of Haitian officials and students interested in learning how Rwandans have "built back better" since the genocide. I would be remiss not to single out two individuals: Dr. Agnès Binagwaho, who has advised and shepherded our work in Rwanda from the beginning, and Anne Sosin, who has helped Didi bring the Haiti-Rwanda Commission into being. On a personal note, it was easier for Didi and me to work in the quake zone knowing that our children were in a safe place, which is precisely how our family thought—and still thinks—of Rwanda. I am deeply grateful for our oldest daughter Catherine's discerning contribution to this book. Her efforts have been felt in our work in Haiti and Rwanda too. I can only hope this testament will help our other children (Elizabeth, Charles-Sebastien, Rick Ryan, and Richard) understand our long absences.

Finally, writing requires protected time and protected spaces, and these were very hard for me to find. My deepest gratitude goes to Jennie Block, who insisted on both; Jon Weigel, who did more than anyone else to help me finish my part of this volume; Maryse Penette-Kedar, who offered me safe haven within the quake zone, Todd and Anne McCormack, who as ever provided safe haven in Boston; and my brother Jeff, who not only helped me carve out a few days to write but also read parts of the book and discussed most of it. Writing also requires editors of the more informal sort: friends who read drafts or just listened to arguments. This past year, Claire Pierre and Louise Ivers, much mentioned in this book, and also Jean-Renold Réjouit, Abbey Gardner, and Cassia Holstein, helped me to understand things about the quake and about development assistance that I might not otherwise have grasped. As ever, and for almost thirty-five years, Haun Saussy has helped me to understand and better describe complex events.

2010–2011 has been a grim season of loss. In addition to those lost on January 12, we all miss Tom White, Yolande "Mamito" Lafontant, Patricia Neal, Alix Chipps, Joan Kleinman, and many others. The dedication page allows me to thank Al and Diane Kaneb, who, like Tom, have supported our efforts unstintingly and generously for long years. Love is good, but unconditional love is better, and it's for this reason I dedicate this volume to two friends who are still very much with us, and still standing with Haiti.

The longer (though necessarily incomplete) list of friends, family, volunteers, and donors who contributed in countless ways to our efforts after the earthquake can be found at http://www.pih.org/eqgratitude.

# INDEX

**Paul Farmer,** MD, PhD, is Kolokotrones University Professor at Harvard University and Chair of the Department of Global Health and Social Medicine at Harvard Medical School. He is Chief of the Division of Global Health Equity at Brigham and Women's Hospital in Boston, and co-founder of Partners In Health. He also serves as UN Deputy Special Envoy for Haiti, under Special Envoy Bill Clinton. Dr. Farmer and his colleagues have pioneered novel, community-based treatment strategies that demonstrate the delivery of high-quality health care in resource-poor settings. He has written extensively on health, human rights, and the consequences of social inequality; his clinical interests include the management of drug-resistant infections. His titles include *Partner to the Poor: A Paul Farmer Reader; Pathologies of Power: Health, Human Rights, and the New War on the Poor; The Uses of Haiti; Infections and Inequalities: The Modern Plagues;* and *AIDS and Accusation: Haiti and the Geography of Blame.* He is a member of the Institute of Medicine of the National Academy of Sciences and of the American Academy of Arts and Sciences.

PublicAffairs is a publishing house founded in 1997. It is a tribute to the standards, values, and flair of three persons who have served as mentors to countless reporters, writers, editors, and book people of all kinds, including me.

I. F. STONE, proprietor of *I. F. Stone's Weekly*, combined a commitment to the First Amendment with entrepreneurial zeal and reporting skill and became one of the great independent journalists in American history. At the age of eighty, Izzy published *The Trial of Socrates*, which was a national bestseller. He wrote the book after he taught himself ancient Greek.

BENJAMIN C. BRADLEE was for nearly thirty years the charismatic editorial leader of *The Washington Post*. It was Ben who gave the *Post* the range and courage to pursue such historic issues as Watergate. He supported his reporters with a tenacity that made them fearless and it is no accident that so many became authors of influential, best-selling books.

ROBERT L. BERNSTEIN, the chief executive of Random House for more than a quarter century, guided one of the nation's premier publishing houses. Bob was personally responsible for many books of political dissent and argument that challenged tyranny around the globe. He is also the founder and longtime chair of Human Rights Watch, one of the most respected human rights organizations in the world.

. . .

For fifty years, the banner of Public Affairs Press was carried by its owner Morris B. Schnapper, who published Gandhi, Nasser, Toynbee, Truman, and about 1,500 other authors. In 1983, Schnapper was described by *The Washington Post* as "a redoubtable gadfly." His legacy will endure in the books to come.

Peter Osnos, *Founder and Editor-at-Large*